ORTHOPAEDICS

Principles of Basic and Clinical Science

ORTHOPAEDICS

Principles of Basic and Clinical Science

edited by

Felix Bronner
Richard V. Worrell

CRC Press
Boca Raton London New York Washington, D.C.

Library of Congress Cataloging-in-Publication Data

Orthopaedics : principles of basic and clinical science / Felix
Bronner and Richard V. Worrell, editors.
p. cm.
Includes bibliographical references and index.
ISBN 0-8493-9237-3 (alk. paper)
1. Orthopedics. I. Bronner, Felix. II. Worrell, Richard V.
[DNLM: 1. Bone and Bones--physiology. 2. Bone Diseases--diagnosis. 3. Bone Diseases--therapy. WE 200 077 1999]
RD731.0783 1999
616.7—dc21
DNLM/DLC 99-20513
For Library of Congress CIP

International Standard Book Number 0-8493-9237-3
Library of Congress Card Number 99-20513
Printed in the United States of America 1 2 3 4 5 6 7 8 9 0
Printed on acid-free paper

Preface

Knowledge of the biology of bone and of skeletal diseases has increased significantly in recent years. The availability of bone cell culture systems and the application of powerful contemporary techniques have led to new and broader insights of skeletal metabolism and its disorders. Three professional journals, and many conferences, both general and specialized, are dedicated to recording new knowledge on bone. The amount of information, therefore, that practitioners and scientists entering the field must master is very large, and often dispersed; moreover, available texts tend to be exhaustive and comprehensive. It occurred to us that a text that summarizes and classifies contemporary knowledge of the skeletal system, yet takes into account the broad body of knowledge accumulated in the past 50 years will, if concise and didactically clear, contribute to the professionalization of the many individuals attracted to the field.

The current book comprises three sections: *Bone as a Tissue*, *Mineral Metabolism of Bone*, and selected *Clinical Topics*. In Section I, *Bone as a Tissue*, the structure and function of bone and connective tissue are discussed in Chapter 1 by Webster S.S. Jee and Chapter 2 by Joel Rosenbloom. Jee describes bone morphology, identifies a basic multicellular unit of bone in terms of which he later discusses bone turnover, and describes the four types of bone cells, followed by an analysis of how the tissue ossifies, grows, models and remodels. The development of a typical long bone is then described, as is how bone adapts to mechanical usage, and how age-related bone losses can be modeled. Rosenbloom, in Chapter 2, analyzes collagens, the elastic fiber of connective tissue; describes the major groups of the matrix proteins and of the proteoglycans; and provides the chemical information needed to understand the multitude of compounds that make up the connective tissues and how they might function. The third chapter, by J. Edward Puzas, provides a more detailed analysis of the two major cells of bone, osteoblasts and osteoclasts, and of the detailed signaling pathways that lead to their differentiation and function, information that can lead to better understanding and ultimately better therapy of osteoporosis and other skeletal diseases. The fourth chapter, by Deborah A. Redford-Badwal and David W. Rowe, deals with the heritable diseases of bone and connective tissue. It provides information and concepts needed to understand mutations. It also describes the major heritable diseases in terms of their molecular defects, knowledge of which should lead to better diagnosis and therapy. In Chapter 5, Felix Bronner, one of the editors of the book, summarizes current biological understanding of osteoporosis, the condition that afflicts postmenopausal women and ultimately all elderly.

Section II, *Mineral Metabolism of Bone*, is made up of five chapters, four of which are written by Bronner. Chapter 6 is a detailed analysis of the metabolism and homeostasis of calcium, the major cation of bone mineral, whose plasma concentration is more closely regulated than that of almost all other plasma ions. Chapter 7 discusses phosphate metabolism and that of a number of metals that are found in bone and can give rise to significant health concerns, as is true for lead and cadmium. The next two chapters, 8 and 9, deal with the systemic hormones and local modifiers of bone metabolism, providing functional descriptions of major hormones like parathyroid hormone and of significant signal molecules like the cytokines. In Chapter 10, Michael Kleerekooper discusses metabolic bone diseases in terms of case histories, an effective instructional tool for students and practitioners and one that can teach the basic scientist how disciplinary knowledge is applied to diagnosis and therapy.

The third section, *Clinical Topics*, will be of special interest to orthopaedic residents; it also provides students and biomedical scientists with applications of direct clinical relevance. In Chapter 11, William L. Sibbitt describes in detail normal and diseased joints; their histological appearance, important for diagnostic purposes; and the major disease conditions encountered in practice. He also refers to treatment. In this and subsequent *Clinical Topics* chapters, treatment is discussed, but does not constitute the main thrust.

The importance of nerves and muscles for proper skeletal function cannot be understated and, in Chapter 12, George E. Omer describes how nerve and muscle cells interact in the skeleton, and how injured nerves and denervated skeletal muscles can be repaired to restore function.

Biomechanics as applied to the skeleton has become an important field of research and orthopaedic practice. In Chapter 13, Thomas A. DeCoster and Brian Robinson review biomechanical principles as they apply to the musculoskeletal system, provide definitions of relevant terminology, and discuss nails, plates, plus external and internal fixation from a biomechanical viewpoint. In Chapter 14, Andrew E. Caputo discusses ligament, tendon and bone healing; how ligaments and tendons respond to immobilization; and how they react to subsequent exercise. Caputo also analyzes the various stages of bone healing, and how bone grafting and electrical stimulation can be utilized to effect bone union.

Richard V. Worrell, co-editor of this book, describes bone tumors and tumor-like lesions in Chapter 15, illustrating the various conditions with a series of photographs. Continuing as author of Chapter 16, Worell treats pyogenic and nonpyogenic osteomyelitis as major topics in his discussion of infectious diseases of bone.

The next two chapters, 17 and 18, deal with two specialized orthopaedic topics: The Foot, authored by Richard A. Miller and David M. Bloome, and The Hand, by Charles R. Prybil and Moneb S. Monheim. Both chapters describe the intricate anatomy of these two extremities, their disorders and appropriate treatments. The last chapter, again authored by Richard V. Worrell, discusses implants and their biology, a topic that is becoming increasingly current.

In structuring the book, we as editors wanted to develop a logical sequence, but are aware that few will read the book from cover to cover. Instead we believe each chapter can stand on its own, with related chapters providing complementary information. We thank our colleagues for their effort, patience and willingness to accept editorial suggestions and are grateful to CRC Press for helping to bring this project to realization.

Felix Bronner
Farmington, Connecticut

Richard V. Worrell
Albuquerque, New Mexico

Editors

Since his days as a graduate student at MIT, **Felix Bronner, Ph.D.,** Professor emeritus of BioStructure and Function and of Nutritional Sciences at the University of Connecticut, has studied calcium and mineral metabolism. Among the first investigators to have been able to use radioactive calcium, he elaborated the fate of calcium in the body of both humans and animals. Subsequently, Dr. Bronner began a detailed study of how calcium is absorbed in the intestine, then handled in the kidney and in bone. Based on these studies, he was able to formulate a general theory of calcium homeostasis. Recently, in collaboration, Dr. Bronner was able to extend his early studies on the regulation of calcium metabolism by making use of extensive findings in children studied with stable calcium isotopes.

Author of over 100 research papers, 67 chapters in books, and editor of 58 books and treatises, including founding editor of *Current Topics in Membranes and Transport*, Dr. Bronner has also organized many scientific meetings and symposia. He has trained graduate students and postdoctoral fellows and is the 1975 recipient of the André Lichtwitz prize awarded by the French National Institutes for Medical Research (INSERM) for excellence in calcium and phosphate metabolism research. In 1996, he was awarded an honorary doctorate by France. He is a fellow of the American Association for the Advancement of Science and of the American Society for Nutritional Sciences and member of numerous professional societies, including the Orthopaedic Research Society. He was the founder and first chair of the Gordon Research Conference on Bones and Teeth.

Dr. Richard Worrell is Professor and Vice Chairman of the Department of Orthopaedics of the University of New Mexico School of Medicine. After completing residency and post-residency training in orthopaedic surgery and pathology at the State University of New York at Buffalo School of Medicine and affiliated hospitals and Temple University School of Medicine, his first full-time academic position was at the University of Connecticut School of Medicine. He was appointed as the first head of the Division of Orthopaedic Surgery in 1968. In 1969, he established the residency training program in Orthopaedic Surgery at the University of Connecticut Health Center. His primary academic interests are in the fields of orthopaedic pathology and oncology. He has a private collection of over 70,000 orthopaedic pathology and oncology teaching slides. He currently teaches pathology of the musculoskeletal system to both orthopaedic and pathology residents at the University of New Mexico.

Dr. Worrell is a member of the American Orthopaedic Association, the American Academy of Orthopaedic Surgeons, the Academic Orthopaedic Society, the Orthopaedic Research Society, the American College of Surgeons, the American Society of Clinical Pathologists, the American Society of Clinical Oncology, and many other professional organizations. He is listed in *Who's Who in America*, *Who's Who in Medicine and Healthcare* and *The Best Doctors in America*.

Contributors

David M. Bloome, M.D.
Department of Orthopaedic Surgery
University of New Mexico
Health Sciences Center
Albuquerque, New Mexico

Felix Bronner, Ph.D.
Department of BioStructure & Function
University of Connecticut Health Center
Farmington, Connecticut

Andrew E. Caputo, M.D.
Department of Orthopaedic Surgery
University of Connecticut Health Center
Farmington, Connecticut

Thomas A. DeCoster, M.D.
Department of Orthopaedics
University of New Mexico
Health Sciences Center
Albuquerque, New Mexico

Webster S. S. Jee, Ph.D.
Division of Radiobiology
University of Utah
Salt Lake City, Utah

Michael Kleerekoper, M.D., F.A.C.E.
Department of Internal Medicine
Wayne State University
Detroit, Michigan

Gregory D. Lewis, Ph.D.
Department of Orthopaedics
University of Rochester
Rochester, New York

Richard A. Miller, M.D.
Department of Orthopaedics
University of New Mexico
Health Sciences Center
Albuquerque, New Mexico

Moheb S. Moneim, M.D.
Department of Orthopaedics
University of New Mexico
Health Sciences Center
Albuquerque, New Mexico

George E. Omer, Jr., M.D.
Department of Orthopaedics
University of New Mexico
Health Sciences Center
Albuquerque, New Mexico

Charles R. Pribyl, M.D.
Department of Orthopaedics
University of New Mexico
Health Sciences Center
Albuquerque, New Mexico

J. Edward Puzas, Ph.D.
Department of Orthopaedics
University of Rochester
Rochester, New York

Deborah A. Redford-Badwal, D.D.S., Ph.D.
Department of Pediatric Dentistry
University of Connecticut Health Center
Farmington, Connecticut

Brian Robinson, M.D.
Department of Orthopaedics
University of New Mexico
Health Sciences Center
Albuquerque, New Mexico

Joel Rosenbloom, M.D., Ph.D.
Department of Anatomy & Histology
University of Pennsylvania
School of Dental Medicine
Philadelphia, Pennsylvania

David W. Rowe, M.D.
Department of Genetics and
Developmental Biology
University of Connecticut Health Center
Farmington, Connecticut

Wilmer L. Sibbitt, Jr., M.D.
Department of Medicine
University of New Mexico
Health Sciences Center
Albuquerque, New Mexico

Richard V. Worrell, M.D.
Department of Orthopaedics
University of New Mexico
Health Sciences Center
Albuquerque, New Mexico

Can these bones live? ... and they came together,
bone to matching bone... and they came to life.
— Ezekiel: 37

To our families and the many teachers, colleagues, and students who shared with us their knowledge, insights, and questions.

Table of Contents

Section I

Bone as a Tissue

1 Structure and Function of Bone Tissue

Webster S. S. Jee

CONTENTS

0-8493-9237-3/99/$0.00+$.50

1.1 INTRODUCTION

The skeletal system, important to the body both biomechanically and metabolically, is made up of individual bones and the connective tissue that joins them. Bone is the main constituent of the system and differs from the connective tissues in rigidity and hardness. These characteristics of bone result from inorganic salts impregnating the matrix, which consists of collagen fibers, a large variety of non-collagenous proteins, and mineral. The rigidity and hardness of bone enable the skeleton to maintain the shape of the body; to protect the soft tissues of the cranial, thoracic, and pelvic cavities; to supply the framework for the bone marrow; and to transmit the force of muscular contraction from one part of the body to another during movement. The mineral content of bone serves as a reservoir for ions, particularly calcium, and also contributes to the regulation of extracellular fluid composition (Table 1.1), particularly ionized calcium concentration. In addition, bone is a self-repairing structural material, able to adapt its mass, shape, and properties to changes in mechanical and metabolic requirements.

The skeleton has been divided into axial and appendicular subdivisions. This separation is important because composition and functions of the skeleton are divided differently between axial and appendicular components (Table 1.1).

1.2 MORPHOLOGY: MACROSCOPIC AND MICROSCOPIC STRUCTURES[1,2]

The long bones (e.g., humerus, femur, and tibia) serve as the classical model for the macroscopic structure of bone (Figure 1.1). A typical adult long bone consists of a central cylindrical shaft, or diaphysis, and two wider and rounded ends, the epiphyses. Conical regions called the metaphysis connect the diaphysis with each epiphysis.

TABLE 1.1
Subdivision of the Skeleton

Feature	Axial	Appendicular
Main bone tissue	Cancellous	Cortical
Adjacent soft tissue	Viscera	Muscle
Cortices	Thin	Thick
Marrow	Hematopoietic	Fatty
Turnover	High	Low
Main Function		
Cortical	Mechanical	Mechanical
Cancellous*	Metabolic	Mechanical

* Metabolic activity such as uptake and release of calcium occurs in all cancellous bone in red marrow sites throughout the skeleton.

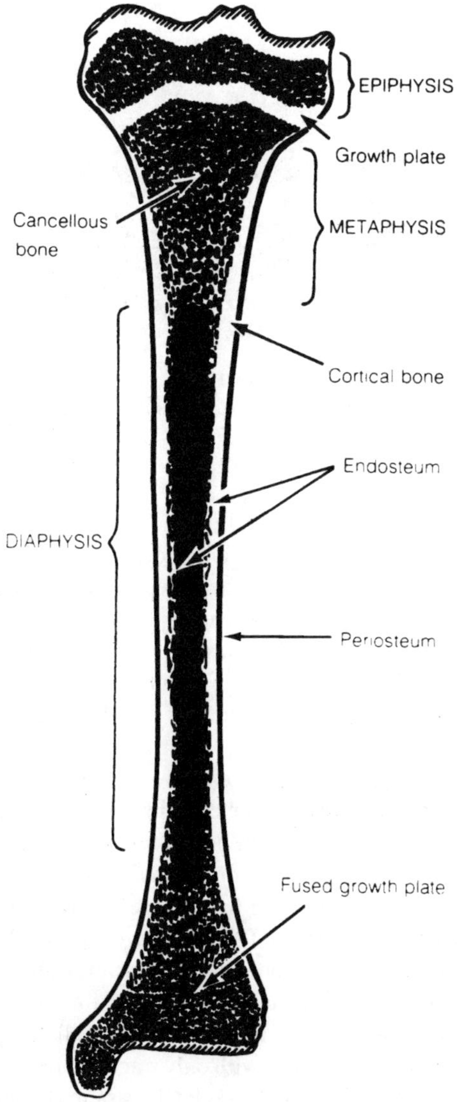

FIGURE 1.1 Diagram of a typical long bone, the tibia. The black space is filled with hematoporetic and/or fatty marrow. (From Weiss, L., *Cell and Tissue Biology, a Textbook of Histology*, Urban and Schwarzenberg, Baltimore, 1988. With permission.)

1.2.1 Cortical and Cancellous Bone

The diaphysis is composed mainly of cortical bone, while the epiphysis and metaphysis contain mostly cancellous bone with a thin shell of cortical bone. In the growing animal, the epiphysis is separated from the metaphysis by a plate of hyaline cartilage known as the growth plate-metaphyseal complex, or the epiphyseal plate.

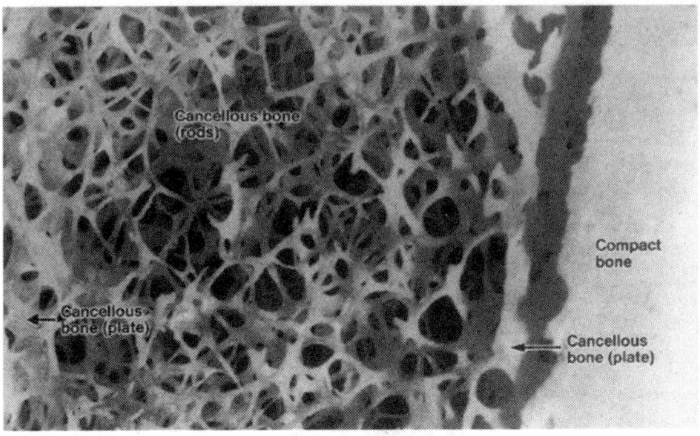

FIGURE 1.2 Morphology of cancellous and cortical bone. Cancellous bone made of a network of trabecular rods and bars and its adjacent "solid" part of compact or cortical bone. (From Weiss, L., *Cell and Tissue Biology, a Textbook of Histology*, Urban and Schwarzenberg, Baltimore, 1988. With permission.)

The growth plate and the adjacent cancellous bone of the metaphysis constitute a region where cancellous bone production and elongation of the cortex occur. In the adult, the cartilaginous growth plate has been replaced by cancellous bone, which causes the epiphysis to become fused to the metaphysis. Obliteration of this cartilage by the fusion of the two cancellous bone masses is called the closure of the epiphysis and forms a synostosis. On the articulating (joint) surfaces at the ends of the long bone, or the ends of the epiphysis, the shell of subchondral bone is covered by a thin layer of specialized hyaline cartilage, the articular cartilage.

The outer surface of most bone is covered by the periosteum, a sheet of fibrous connective tissue and an inner cellular or cambium layer of undifferentiated cells. The periosteum has the potential to form bone during growth and fracture healing. It is not present in areas where tendons or ligaments insert in bone, on bone ends that are lined with articular cartilage, on the surface of sesamoid bones, in subscapular areas, and the neck of the femur. The marrow cavity of the diaphysis and the cavities of cortical and cancellous bone are lined with a thin cellular layer called the endosteum. The endosteum (an internal periosteum) is a membrane of bone surface cells (osteoclasts, osteoblasts, and bone lining cells).

Cortical bone is a dense, solid mass with only microscopic channels (Figures 1.2, 1.3, and 1.5). Approximately 80% of the skeletal mass in the adult human skeleton is cortical bone, which forms the outer wall of all bones and is largely responsible for the supportive and protective function of the skeleton. The bulk of cortical bone is in the shaft of long bones of the appendicular skeleton. The remaining 20% of the bone mass is cancellous bone, a lattice of large plates and rods known as the trabecula, found in the inner parts of bones (Figures 1.1 and 1.2). The distribution of cortical and cancellous bone varies greatly between individual bones. For example, the ulna is 92% cortical and only 8% cancellous bone, while a typical vertebra consists of 62% cortical and 38% cancellous bone. In addition, cortical and cancellous bone differ in their development, architecture, proximity to the bone marrow, blood supply, rapidity of turnover, time, and magnitude of age-dependent changes and fractures (Table 1.2).

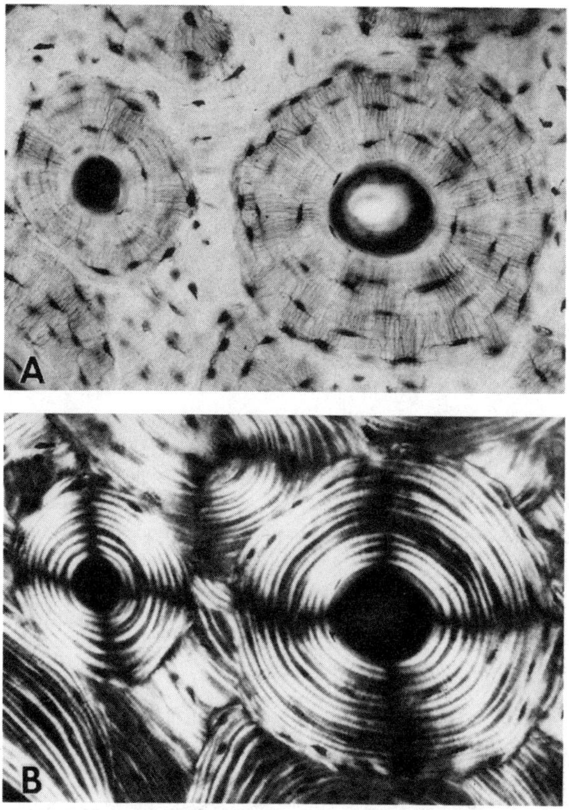

FIGURE 1.3 (A) Cross-section of cortical bone showing osteon with its lacunae and canaliculi and Haversian canal. Note intervening interstitial lamella between osteons. (B) Same section in polarized light. (From Royce, P. M. and Steinmann, B., *Connective Tissue and its Heritable Disorders, Molecular, Genetic and Mineral Aspects*, John Wiley & Sons, Inc., New York, 1993. With permission.)

1.2.2 Woven and Lamellar Bone

Mammalian cortical or cancellous bone is of two main types, woven or lamellar. Bone tissue in the developing embryo is the woven type. Cancellous woven bone is formed by endochondral and intramembranous ossification. In postfetal osteogenesis that occurs when fractures heal, or in ectopic ossification or osteosarcoma, new bone is deposited in woven form. Woven bone, a matrix of interwoven coarse collagen fibers with osteocytes distributed more or less at random, is less organized and shorter-lived than lamellar bone. It is provisional material that is eventually resorbed and replaced by lamellar bone. In human long bones, woven bone is replaced by lamellar bone at age two and three years. Lamellar bone is built up of unit layers (lamellae), like plywood. Each lamella is approximately three to seven microns thick and contains fine fibers that run in approximately the same direction, but whose axes can differ by as much as 90 degrees in adjacent units. In histological preparations,

TABLE 1.2
Differences in Cortical and Cancellous Bone

	Cortical	Cancellous
Skeletal mass	80%	20%
Bone surface	33%	67%
Surface/volume ratio (mm^2/mm^3)	2.5	20
Soft tissue	10%	75%
Adult tissue	Secondary osteon (Haversian systems) Interstial lamellae Circumferential lamellae	Curved plates, rods Bone structural unit Interstitial lamellae
Porosity	Low	High
Marrow	Fatty	Hematopoietic
Main soft tissue	Viscera	Marrow
Developmental	Intramembranous ossification	Endochondral ossification
Turnover	Slow	Rapid
Function	Mainly biomechanical also supportive and protective	Mainly mineral homeostasis, also supportive

the laminations are best seen under polarized light. They appear as alternating light and dark layers, the result of differing orientations of collagen fibers within adjacent lamellae (Figures 1.3 and 1.5).

The lamellae of adult cortical bone appear in three major patterns: (a) circular rings of lamellae (concentric lamellae) surrounding a longitudinally vascular channel that together form a structural cone, the osteon or Haversian system; (b) several layers of lamellae extending uninterrupted around part or all of the circumference of the shaft to form what is known as the circumferential lamellae; and (c) angular fragments of what formerly were concentric or circumferential lamellae filling the gaps between the Haversian systems, known as the interstitial lamellae (Figure 1.5). The lamellae of adult cancellous bone consist of two major types: trabecular packets shaped like shallow crescents and interstitial lamellae (Figure 1.4).

Small cavities (lacunae) connected by their tubular canals (canaliculi) are found throughout woven and lamellar bone. Entrapped bone cells (osteocytes) and their long cytoplasmic processes occupy the lacunae and canaliculi, respectively. The cell processes communicate by gap junctions with the processes of osteocytes lying in adjacent lacunae. Canaliculi that open to the extracellular fluid and bone surfaces form an anastomosing network for the nutrition and metabolic activities of the osteocytes (Figures 1.3 and 1.5).

1.2.3 Composition of Bone[3]

Bone consists of 65% mineral, 35% organic matrix, cells, and water. The bone mineral is in the form of small crystals in the shape of needles, plates and rods

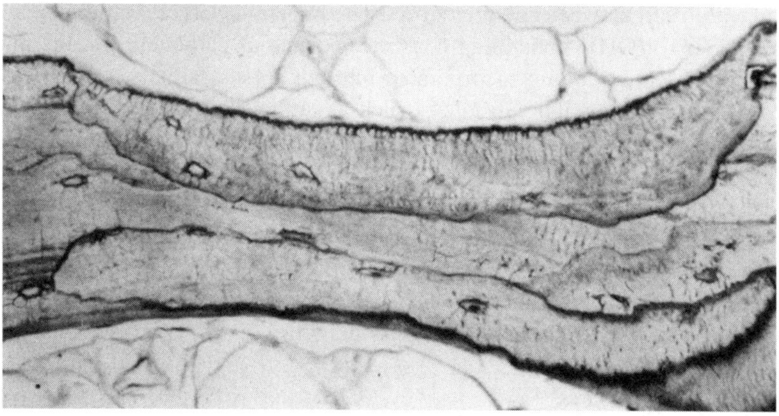

FIGURE 1.4 A part of a trabecula showing individual packet separated by cement lines. (From Fleisch, H., *Bisphosphonates in Bone Disease. From the Laboratory to the Patient,* Parthenon Publishing Group, New York, 1997. With permission.)

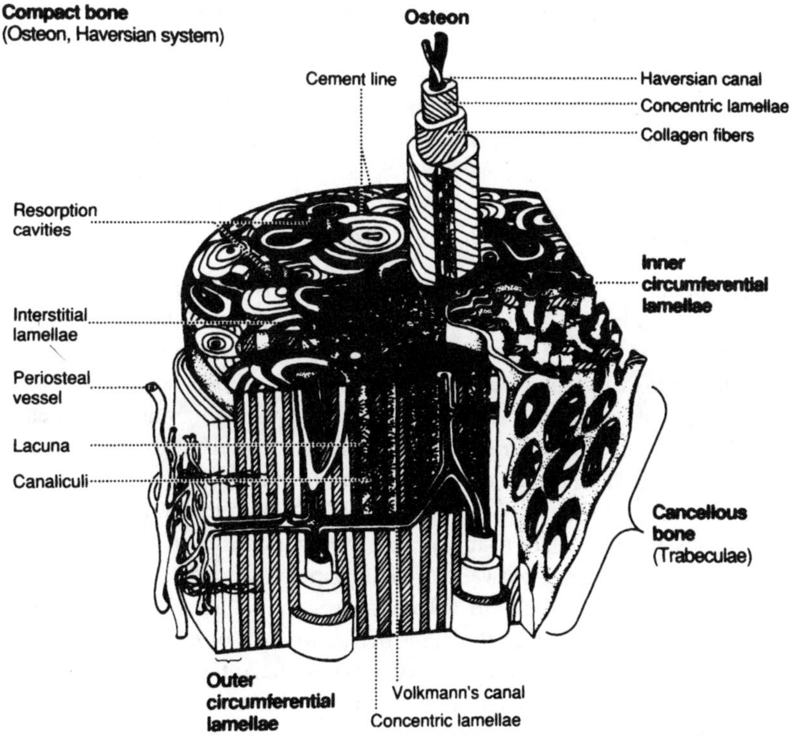

FIGURE 1.5 Diagram of a portion of a long bone shaft containing histological details. (From Weiss, L., *Cell and Tissue Biology, a Textbook of Histology*, Urban and Schwarzenberg, Baltimore, 1988. With permission.)

located within and between collagen fibers. The mineral is largely impure hydroxyapatite, $Ca_{10}(PO_4)_6(OH)_2$, containing constituents such as carbonate, citrate, magnesium, fluoride and strontium incorporated into the crystal lattice or adsorbed onto the crystal surface. Foreign substances such as tetracyclines, polyphosphates, bisphosphonates, and bone seeking radionuclides can also be incorporated with high affinity.

The organic matrix consists of 90% collagen and about 10% of various non-collagenous proteins. The roles of non-collagenous proteins are unclear. The most abundant ones are osteocalcin, osteonectin, osteopontin, and bone sialoprotein. The urinary excretion and plasma or serum levels of some of the non-collagenous proteins unique to bone are used clinically to assess bone turnover.[4]

1.2.4 Bone Surfaces[1,5]

Bone tissue has two major surfaces, periosteal and endosteal. The endosteal surface subdivides into the intracortical, endocortical, and cancellous or trabecular surfaces. Cancellous bone surface contributes more than 66% of the total bone surface because the mean trabecular surface to volume ratio is eight times greater in cancellous than in cortical bone (20 mm^2/mm^3 vs. 2.5 mm^2/mm^3).

At any time the bone surface may be in one of three states: forming, resorbing or quiescent. Bone-forming surfaces are characterized by the presence of osteoid and a covering of osteoblasts. In contrast, the resorbing surfaces contain scalloped concavities (Howship's lacunae) that frequently contain osteoclasts or have osteoclasts located nearby. Quiescent, or resting, bone surfaces are lined by bone-lining cells (Figure 1.6).

1.2.5 Basic Multicellular Unit — BMU[5-7]

In cortical bone the main structural unit is the osteon or Haversian system (Figures 1.3, 1.5, and 1.7). Osteons form approximately two thirds of the cortical bone volume, the remaining one-third is interstitial bone composed of the remnants of past generations of osteons and subperiosteal and subendosteal circumferential lamellae. A typical osteon is a cylinder about 200 or 250 microns in diameter; the canals are interconnected by transverse Volkmann's canals that divide to form a branching network. Within the central canal run blood vessels, lymphatics, nerves, and loose connective tissue, all of which continue through the bone marrow and the periosteum. The total length of a single canal from periosteum to endosteum is about 1 cm, with a mean distance between branch points of about 2.5 mm. The wall of the osteon is made up of 20 to 30 concentric lamellae approximately 70 to 100 microns thick. Surrounding the outer border of each osteon is a cement line, a 1 to 2 micron-thick layer of mineralized matrix deficient in collagen fibers. Two types of cement lines are apparent: reversal lines, which are irregular or scalloped, and arrest lines, which have a smooth contour.

In cancellous or trabecular bone the structural unit is the trabecular packet, a hemiosteon (Figures 1.4, 1.6, and 1.8). The ideal trabecular packet is shaped like a shallow crescent with a radius of 600 microns and is about 50 microns thick and

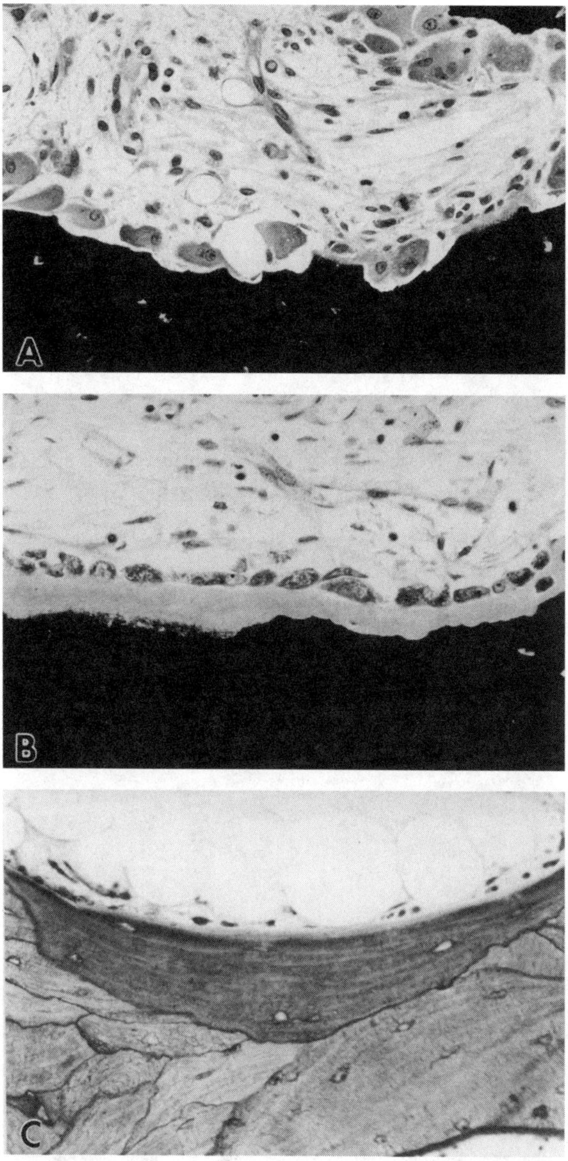

FIGURE 1.6 Cancellous bone remodeling to form a trabecular packet. The osteoclasts erode a burrow (A) which is then refilled by osteoblasts (B) that form a new trabecular packet or pack of new bone (C). (From Royce, P. M. and Steinmann, B., *Connective Tissue and its Heritable Disorders, Molecular, Genetic and Mineral Aspects*, John Wiley & Sons, Inc., New York, 1993. With permission.)

1 mm long. As with cortical bone, cement lines hold the trabecular packets together. Table 1.3 summarizes differences between bone structural units in cortical and cancellous bone.

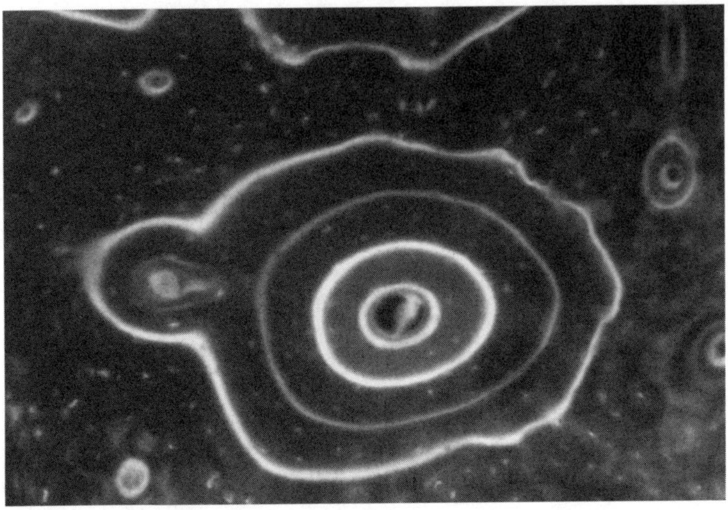

FIGURE 1.7 A fluorescence labeled bone structural unit of cortical bone, the osteon or Haversian system. The osteon is labeled with four different fluorescent bone markers. (From Weiss, L., *Cell and Tissue Biology, a Textbook of Histology*, Urban and Schwarzenberg, Baltimore, 1988. With permission.)

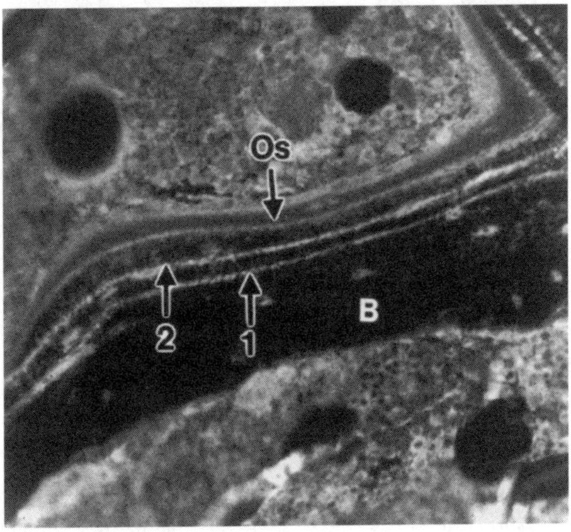

FIGURE 1.8 Double tetracycline labeling of a forming trabecular packet. The first label (1) was given 10 days before the second (2) and the dog was killed 72 hours later. This labeling schedule allows for dynamic histomorphometric analysis of bone tissue. (From Weiss, L., *Cell and Tissue Biology, a Textbook of Histology*, Urban and Schwarzenberg, Baltimore, 1988. With permission.)

TABLE 1.3
Comparison of Adult Cortical and Cancellous Bone Structural Units

Parameter	Cortical (Osteonal)	Cancellous (Trabecular Packet)
Length (mm)	2.5	1.0
Circumference (mm)	0.6	0.6
Wall thickness (mm)	0.075	0.040
Number/mm^3 bone volume	15	40
Total number in skeleton	21×10^6	14×10^6
Duration of resorption (days)	24	21
Duration of formation (days)	124	91
Remodeling period (days)	148	112
Bone turnover rate (%/yr)	3	26

Modified from Recker, R. R., *Bone Histomorphometry: Techniques and Interpretation*, CRC Press, Boca Raton, Florida, 1983. (With permission.)

1.2.6 Cells of Bone

The major cellular elements of bone include osteoclasts, osteoblasts, osteocytes, bone-lining cells, the precursors of these specialized cells, cells of the marrow compartment, and an immune regulatory system that supplies the precursor cells and regulates bone growth and maintenance.

1.2.6.1 The Osteoclasts[1,8,9]

Osteoclasts, the bone resorbing cells, are multinucleated giant cells that contain from one to more than 50 nuclei and range in diameter from 20 to over 100 microns (Figure 1.6A). Their role is to resorb bone. Actively resorbing osteoclasts are usually found in cavities on bone surfaces, called resorption cavities or Howship's lacunae. The cytoplasm of the osteoclasts tends to be foamy in appearance and is acidophilic in its staining characteristics. The surface of osteoclasts adjacent to bone surface has a striated appearance and a ruffled border, an area of extensive membrane enfolding. The ruffled border is surrounded by an ectoplasmic zone, devoid of organelles but containing many active filaments, called the clear or filamentous zone. Osteoclasts adhere to the bone surface at the clear zone, which acts as a permeable seal to maintain the microenvironment needed for bone resorption to occur. The ruffled border secretes products leading to bone destruction.

The osteoclasts originate from the hemopoietic compartment, the granocyte-macrophage colony-forming unit (GM-CFU). The life span *in vivo* appears to be seven weeks, with a half-life for each nucleus of six to seven days in growing rats. Cessation of bone resorption is associated with the migration of osteoclasts from the endosteal surface into adjacent marrow spaces, where it is believed they either degenerate and disintegrate or hibernate.

1.2.6.2 The Osteoblasts[1,10,11]

Osteoblasts are bone-forming cells that synthesize and secrete unmineralized bone matrix (the osteoid), participate in the calcification and resorption of bone, and regulate the flux of calcium and phosphate in and out of bone (Figure 1.6B). Osteoblasts occur as a layer of contiguous cells which in their active state are cuboidal (15 to 30 microns thick). They contain an abundance of alkaline phosphatase and osteo-inductive cell markers in their plasma membrane.

Bone formation occurs in two stages, matrix formation and mineralization. Matrix formation, which precedes mineralization by about 15 days, occurs at the interface between osteoblasts and osteoid. Columnar preosteoblasts have been present for nine days before matrix synthesis occurs. During the period of bone formation, the height of an average osteoblast nucleus declines from about 7 microns to 1 micron at the end of bone formation. Extracellular mineralization occurs at the junction of osteoid and newly formed bone; this region is known as the mineralization front. Because mineralization occurs some time after matrix production, a layer of unmineralized matrix called the osteoid seam remains. The mineralization lag time is normally 10 days in the adult, resulting in a osteoid seam of 8 to 10 microns. In contrast to adult bone, embryonic or woven bone formation has a very short mineralization lag time; as a result, the osteoid seam is either absent or very thin.

The rate of bone formation can be readily determined in man and animals by administering tetracycline or other types of fluorescent bone markers.[12] Tetracycline is an antibiotic that localizes at the mineralization front, thereby causing the newly deposited bone to appear as a tetracycline-labeled band. A labeled bone fluoresces under ultraviolet light and thus marks the location of bone formation at the time of tetracycline administration (Figures 1.7 and 1.8).

The osteoblasts are derived from mesenchymal progenitors. Osteoblast precursors are located near bone surfaces: the periosteum, the endosteum, and the adjacent marrow stroma (perivascular parenchymal cells). They arise from local, undifferentiated intraskeletal mesenchymal cells that are capable of mitosis. The identity of cell types that may transform into an osteoblast progenitor is not known. There is overwhelming evidence that postnatal marrow stroma, but not functioning hematopoietic tissue, can differentiate into osteoblasts. Also, there is a good possibility that precursors of osteoblasts are undifferentiated mesenchymal cells of a potential similar to that found in the early stages in the embryo.

The complete life cycle of an osteoblast involves (a) birth from a precursor cell, (b) differentiation and participation in matrix elaboration and extracellular mineralization, and (c) either reentry into the preosteoblast pool, transformation to bone-lining cells or burial as osteocytes, or death.

1.2.6.3 The Osteocytes[1,9-11]

When osteoblasts stop synthesizing matrix and become embedded within bone, they are called osteocytes. Osteocytes are housed in lacunae, do not divide, and only a single cell is found in a lacuna. Osteocytes maintain contact with one another and with cells lining the bone surface by means of slender processes that traverse the canaliculi of bone via gap junctions. The osteocytes may (1) stabilize bone mineral by maintaining an appropriate local ionic milieu, in collaboration with the bone-lining cells (the bone-lining-osteocyte complex); this milieu controls the efflux of calcium ions; (2) detect microfractures, and (3) respond to the amount and distribution of strain within bone tissue that influence adaptive modeling and remodeling behavior through cell: cell interaction. Thus, osteocytes play a key role in homeostatic, morphogenetic, and restructuring processes that regulate the mineral content and architecture of the bone mass.

1.2.6.4 The Bone-lining Cells[1,9,12-14]

When the osteoblasts are not in the process of forming bone they are flattened, elongated cells covering quiescent bone surfaces and are called resting osteoblasts or bone-lining cells (Figure 1.6C). The bone-lining cell has a distinct morphological phenotype: direct apposition to the bone surface, a thin, flat nuclear profile with attenuated (1 micron thick and up to 12 microns long) cytoplasm extending along the bone surface. Gap junctions are seen between adjacent bone-lining cells and between bone-lining cells and osteocytes. The surface density of bone-lining cells is about 19 cells per millimeter bone surface perimeter in fatty marrow sites of young adult dogs, and decreases somewhat with age. Their density seems greater in hemopoietic marrow.

Bone-lining cells are believed to be derived from osteoblasts that have become inactive, or osteoblast precursors that have ceased activity or differentiated and flattened out on bone surfaces. They occupy the majority of the adult bone surface. Little is known of their history. They may be a mixed population of cells, possibly returning to the stem cell or preosteoblast pool. The prolific capacity and differentiation potential of bone-lining cells under normal physiological condition is poorly understood.

The bone-lining cells are capable of forming bone, without prior bone resorption (formation drift) in response to bone anabolic agents[13] and may regulate mineral homeostasis with the complex of osteoblasts and osteocytes.[14] Perhaps bone-lining cells, like osteocytes, may be influenced by functional strain within bone tissue that influences adaptive changes. Thus, bone-lining cells may be involved in homeostatic, morphogenetic, and restructuring processes that constitute regulation of bone mineral, mass, and architecture, as well as the hematopoietic process.

1.3 SKELETAL DEVELOPMENT[1,2]

Skeletal development begins as mesenchymal condensations that appear early in the fetal period. These condensations ossify to form membrane (dermal) bones through intramembranous ossification, and cartilage bones through endochondral ossification. The latter become chondrified and form hyaline cartilage in the shape of future bones. However, in both types of ossification, bone formation is similar, beginning with an increase in the number of cells and fibers. The cells differentiate into osteoblasts, which lay down an unmineralized matrix, the osteoid that mineralizes almost immediately. Some osteoblasts are trapped in the matrix around them and become osteocytes. The shape and manner of growth of this new bony tissue depend on the individual bone and are genetically determined. Embryonic bone formation involves woven bone formation, and fine-bundled lamellar bone that replaces woven bone through bone remodeling is not formed until after birth.

1.3.1 Intramembranous Ossification[1]

Intramembranous ossification or membrane bone formation forms the bulk of the future cortical bone shell. This forms most of the bones of the vault of the skull, many of the bones of the sense organs and of the facial skeleton, and parts of the clavicle and mandible. Fibrocellular condensations during the embryonic period constitute the first indication of membrane bones. Then the primary center of ossification of each bone appears as an increase in cells and fibers, and bone is apposed. Loose spicules or trabeculae are formed by osteoblasts and interconnect to form the primary cancellous bone (spongiosa). Trabeculae continue to increase in thickness and enlarge by addition to their free ends. Compact bone is formed when the spaces between the primary spongiosa are filled in by the primary osteons (compaction). This bone is then gradually replaced by secondary osteons.

1.3.2 Endochondral Ossification[1]

Endochondral ossification or cartilage bone formation forms the bulk of the future cancellous bone. It forms most of the bones at the base of the skull, the vertebral column, the pelvis, and the extremities. A cartilage bone begins as a mesenchymal condensation or blastema, which usually appears during the embryonic period. Cartilage cells (chondrocytes) proliferate and deposit matrix until a cartilage model of the future bone is formed. The cartilage cells mature, grow, and its matrix subsequently calcifies. Unresorbed calcified cartilage cores form the substrate in which osteoblasts appose woven bone to form the primary spongiosa. The spicules in the primary spongiosa are composed of mosaic pieces of calcified cores surrounded by woven bone tissue. This is later either lost or replaced with a lamellar trabecular packet as the secondary spongiosa, i.e., the future adult spongiosa, is formed.

1.3.3 Growth[1]

It is the combination of genetic and circulating systemic factors that controls general growth, while regional factors, especially mechanical usage, can modulate it locally. Longitudinal bone growth adds new spongiosa to preexisting spongiosa and new length of cortical bone to preexisting cortex, whereas radial or periosteal bone growth adds new width by apposing subperiosteal bone to the cortex.

1.3.4 Modeling[1,5]

Growth and modeling go hand in hand. Local influences modulate growth to produce functionally and mechanically purposeful architecture. Modeling involves resorption drifts and formation drifts that remove or add bone over wide regions of bone surfaces

TABLE 1.4
Comparison of Modeling and Remodeling

	Remodeling	Modeling
Occurrence	Adult skeleton	Growing
Location	Spatially related	Different surfaces
Coupling	A→R→F[a]	A→F; A→R[a]
Timing	Cyclical	Continuous
Extent	Small (<20%)	Large (>90%)
Apposition rate	Slow (0.3 to 1.0 μm/day)	Fast (2 to 10 μm/day)
Balance	Net loss	Net gain

[a] A, activation; R, resorption; F, formation.

Modified from Parfitt, A.M., The physiologic and clinical significance of bone histomorphometric data., in *Bone Histomorphometry: Techniques and Interpretation*, Recker, R. R., Ed., CRC Press, Boca Raton, Florida, 1983.

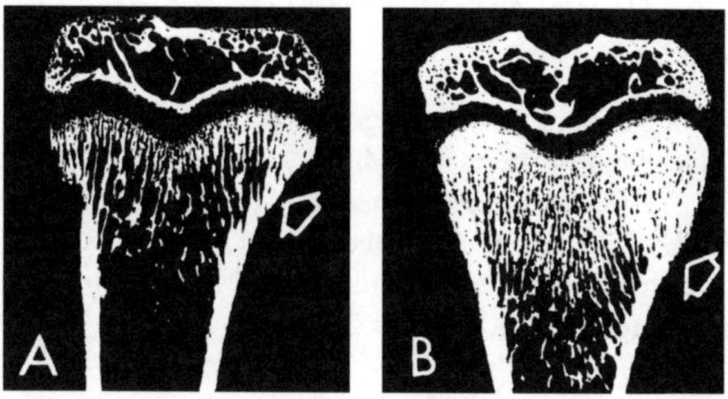

FIGURE 1.9 Normal (A) and abnormal (B) modeling of the proximal tibial metaphysis. (A) Normal funnel shaping of the metaphyses by resorption drift. (B) A convex metaphysis formed from the inhibition of bone resorption by a bisphosphonate. (From Weiss, L.,*Cell and Tissue Biology, a Textbook of Histology*, Urban and Schwarzenberg, Baltimore, 1988. With permission.)

(Table 1.4; Figure 1.9). During growth, formation drifts add periosteal bone faster than resorption drifts remove endosteal bone. Modeling controls the growth, shape, size, strength, and anatomy of bones and joints. Collectively, modeling leads to increasing the cortical outside and marrow cavity diameters, the shaping of the ends of long bone, drifting trabeculae and cortices, enlarging the cranial vault, and changes in cranial vault curvature.

1.3.5 Remodeling and Bone Turnover[1,2,4,5,7,15]

Bone remodeling produces and maintains bone that is biomechanically and metabolically competent. Immature (woven) bone formed at the metaphyses is structurally inferior to mature bone. Moreover, the quality of adult bone deteriorates with time. Therefore, bone must replace or renew itself. The replacement of immature (primary) and old bone occurs by resorption, followed by formation of new lamellar bone, a process called remodeling (Table 1.4). The products of bone remodeling are reversal (scalloped cement) lines, secondary osteons or Haversian systems, trabecular packets, and interstitial lamellae (persisting fragments of bone units that have been partially resorbed by continual bone remodeling).

In humans, after two to three years of age, the immature bone during infancy is resorbed and replaced by secondary bone. A drastic reduction in the amount of bone occurs during the conversion of primary to secondary spongiosa. Changes in number and shape of bone trabeculae during the conversion of primary to secondary spongiosa are dramatic. Remodeling does not end with the replacement of primary bone, but continues throughout life. The secondary bone is continuously destroyed and replaced by new generations of bone. Assuming normal rates of adult bone turnover, cortical bone has a mean age of 20 years and cancellous bone one of 4 years. The periodic replacement of bone (bone turnover) helps to maintain load bearing, to repair microscopic structural damage, and to replace old bone, thereby maintaining the capacity of the skeleton to regulate calcium homeostasis.

1.3.6 Basic Multicellular Unit (BMU) or Bone Remodeling Unit (BRU)[1,2,5-7,15]

The operational group of bone cells that accomplishes one quantum of bone turnover — removal and replacement of pre-existing bone with a new structural unit (the osteon or hemiosteon) — is referred to as a bone remodeling unit (BRU) or basic multicellular unit (BMU). The life cycle of the unit includes six consecutive stages of resting, activation, resorption, reversal (coupling), formation, mineralization, and back to resting (Figures 1.6 and 1.10-1.13).

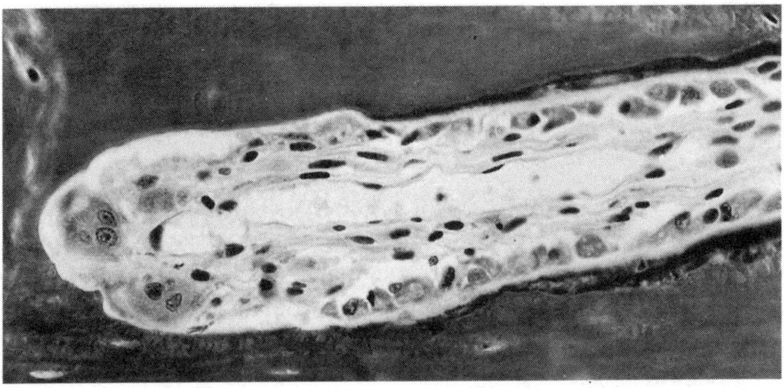

FIGURE 1.10 Cortical bone remodeling. Osteoclast resorbing a tunnel and osteoblast filling it. (From Royce, P. M. and Steinmann, B., *Connective Tissue and its Heritable Disorders, Molecular, Genetic and Mineral Aspects*, John Wiley & Sons, Inc., New York, 1993. With permission.)

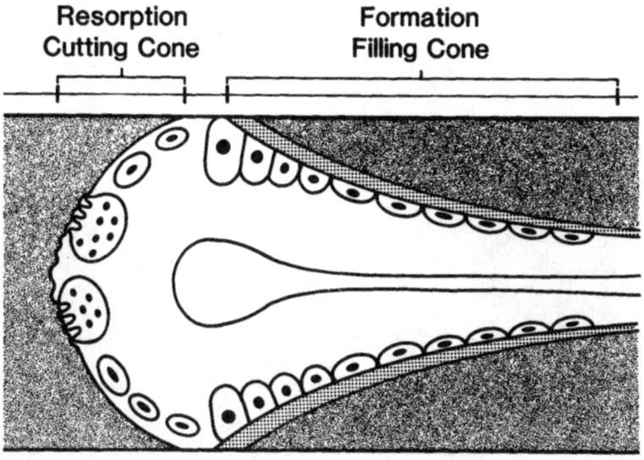

FIGURE 1.11 Diagram of a longitudinal osteonal bone, bone remodeling or basic multicellular unit forming an osteon or Haversian system. (From Bronner, F. and Worrell, R.V., Eds., *A Basic Science Primer in Orthopaedics*, Williams & Wilkins, Baltimore, 1991. With permission.)

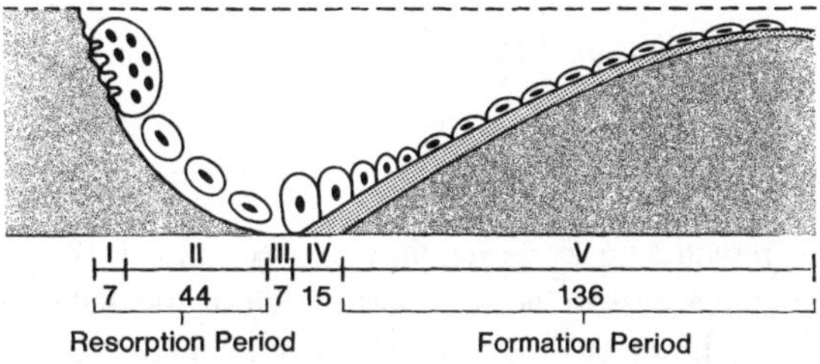

FIGURE 1.12 A cancellous bone remodeling unit, or BMU, divided into the osteoclastic resorption (I), mononuclear resorption (II), coupling or reversal phase (III), initial mineralization phase (IV), and formation and mineralization (V) phases. (From Bronner, F. and Worrell, R.V., Eds., *A Basic Science Primer in Orthopaedics*, Williams & Wilkins, Baltimore, 1991. With permission.)

1.3.6.1 Resting

In large adult animals, including humans, about 80% of the cancellous and cortical bone surfaces (periosteal and endosteal) and about 95% of the intracortical surface are inactive with respect to bone remodeling at any given time. These inactive surfaces are in the resting stage. They are covered by bone-lining cells that may function as osteogenic precursor cells and an endosteal membrane, a thin 0.1 to 0.5 micron layer of unmineralized connective tissue with fewer collagen fibers and less amorphous ground substance than found in bone.

1.3.6.2 Activation

The conversion of the quiescent bone surface to resorption activity is referred to as activation. The factor that initiates this process is unknown, but activation is believed to occur at random and partly in response to focal structural or biomechanical

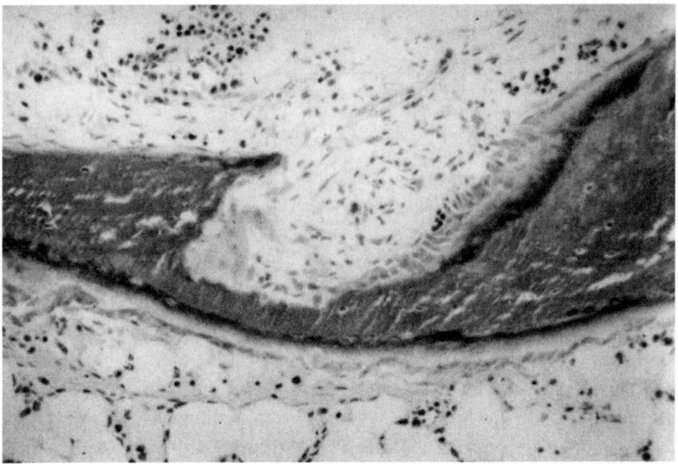

FIGURE 1.13 Cancellous bone remodeling, or BMU, in a renal osteodystrophy patient. The osteoclastic resorption is abnormally deep and may sever the trabecula. (From Weiss, L., *Cell and Tissue Biology, a Textbook of Histology*, Urban and Schwarzenberg, Baltimore, 1988. With permission.)

requirements. The remodeling cycle requires the recruitment of osteoclasts and the means for them to gain access to the bone surface (attraction and attachment). Briefly, bone-lining cells are believed to digest the endosteal membrane and to retract, thereby exposing the mineralized bone surface, which is chemotactic for osteoclast precursor cells. This insulated behavior of osteoblast-lineage cells may explain why receptors of many of the known bone-resorbing agents are found in osteoblasts and not in osteoclasts.

1.3.6.3 Resorption

Where osteoclasts come in contact with the surface of bone, they begin to erode the bone, forming cavities referred to as Howship's lacunae in cancellous bone, and as cutting cones or resorption cavities in cortical bone. In the cortical bone of dogs, the osteoclasts in the cutting cone travel in a direction roughly parallel to the long axis of the bone at a speed of about 20 to 40 microns per day and radially about 5 to 10 microns per day. The mean depth of erosion is about 60 microns in trabecular bone and about 100 microns in cortical bone. This phase takes about 1 to 3 weeks.

1.3.6.4 Reversal (Coupling)

This term refers to a 1- to 2-week interval between the completion of resorption and the commencement of formation. The histological counterpart of the reversal period is the point in time when the Howship's lacunae and the cutting cones lack osteoclasts, but contain mononuclear cells of unknown origin and function. Exactly what triggers the coupling process is not known.

1.3.6.5 Formation and Mineralization

Bone formation occurs in two stages, matrix synthesis followed by extracellular mineralization. Soon after the deposition of cement substance (the reversal line), the new osteoblasts begin to deposit a layer of bone matrix referred to as the osteoid seam. The osteoid seam will have reached a level of approximately 70% of its final mineralization after about 5 to 10 days. Complete mineralization takes about 3 to 6 months in both cortical and trabecular bone.

In the adult skeleton, the usual BMU resorbs 20 parts of bone but replaces 19, creating a negative bone balance. This has led to the term "bone remodeling-dependent bone loss." Increased mechanical usage (MU) depresses the number of new remodeling packets. It may also cause each completed packet to become less negative, thus conserving trabecular and endocortical bone next to marrow. Remodeling increases as a result of disuse. This accelerates trabecular and endocortical bone loss, with the spongiosa becoming osteopenic and the marrow cavity enlarging.

1.3.6.6 Bone Turnover[15]

Bone turnover depends on the surface-restricted activation frequency and on the surface-to-volume ratio. Activation frequency is the intensity of remodeling, the reciprocal of the average time interval between the start of consecutive cycles of remodeling at the same site. The surface-to-volume ratio of typical cancellous and cortical bone differs by a factor of at least 10 (Table 1.2). Site measurements of turnover in the human skeleton have been limited to the rib and ilium. Cortical bone turnover in the rib is about 4%/year. In the ilium, activation frequency is about the same in cancellous, endocortical, and intracortical subdivisions of the endosteal surfaces, so the difference in bone turnover is related entirely to the difference in surface-to-volume ratio.

Direct measurements of turnover in axial and appendicular cancellous bone in the adult beagle dog and their relationship to hematopoietic (red) and fatty (yellow) marrow are listed in Table 1.5.

1.3.6.7 The Remodeling Space

The remodeling space consists of the hole made by the remodeling process. Accordingly, an increase in the number of BMUs and in the time required to fill the hole will increase remodeling space.

TABLE 1.5
Cancellous Bone Turnover in Adult Beagle Dogs

Site	Marrow	Turnover (%/year) Rate
Lumbar vertebra	Red	205
Proximal femur	Red	138
Ilium	Red	164
Distal radius	Yellow	85

1.4 DEVELOPMENT OF A TYPICAL LONG BONE[1]

The sequence of growth and development in a long bone is outlined below. Briefly: (1) a hyaline cartilage model is laid down, and grows by apposition from the perichondrium and by proliferation of the cells at the ends; (2) a subperiosteal ring of bone is laid down by intramembranous ossification; (3) the central portion of cartilage anlage calcifies, and vascular mesenchyme enters to form the primary endochondral ossification center; (4) the zone of ossification spreads toward the ends of the bone; (5) blood vessels and mesenchyme enter the superior and inferior epiphyseal ossification centers to form articular cartilage and growth plate; (6) the growth plate, responsible for bone elongation, consists of cartilage cells that multiply, hypertrophy, die, and calcify their matrix in the form of cell columns; (7) blood vessels and osteogenic cells invade and selectively destroy about 2/3 of the calcified cartilage matrix and deposit bone around the remaining deposits to form the primary spongiosa that subsequently is remodeled into secondary spongiosa; (8) the shaft of cortical bone increases in width, with periosteal bone formation exceeding endocortical bone resorption; and (9) bone elongation stops when the growth plate ossifies (epiphyseal closure) to form the continuous bone marrow cavity. A more detailed description of this process can be found in any basic histology textbook.

1.5 SKELETAL MASS AND ITS CHANGES

A child's bone bank represents the difference between bone added by growth and by modeling-dependent bone gain on one hand, and bone removed by remodeling-dependent bone loss on the other. In adults, however, where growth no longer goes on and where modeling comes to a near-standstill, remodeling-dependent bone loss controls most of the adult bone bank. This means the bone bank depends mostly on the activation frequency (a histologic index of the intensity of bone remodeling), or the bone balance at a given moment on the bone mass accumulated during growth, i.e., the peak bone mass. In other words, accumulating bone mass in children depends on controlling longitudinal bone growth, modeling, and remodeling. Managing bone mass in adults depends on the peak bone mass and how remodeling converts it thereafter.

1.5.1 Skeletal Adaptation to Mechanical Usage[16-21]

Mechanical usage plays an important role in skeletal development and maintenance. Mechanical regulation of bone biology begins at about 5 to 7 weeks of prenatal life when most of the adult skeletal elements and soft tissue have formed. Intermittent skeletal tissue strains caused by muscular contraction modulate cartilage growth, ossification, plus bone modeling and remodeling, throughout the skeleton. After birth, growth and ossification of the skeleton are strongly influenced by externally applied forces.

How mechanical usage regulates bone mass and architecture introduces a new concept of bone response to mechanical usage and can best be explained by Frost's mechanostat hypothesis.[19] The hypothesis helps to explain many clinical and experimental observations that previously did not make sense. Nevertheless, no matter how logical it is, it is still a hypothesis. Frost, building on earlier work by Curry and Lanyon, proposed the mechanostat as a name for the biologic mechanisms that fit skeletal mass and architecture to the needs of one's normal physical activities. It is well recognized that bone mass adapts to mechanical usage (MU) in a special way: The MU makes its biologic mechanisms correct errors between the mass and its MU. The mechanism would behave like a home thermostat in that it would turn "on" in response to error and "off" in its absence, so that is why it was named the mechanostat. The relationship can be encoded thus:

MU → bone → mechanostat → bone mass effect

The mechanostat has been proposed to consist of at least these tissue-level biologic mechanisms: growth, modeling and remodeling mechanisms, the minimum effective strain (MES) mechanisms that control the latter two, including their location and rates, plus the mechanical transducers (mechanical signals and relay stations) in bone that pass that information to the biologic side of the MES mechanisms. That relation could be written thus:

MU → bone → MES mechanics → responding growth/modeling/remodeling systems

The mechanostat concept is based on the idea that there exists an effective strain (MES) set point. With a mechanical overload, a response will occur which increases muscle and bone mass and strength (Figure 1.14). If there is a persistent underload,

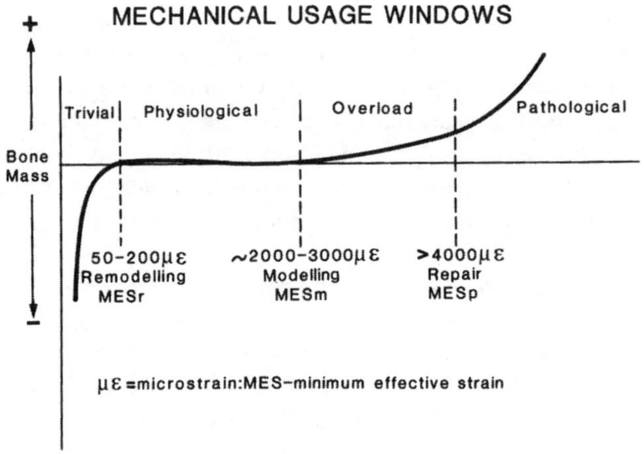

FIGURE 1.14 Mechanical usage windows (Adapted from Frost, H. M., *J. Bone and Mineral Research*, 12, 1539, 1997.)

TABLE 1.6
Proposed Effects of Mechanical Usage (MU), Disease, Drugs, and Hormones on the Set Point Range for Bone and Resulting Effects on Bone Mass in the Adult Skeleton[a]

	Set Point	Annual Net Bone Loss, Global	Annual Remodeling
Mechanical usage, normal	O[b]	N	N
Mechanical usage, deficient	I	I	I
Oophorectomy	I	I	I
Paralysis	I	I	I
Adrenal steroids	I	I	I
1^0 Hyperparathyroidism	I	I	I
Calcium deficiency	I	I	I
Mechanical usage, increased	D	D	D
Estrogen	D	D	D
Thyroidectomy	D	D	D
Calcitonin	D	D	D
Weightlifting	D	D	D

[a] Modified from Frost, H. F., *Anat. Rec.* 219, 1, 1987.
[b] O, no change; N, normal; D, decreased; I, increased.

as in hypogravity situations, muscle and bone mass will diminish to a level corresponding to the lower load. The set point is defined as a range of strain values that will produce no response. Strains above the set point (or set point range), i.e., beyond 2,000 to 3,000 microstrain, will evoke a positive response leading to an increased bone mass. Strains below the physiological set point range, i.e., below 200 microstrain, will trigger a response that causes bone loss. Thus, modeling-dependent bone gain is stimulated at strains above 2,000 microstrain and remodeling is stimulated at strains below 200 microstain. When modeling is "on", remodeling is "off" and vice versa, because modeling-dependent bone gain and remodeling-dependent bone loss take place within different strain ranges.[20] Non-mechanical agents can evoke changes or errors in the setpoint range, leading in turn to changes in modeling and remodeling activities, even though there has been no effective change in the strain environment.

The non-mechanical agents (e.g., hormones, growth factors, nutrition, diseases, genetics, toxic agents, etc.) can either act directly on the mechanical regulation of bone cells or on biologic mechanisms that are independent of the mechanical stimuli. In either case interaction would occur between mechanical and non-mechanical factors. Such additive or synergistic influences have been reported; this indicates mechanical stimuli that modulate controlling bone mass in turn are subject to modulation by endocrine states, diet, or drugs (Table 1.6). Thus, the relationship between mechanical usage and nonmechanical agents in the control of bone mass can be encoded as thus:

```
                ------------mechanical usage feedback loop ← -------
                ↓                                                    |
Load   →   bone mass   →   signals-biologic mechanisms-bone mass
                ↑                    ↑                    ↑
           set point   ←   systemic local non-mechanical agents
```

1.5.2 Age-Related Bone Loss[18,21,22]

Two distinct phases of age-related bone loss have been described: a slow age-related phase that occurs in both sexes, and a transient accelerated phase that occurs in postmenopausal women. The slow phase begins about age 40 and continues throughout life. Its rate is similar in both sexes and leads to a comparable loss of cortical and cancellous bone. The accelerated phase of postmenopausal bone loss is due to estrogen deficiency and results in much greater relative loss of cancellous than cortical bone, with most of the bone lost during the first 4 to 8 years after the menopause (Figure 1.15). The accelerated postmenopausal phase is the result of increased osteoclastic resorption. This, in turn, causes greater bone loss (deeper bone cavitation) than can be overcome by osteoblastic activity. The high level of osteoclastic activity results in perforation of trabecular plates and the loss of architectural elements in cancellous bone. These cannot be replaced. In contrast, the slow phase of bone loss is associated mainly with impaired osteoblastic activity at the cellular level, that is, each osteoblast does less work and collectively the osteoblasts fail to refill the cavity completely. This leads to a progressive thinning of whatever trabecular bone is left in women and of trabecular bone in men, as well as to a decrease in the width of the cortex.

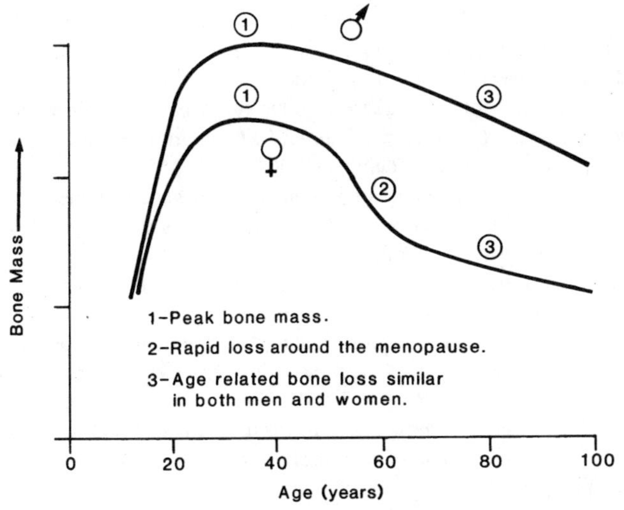

FIGURE 1.15 Pattern of age-related bone loss in men and women.

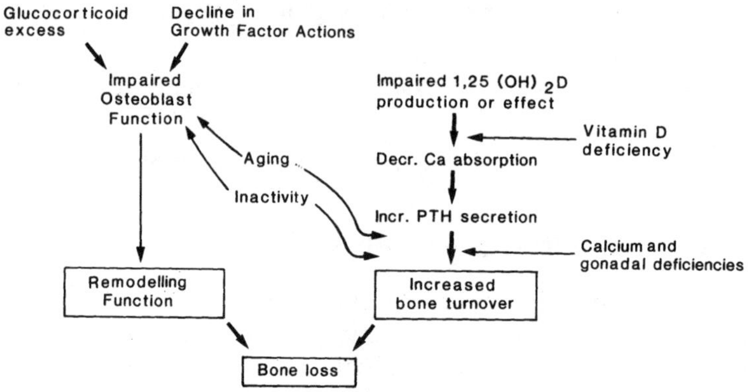

FIGURE 1.16 Model of age-related bone loss.

The causes of age-related bone loss are believed to be multifactorial. Some of the factors include a decline in hormonal activity (gonadal hormones, growth hormones, thyroxin, etc.), nutritional deficiency, especially of calcium and vitamin D, and inactivity. A proposed model for age-related bone loss is shown in Figure 1.16.

REFERENCES

1. Jee, W.S.S., The skeletal tissues, in: *Cell and Tissue Biology, A Textbook of Histology,* Weiss, L., Ed., Urban and Schwarenberg, Baltimore, 1988, Chapter 7.
2. Baron, R., Anatomy and ultrastructure of bone, in: *Primer on the Metabolic Bone Diseases and Disorders of Mineral Metabolism*, Third Edition, Favus, M.J., Ed., Lippencott-Raven, Philadelphia, 1996, 3.
3. Termine, J.D. and Robey, P.G., Bone matrix proteins and the mineralization process, in: *Primer on the Metabolic Bone Diseases and Disorders of Mineral Metabolism,* Third Edition, Favus, M.J., Ed., Lippincott-Raven, Philadelphia, 1996, 24.
4. Eyre, D.R., Biochemical markers of bone turnovers, in: *Primer on the Metabolic Bone Diseases and Disorders of Mineral Metabolism,* Third Edition, Favus, M.J., Ed., Lippincott-Raven, Philadelphia, 1996, 114.
5. Parfitt, A.M., The physiologic and clinical significance of bone histomorphometric data, in: *Bone Histomorphometry: Techniques and Interpretation*, Recker, R.R., Ed., CRC Press, Boca Raton, 1983, 143.
6. Hattner, R., Epker, B.N., and Frost, H.M., Suggested sequential mode of control of changes in cell behavior in adult bone remodeling, *Nature*, 206, 489, 1965.
7. Ericksen, E.F., Normal and pathological remodeling of human trabecular bone: Three dimensional reconstruction of the remodeling sequence in normals and in metabolic bone disease, *Endocrine Review,* 7, 179, 1986.
8. Mundy, G.R., Bone resorbing cells, in: *Primer on the Metabolic Bone Diseases and Disorders of Mineral Metabolism*, Third Edition, Favus, M.J., Ed., Lippincott-Raven, Philadelphia, 1996, 16.
9. Teitelbaum, S.L., Tondravi, M.M., and Ross, F.P., Osteoclast Biology, in: *Osteoporosis*, Marcus, R., Feldman, D., and Kelsey, J., Eds., Academic Press, San Diego, 1996, Chapter 3.

10. Lian, J.B. and Stein G.S., Osteoblast biology, in: *Osteoporosis*, Marcus, R., Feldman, D., and Kelsey, J., Eds., Academic Press, San Diego, 1996, Chapter 2.
11. Puzas, J.E., Osteoblast cell biology — lineage and functions, in: *Primer on the Metabolic Bone Diseases and Disorders of Mineral Metabolism,* Third Edition, Favus, M.J., Ed., Lippincott-Raven, Philadelphia, 1996, 11.
12. Recker, R.R., Ed., *Bone Histomorphometry: Techniques and Interpretation*, CRC Press, Boca Raton, 1983.
13. Jee, W.S.S. and Ma, Y.F., The *in vivo* anabolic actions of prostaglandins in bone, *Bone*, 21, 297, 1997.
14. Miller, S.C. and Jee, W.S.S., The bone lining cell: A distinct phenotype?, *Calcif. Tissue Int.*, 41,1, 1992.
15. Parfitt, A.M., The skeletal heterogeneity and the purposes of bone remodeling: Implications for the understanding of osteoporosis, *Osteoporosis,* Marcus, R., Feldman, D., and Kelsey, J., Eds. Academic Press, San Diego, 1996, Chapter 12.
16. Martin, R.B. and Burr, D.B., Mechanical Adaptation, *Structure, Function and Adaptation of Compact Bone*, Raven Press, New York, 1989, Chapter 4.
17. Jee, W.S.S., Li, X.J., and Ke, H.Z., The skeletal adaptation to mechanical usage in the rat, *Cells and Materials*, Supplement 1, 131, 1991.
18. Burr, D.B., Muscle strength, bone mass and age-related bone loss, *J. Bone and Mineral Research*, 12, 1547,1997.
19. Frost, H.M., The mechanostat: A proposed pathogenic mechanism of osteoporoses and the bone mass effects of mechanical and nonmechanical agents, *Bone and Mineral*, 2, 73, 1987.
20. Frost, H.M., A vital biomechanical model of synovial joint design, *Anatomic Record*, 240, 1, 1994.
21. Frost, H.M., On our age-related bone loss: Insights from a new paradigm, *J. Bone and Mineral Research*, 12, 1539, 1997.
22. Kassem, M., Melton, L.J., and Riggs, B.L., The type I/type II model for involuntional osteoporosis, *Osteoporosis*, Marcus, R., Feldman, D., and Kelsey, J., Eds., Academic Press, San Diego, 1996. Chapter 34.

2 Structure and Function of Connective Tissue

Joel Rosenbloom

CONTENTS

Abbreviations used: bp, base pairs; BSP, bone sialoprotein; FACIT, fibril-associated collagen; FBLN, fibulin; FBN, fibrillin; LTBP, latent TGF-β binding protein; MFAP, microfibril associated protein; MAGP, microfibril associated glycoprotein; OPN, osteopontin; RGD, Arg-Gly-Asp; SLRPs, small leucine-rich proteoglycans.

0-8493-9237-3/99/$0.00+$.50

2.1 THE COLLAGENS

2.1.1 General Structure

The connective tissues of the musculo-skeletal system consist of fibrous and nonfibrous components. The fibrous components include those composed of the collagens and elastin while a much wider variety of macromolecules constitutes the nonfibrous group.

The collagens are the most abundant proteins in the vertebrate body and are major proteins in bone and cartilage extracellular matrices. They play important roles in determining the size, shape, and strength of these tissues. Several unique features distinguish the collagens from other proteins. They are composed of three polypeptide chains which are called α chains and form characteristic left-handed helices. These in turn assemble into a relatively rigid right-handed triple helix, well-suited to its function as a major structural component. The primary structure of individual α chains can be represented by a repeating Gly-X-Y tripeptide.[27,37,38] While several other proteins, including the complement component C1q, contain relatively short stretches of Gly-X-Y repeats, they are not considered collagens because they do not function as part of the extracellular matrix. Proline is frequently found in the X position and 4-hydroxyproline in the Y position, and these two imino acids serve to limit the rotation of the chains. Hydroxyproline is required for stabilization of the triple helix. Steric limitations in the conformation of the triple helix require that glycine occur at every third residue in the center of the helix and place the side chains of the other amino acids on the periphery of the molecule. This latter arrangement permits interaction between residues of different molecules and facilitates their self assembly into fibers. The fibers are stabilized by lysine- and hydroxylysine-derived crosslinks of individual collagen molecules.[21]

Presently, 20 types of collagen molecules have been identified, which are formed from the products of approximately 30 different genes. Each collagen type has been assigned a Roman number and individual α chains are designated α1, α2, etc., followed by the Roman numeral of the collagen type and the complete designation of a molecule includes the ratio in which the chains occur. Thus, the α chains of type I collagen are α1(I) and α2(I), and the molecular designation is $[\alpha1(I)]_2\alpha2(I)$. For type II collagen which is a homotrimer the designation would be $[\alpha1(II)]_3$.

2.1.2 Classification of Collagens

Based on their structure, the collagens can be grouped into distinct categories (Table 2.1).[27,37,38] The first group forms banded fibers and includes types I, II, III, V, and XI. These collagens have uninterrupted triple-helical domains in which each α chain contains 338 to 343 Gly-X-Y triplets. These molecules aggregate in a characteristic packing pattern in which the individual molecules are approximately 4.4 times the length of the 67 nm repeat period, called the D period. They are staggered about one-quarter their length, leaving a small space between the amino terminal of one molecule and the carboxy terminal of the next (Figure 2.1). Recent evidence suggests that fibrils in some instances are heterotypic, that is, composed of more than one fibrillar collagen type.[5] Differences in molecular composition then

TABLE 2.1
Classification of the Collagens

Type	Comment
	Fibrillar
I	• Most abundant, widespread in many connective tissues
II	• Cartilage, vitreous humor
III	• Widespread, particularly in skin, lung, and blood vessels
V	• Often associated with type I as a minor constituent
XI	• Often associated with type II in heterotypic fibrils
	Fibril Associated (FACIT)
IX	• Surface of type II Fibrils
XII	• Found with type I
XIV	• Found with type I
	Network Forming
IV	• Found in basement membranes
VIII	• Descemet's membrane in the cornea, subendothelial matrices
X	• Found in hypertrophic cartilage
	Anchoring
VII	• Provides link between epidermal basement membrane and underlying dermis
	Beaded Filament
VI	• Widely distributed
	Miscellaneous
XIII	• Contains transmembrane domain
XVII	• Contains transmembrane domain
XV	• Many tissues
XVI	• Many tissues
XVIII	• Found in liver and kidney

give rise to different properties. Analysis of the genes encoding the fibrillar collagens strongly suggests that all were derived from a prototypic ancestral gene.[35] The triple helical domains of most of the chains are encoded in 42 exons which are usually 54 base pairs (bp) and less frequently twice or three times 54 bp. Each exon begins with a glycine codon and thus encodes a fixed number, usually six, of Gly-X-Y repeats.

The second group is called fibril-associated collagens with interrupted triple helices (FACIT), and includes types IX, XII, and XIV. These collagens associate with the first group, and are localized to the surface of banded fibrils. For example, in cartilage, type IX collagen molecules are arranged on the surface of fibrils in register with the D periodicity.[37,38] This permits covalent crosslinking between type IX and type II molecules. A non-collagenous globular domain of the type IX molecule functions as a hinge allowing other type IX domains to extend outwards from the fibril surface where they may interact with other matrix components

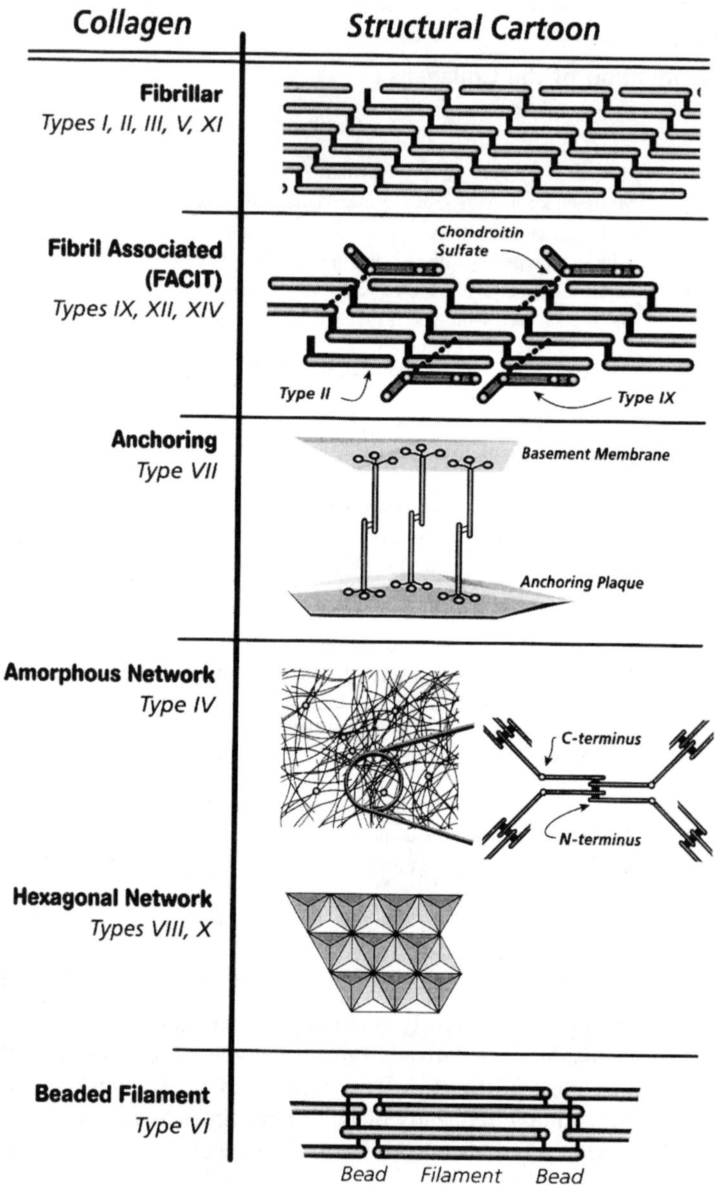

FIGURE 2.1 Diagrammatic representation of the various types of collagen. In the fibrillar collagens, individual molecules are organized in a staggered array and are bound together by crosslinks derived from the oxidation of lysyl and hydroxylysyl residues. FACIT collagens are localized to the surface of fibrils. The dotted line in the FACIT collagen represents an attached chondroitin sulfate side chain.

(Figure 2.1). Interestingly, a glycosaminoglycan side chain is often attached to this non-collagenous domain, but its function is unknown. Type XII and type XIV collagens, which have some structural similarity to type IX, also contain glycosaminoglycan side chains in their large amino terminal globular domains. Type XII is often associated with type I collagen.

The network-forming group is composed of type IV, the first non-fibrillar collagen to be identified and studied, and types VIII and X collagens. Although designated as a single collagen, type IV consists of six different α chains that contain collagenous as well as non-collagenous domains. These chains can form a variety of molecular combinations. The basic unit of the supramolecular organization of type IV collagen is thought to consist of four molecules joined at their amino termini by disulfide bridges and each individual molecule is bound at its carboxy terminal to the carboxy terminal of another molecule. These basic units assemble into an extended network (Figure 2.1).[38,41]

The other two collagen types found in this class, types VIII and X, while similar to each other in gene and domain structure, are quite different from type IV. They consist of a nonhelical amino terminus, a globular carboxy terminus, and a central single triple-helical domain which is only about half as big as the fibrillar collagens and contains eight imperfections. The type X collagen molecule, $[\alpha 1(X)]_3$, is found only in hypertrophic cartilage that is undergoing endochondral bone formation. Unlike the fibrillar collagens, the intact type X molecule is incorporated without proteolytic processing into the hypertrophic cartilage extracellular matrix where it forms distinct hexagonal arrays. It may regulate mineralization or vascular invasion.

The anchoring class consists solely of the long-chain homotrimeric type VII collagen, whose individual chains contain a central triple-helical domain that is about one-third larger than that of the fibrillar collagens.[37,38] Type VII collagen has a small amino terminal globular domain and a relatively large complex carboxy terminal domain. The collagen is found only in subepithelial structures that anchor the underlying matrix to the basement membrane of stratified epithelia (Figure 2.1). Two type VII molecules are aligned antiparallel to one another, with the overlap at their amino termini stabilized by disulfide crosslinks. The carboxy ends are thus available to insert into the lamina densa of the basement membrane at one end and into anchoring plaques within the stroma at the other end. This stabilizes the epidermis to the underlying dermis.

The beaded filament class consists of type VI collagen.[36] These molecules are composed of three different α chains with a central collagenous domain and large noncollagenous domains at either end. Based upon a model of the supramolecular assembly of type VI collagen, two type VI molecules appear to form antiparallel dimers. Two of these then associate laterally to form tetramers that in turn assemble into the beaded filaments as illustrated in Figure 2.1.

2.1.3 Biosynthesis

The fibrillar collagens are synthesized as larger precursor molecules, designated as procollagens, which undergo a number of reactions before incorporation into the fiber.[25] Intracellularly, signal peptides are cleaved and Y-position proline and lysine residues are hydroxylated to 4-hydroxyproline and hydroxylysine, while a few

X-position prolines are hydroxylated to 3-hydroxyprolines. Galactose or galactose and glucose are added to some of the hydroxylysine residues and more complex mannose-containing carbohydrates are added to the C-terminal propeptide. Disulfide bonds form between the associated C-terminal propeptides. After about 100 4-hydroxyprolines are formed per α chain, triple helix formation begins in the carboxy portion and proceeds to the amino terminus. After secretion, the N- and C-propeptides are cleaved by distinct propeptidases, and the molecules then self-assemble into fibers. Some lysine and hydroxylysine residues are then oxidized to aldehyde derivatives which condense to form a family of complex crosslinks stabilizing the fiber.

Synthesis and assembly of non-fibrillar collagens are often but not always similar. Frequently (as in type IV), N- and C-propeptides are not removed, and, as noted above, glycosaminoglycans may be added to some chains (types IX, XII, and XIV).

2.2 ELASTIC FIBERS

The function of tissues such as the dermis, lung, and large blood vessels requires that they possess elastic properties.[31] In vertebrates, this property is achieved largely through the presence of elastic fibers that are composed of two distinct components: (i) a more abundant amorphous component made up of the protein elastin, and (ii) a 10 to 12 nm microfibrillar component that is located primarily around the periphery of the fiber.[32,35] Some characteristics of non-collagenous matrix proteins are given in Table 2.2.

2.2.1 Elastin

Consistent with its unique physical properties, elastin has an unusual amino acid composition, rich in glycine (33%) and proline (10 to 13%), and in hydrophobic amino acids that constitute approximately 44% of the total residues. Elastin is synthesized via a soluble 72 kDa precursor, tropoelastin; significant synthesis occurs only in embryonic and rapidly growing tissues. Some of the prolyl residues in tropoelastin are hydroxylated post-translationally. However, unlike collagen where hydroxproline stabilizes the triple helical structure, the function of hydroxyproline in tropoelastin is unknown. Also unlike the fibrillar collagens, tropoelastin is incorporated without proteolytic cleavage into the insoluble fiber. In several developing embryonic systems, a strong correlation between messenger RNA levels and the rate of elastin synthesis has been demonstrated; this suggests that the rate of synthesis is controlled by the mRNA steady-state level.

A critical feature of the elastin fiber, crucial to its elastic function, is the extensive extracellular crosslinking of tropoelastin. Elastin contains about 4% lysine, most of which is incorporated into crosslinks. There are very few charged residues in the elastin portion of the mature fiber. The enzyme that catalyzes the oxidative deamination and condensation of lysyl side chains, lysyl oxidase, is the same enzyme involved in collagen crosslink formation.[16] Some of the final bifunctional products such as lysinonorleucine and allysine aldol are also found in collagen fibers, but the tetrafunctional ones, the desmosines, are found exclusively in elastin. Positional considerations have suggested that a critical step in the crosslinking pathway is the formation of a bifunctional "within chain" intermediate crosslink, which then condenses with another bifunctional intermediate on a second chain to form the tetrafunctional desmosine crosslinks. All but about 5 of the 34 lysine residues of tropoelastin are incorporated into some form of crosslink. The net result is a highly insoluble polymer in which some type of interchain lysine-derived crosslink occurs about every 65 to 70 residues.

TABLE 2.2
Characteristics of Non-Collagenous Matrix Proteins

Protein	Comment
Elastin	Tropoelastin, 70 kDa biosynthetic intermediate, heavily cross-linked to form fiber. Provides elasticity to tissues. Mutations cause supravalvular aortic stenosis.
Fibrillins (FBN)	Fibrillin family contains two members. Major component of elastic microfibrils, 350 kDa, contains EGF and TGF-β binding protein motifs. Mutations in FBN1 result in Marfan Syndrome and mutations in FBN2 cause contractural arachnodactyly.
Latent TGF-β Binding Proteins (LTBP)	LTBP is a family that contains at least four members ranging in size from 150 to 205 kDa. Contain EGF and TGF-β binding protein motifs. Secreted as a complex with latent TGF-β, but also found as a free protein.
Fibulins (FBLN)	Family consists of FBLN1 and FBLN2, 350 kDa. Contains EGF and anaphylatoxin motifs. Widely distributed.
Microfibril Associated Glycoproteins (MAGP)	A family of proteins: MAGP1 (also called MFAP2) 31 kDa, widely distributed in microfibrils; MAGP2 (also called MP25), 25 kDa has a more restricted distribution.
Microfibril Associated Proteins (MFAP)	Included in this group of proteins is MFAP1 (very acidic), MFAP3, MFAP4 (frequently deleted in Smith-Magenis Syndrome), and MP70/78 (also called Big/h3) associated with type VI collagen; mutations cause corneal dystrophy.
Osteocalcin	~5 kDa, contains γ-carboxyl glutamate (gla) which mediates high affinity Ca^{++} binding. May reuglate osteoclast activity. Gene knockout in mice leads to hypermineralization.
Osteonectin (SPARC)	~40 kDa, multiple low affinity Ca^{++} binding sites, 2 EF hand high affinity Ca^{++} binding sites. May mediate deposition of hydroxyappetite.
Fibronectin	~400 kDa, 2 disulfide linked chains contain RGD integrin-binding sites. Also binds fibrin, heparin, and collagen. Widely distributed.
Osteopontin (OPN)	~44 to 75 kDa, is glycosylated and phosphorylated. Contains RGD cell binding site. May regulate mineralization.
Bone Sialoprotein (BSP)	~46 to 75 kDa, contains polyglutamyl sequences and is heavily glycosylated. Binds to cells and may regulate mineralization.
Laminins	Molecule composed of α (~400 kDa), β (~200 kDa) and γ (~200 kDa) subunits. Major component of basement membranes. Mutations cause forms of epidermolysis bullosa and muscular dystrophy.

2.2.1.1 Basis of Elastic Properties

Elastic recoil is a critical property of several tissues and organ systems. For example, during an average lifetime the elastic fibers in the aortic arch undergo more than a billion stretch/relaxation cycles. Since the turnover of elastin appears to be quite low, individual fibers can conceivably last a lifetime.[22] The rather amazing durability of the elastic fiber suggests that the elastomeric force results not from the stressing of chemical bonds, as this could result in progressive deterioration, but rather from the number of conformations accessible to the crosslinked polypeptide chains. Removal of the stretching force increases the number of available conformational states and provides the free energy for elastic recoil. As is true in rubber, elasticity is the result of an increase in entropy that occurs upon relaxation.

2.2.2 Microfibrillar Proteins

The microfibrils consist of what appear to be tubular structures, about 10 to 12 nm in diameter. Their staining properties and susceptibilities to enzymatic digestion differ from those of amorphous elastin.[9] At high resolution, the microfibrils appear in cross-section as an outer electron-dense shell that surrounds an inner lucid core. In longitudinal section they appear as a beaded chain. This suggests they may be composed of more than one protein. Apparently similar microfibrils are present in many tissues. These include tissues with abundant elastin, as well as those without detectable elastin. Examples of the latter are the ocular ciliary zonule and the periodontal ligament. In the dermis, the microfibrillary bundles that connect the deep dermal elastic plexus with the dermo-epidermal junction region consist of microfibrils that are indistinguishable from those associated with elastic fibers, even though in their superficial distribution no elastin is associated with them.

Because of their insolubility and apparent complexity, chemical characterization of the microfibrils progressed slowly until recently. The structural proteins of the microfibrils can be conveniently divided into two groups: (i) those larger than 125 kDa, and (ii) those smaller than 115 kDa. The larger molecular weight group consists of three gene families: (1) fibrillins, (2) latent TGF-β binding proteins (LTBPs), and (3) fibulins. Significantly, these three families share protein domain motifs as discussed below.

2.2.2.1 Fibrillins

The largest of these proteins and quantitatively the most important are the fibrillins, 350 kDa glyproteins reported to form an integral part of the microfibril structure.[34] These are extended flexible molecules approximately 148 nm long and 2.2 nm wide. Multiple fibrillin molecules probably align in a parallel head-to-tail fashion to form a major portion of the microfibrils. The human gene that encodes fibrillin-1 (FBN1) is located on chromosome 15q15-21 and the gene that encodes FBN2 is on chromosome 5q23-q31.[23,28] Analysis of the deduced fibrillin amino acid sequences has demonstrated that the proteins contain multiple repeats of a sequence motif previously observed in the epidermal growth factor.[8] Many of these repeats contain consensus sequences that have been associated with calcium binding. A second motif, originally found in latent TGFβ binding proteins (LTBPs),[17] has also been identified in the fibrillins (Figure 2.2 compares the structures of the FBNs and LTBPs). Of great interest is the recent report of a protein in jellyfish having extensive

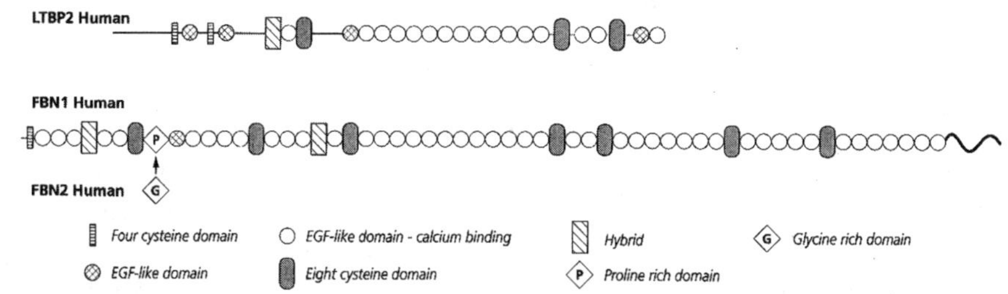

FIGURE 2.2 Diagrammatic representation of the domain structure of the latent TGF-β binding protein and fibrillin gene families. The overall organization of the two fibrillin proteins is very similar and they differ mainly in a segment which is proline-rich in FBN1 and glycine-rich in FBN2. Phylogenetic analysis indicates that the FBN and LTBP gene families are related.

homology to mammalian fibrillin. This suggests that fibrillin is a very ancient protein that evolved long before elastin.[29]

2.2.2.1.1 The Marfan syndrome and congenital contractural arachnodatyly

Inherited as an autosomal dominant disorder with complete penetrance, the Marfan syndrome (MFS) is characterized by a complex and variable phenotype in which disorders in the skeletal, ocular and cardiovascular systems predominate, with dissecting aortic aneurysm the leading cause of premature death of MFS patients. The cloning of the fibrillin genes proved to be a turning point in the identification of the defective protein. It is now certain that mutations in FBN1 are responsible for the vast majority, if not all, cases of MFS and to date more than 75 mutations have been identified.[23,28] The mutations are distributed throughout the molecule, but in general there is no clear genotype/phenotype relationship with the exception that mutations causing the severe, neonatal phenotype cluster in the middle of the molecule. Interestingly, mutations in FBN2 have been linked to a second condition, congenital contractural arachnodactyly, which shares some of the features of MFS, but lacks the cardiovascular and ocular manifestations, and has additional characteristic features including crumpled ears.

2.2.2.2 Latent TGFβ Binding Proteins

Several members of the LTBP family have been cloned and shown to contain repeating domains similar to those found in FBN1 and FBN2 (Figure 2.2). TGF-β is always secreted as a latent complex and in some cases this complex is bound to a LTBP.[3,17] To date, four distinct LTBPs have been cloned and characterized, ranging in size from 125 kDA to 205 kDa. The function of LTBPs remains to be determined, since they are not necessary to maintain TGF-β in an inactive form, nor do they appear to bind mature TGF-β. Although LTBPs may facilitate the secretion of TGF-β or the binding of the inactive complex to the cell surface where activation takes place, they are also found as free proteins associated with components of the extracellular matrix.[13]

2.2.2.3 Fibulins

The fibulins (FBLN) are extracellular matrix and blood glycoproteins that self-associate and can bind fibronectin.[2] Molecular cloning has identified two distinct fibulin genes. The deduced amino acid sequences reveal that the molecules are modular, having several types of repeated cysteine-containing motifs, including EGF-like and anaphylatoxin-like domains. FBLN1 is alternatively spliced and four forms have been identified which differ from one another at their carboxy termini. The fibulins are expressed in all major tissues with the exception of the brain. Fibulin protein is widely distributed in connective tissues such as those in the skin, in embryonic connective tissues, and in association with basement membranes. FBLN1 is particularly evident in the basal lamina that surrounds smooth muscle cells in blood vessels.[30] It also occurs in association with elastic fibers found in the dermal layer of the skin.

2.2.2.4 Other Microfibrillar Proteins

A number of other proteins unrelated to the FBNs, LTBPs, or FBLNs appear to be microfibril constituents. These include 25 kDa and 31 kDa components, designated microfibril associated glycoproteins (MAGPs). Molecular cloning has demonstrated that the two share limited regions of homology.[12,14] The observation that these proteins can be extracted with the help of a strong reducing agent suggests that intermolecular disulfide bonding is an important feature of the association of the polypeptide chains in the fibrils.

Other candidate microfibril components are a 115 kDa protein called emilin,[4] a protein designated βig/h3 and several proteins designated microfibril associated proteins (MFAPs).[1,19,40] One of the latter, MFAP1, is extremely acidic with glutamic acid comprising 23% and aspartic acid 6% of the residues. The acidic nature of the protein suggests that it may have an important function in the assembly of the very basic tropoelastin molecules.

In summary, the available evidence indicates that microfibrillar structures with apparently similar morphology are widely distributed in many tissues in the body. However, a completely satisfactory molecular model of the microfibrils has yet to be developed and the precise relationships between the fibrillins and other components of the microfibril remain obscure.

2.2.3 Fiber Assembly

Information on elastic fiber assembly is limited. The notion that secreted tropoelastin molecules simply diffuse onto the surface of growing fibers where they bind and become crosslinked does not explain the efficiency of the assembly process, the variable form of elastic fibers in different tissues, nor the non-random nature of the crosslinks. Assembly probably requires helper proteins both inside and outside of the cell. Elastin fibrillogenesis takes place at sites close to the cell membrane, generally in infoldings of the cell surface.[35] Microfibrils are the first visible components of elastic fibers that form a plexus upon which elastin appears as an amorphous material. These amorphous areas gradually coalesce and generate the central core of elastin. The majority of microfibrils are progressively displaced to the outer aspect of the fiber, a position they retain in the mature tissue. The observation that microfibrillar aggregates take the form and orientation of presumptive elastic fibers suggests that they direct the morphogenesis of elastic fibers by acting as a scaffold on which elastin is deposited. Microfibrils may serve to align tropoelastin molecules in precise register so that crosslinking regions are juxtaposed prior to oxidation by lysyl oxidase.

How secretion of tropoelastin is targeted to sites of elastic fiber assembly remains unknown. There is some evidence, however, that a 67 kDa protein binds tropoelastin in the endoplasmic reticulum and chaperones its secretion to assembly sites on the cell surface.[24] At the plasma membrane, tropoelastin may remain bound to the 67 kDa protein until an interaction with the microfibril induces the transfer of tropoelastin to the growing fiber. The 67 kDa elastin-binding protein is a galactoside lectin and its affinity for elastin is greatly diminished by interactions with carbohydrate. Galactose sugars on microfibrillar glycoproteins may provide specific signals for release of tropoelastin at sites of fiber assembly. Persuasive evidence exists that the carboxy-terminal end of tropoelastin mediates interactions with microfibrils.[6]

2.3 OTHER MATRIX PROTEINS

2.3.1 OSTEOCALCIN

Osteocalcin or bone gla protein (BGP) seems only expressed by osteoblasts.[11] It is one of a large group of proteins where some of the glutamic residues have been enzymatically γ-carboxylated by a reaction that requires vitamin K as a cofactor. Because of the modification, osteocalcin has a high affinity for Ca^{++} and hydroxyapatite crystals. Although the primary and higher order structure of many matrix proteins are known, elucidation of their function has remained elusive. Osteocalcin can inhibit the growth of hydroxyapatite crystals and increase the adhesion and spreading of osteoclastic cells. The protein might, therefore, modulate bone formation and mineralization. *In vivo* studies have shown that osteocalcin-depleted bone particles are resistant to resorption. Furthermore, mice whose osteocalcin gene had been deleted by homologous recombination exhibited greater bone mass and ectopic calcification, particularly of blood vessels.

2.3.2 OSTEONECTIN

Osteonectin was first isolated from bone, but has subsequently been identified in a number of tissues and has acquired a variety of names (SPARC, culture shock protein, BM40).[21] The protein has a high affinity for Ca^{++} due to the presence of two EF-hand binding sites. Its function is not known. Suggested roles include regulating cell cycle progression, cell-cell interactions, cell-matrix interactions, and modulating cell shape.

2.3.3 Fibronectin

Fibronectin is a major component of many connective tissues where it is synthesized by fibroblasts and other cells.[20,26] It is also synthesized by the liver and secreted into the blood where it is found in relatively high concentration. Many isoforms of the protein exist due to alternative splicing of the mRNA, but the specific forms in bone are not known. The protein is produced early in bone formation and osteoblasts readily adhere through integrin receptors to fibronectin-enriched matrices. Frequently, the tripeptide sequence Arg-Gly-Asp (RGD) in the ligand protein mediates this binding, but there are instances in which binding is independent of this sequence.

2.3.4 Osteopontin

Osteopontin (OPN) is a major non-collagenous bone matrix glycoprotein (M_r 41,500).[7,10] The protein is phosphorylated at many serine and threonine residues, and contains O-linked and one possible N-linked glycosylation site. Many segments of the protein are in an α-helical conformation, with some β-sheet structure in the amino terminal region. OPN contains one RGD sequence that interacts with the cell surface receptor, $\alpha_v\beta_3$ integrin, which mediates adhesion of osteoblasts and osteoclasts. OPN binds to hydroxyapatite and inhibits crystal growth. Because the protein mediates adhesion of osteoblasts and osteoclasts and because it is localized to the interface between both osteoblasts and osteocytes and bone, OPN may well participate in the regulation of bone matrix mineralization and resorption.

2.3.5 Bone sialoprotein (BSP)

BSP has a more limited distribution than OPN and is most characteristically found in mineralizing tissues such as newly forming bone, hypertrophic cartilage, and dentin. The protein is highly glycosylated (50% carbohydrate of which 12% is sialic acid) and contains a stretch of polyglutamic acid (probably responsible for the high Ca^{++} affinity), multiple sulfo-tyrosines and one RGD sequence near the carboxy terminus. Like OPN, BSP can mediate cell attachment and is likely to be involved in matrix mineralization.

2.3.6 Laminins

The laminins are major constituents of basement membranes.[20,23,41] Laminin molecules are composed of three chains: a 400 kDa α chain, a 200 kDa β chain, and a 200 kDa γ chain. These chains are linked together by disulfide bonds to form a cruciform molecule with a large globular domain at the base of the cross, and smaller globular domains at the end of each arm. At least 12 different laminin molecules have been identified. They participate in a variety of processes including cell adhesion, cell migration, and cell differentiation.

2.4 PROTEOGLYCANS

The proteoglycans consist of a growing family of macromolecules that are composed of a protein core to which glycosaminoglycans (GAGs) are covalently bound.[15,18] The GAG side chains are linear polymers of repeating disaccharides that contain a hexosamine and carboxylate and/or sulfate ester. Both the protein cores and GAGs are structurally diverse. The majority of our information with respect to the protein cores has come from molecular cloning. Based largely upon cDNA sequence analysis and their distribution within the extracellular matrix, the proteoglycans can be organized into several groups.

2.4.1 Small Leucine-Rich Proteoglycans (SLRPs)

The SLRPs have relatively small compact protein cores that are composed largely of characteristic repeat segments in the central portion of the molecule. These consist of alternating hydrophobic and hydrophilic amino acid residues with conserved leucines. Presently, five members have been identified: decorin, biglycan, fibromodulin, leumican, and epiphycan. Attached to the core proteins are chondroitin, dermatan, or keratan sulfate chains. The various SLRPs have been shown to interact specifically with several types of collagen (I,II, and VI) as well as fibronectin and TGF-β. These interactions may be important in regulating collagen fibril diameter, since binding of decorin appears to limit fibril dimensions. Through binding of TGF-β, the SLRPs may also regulate overall matrix production.

2.4.2 Large Modular Proteoglycans

These proteins are grouped together based upon their shared content of several modular domains. The group can be subdivided into those that bind and those that do not bind hyaluronan. The first class binds hyaluronan through a characteristic amino terminal region and contains a lectin domain that binds carbohydrates. They are found in a wide variety of connective tissues where they contribute to the elastic properties of cartilage and may serve to connect cell surfaces rich in hyaluronan to other carbohydrate-containing matrix molecules.

REFERENCES

1. Abrams, W.R., Ma, R.-I., Kucich, U., Bashir, M.M., Decker, S., Tsipouras, P., McPherson, J.D., Wasmuth, J.J., and Rosenbloom, J., Molecular cloning of the microfibrillar protein MFAP3 and assignment of the gene to human chromosome 5q32-q33.2, *Genomics* 26, 47, 1995.
2. Argraves, W.S., Tran, H., Burges, W.H., and Dickerson, K., Fibulin is an extracellular matrix and plasma glycoprotein with repeated domain structure, *J. Cell Biol.* 111, 3155, 1990.

3. Bashir, M.M., Han, M.-D., Abrams, W.R., Tucker, T., Ma, R.-I., Gibson, M., Ritty, T., Mecham, R., and Rosenbloom, J., Analysis of the human gene encoding latent transforming growth factor-β-binding protein-2, *Int. J. Biochem. Cell Biol.* 28, 531, 1996.
4. Bressan, G.M., Daga-Gordini, D., Colombatti, A., Castellani, R., Marigo, V., and Volpin, D., Emilin, a component of elastic fibers preferentially located at the elastin-microfibrils interface. *J. Cell Biol.* 121, 201, 1993.
5. Brewton, R.G. and Mayne, R., Heterotypic type II, IX, and XI fibrils: comparison of vitreous and cartilage forms, in *Extracellular Matrix Assembly and Structure,* Yurchenco, P.D., Birk, D.E., and Mecham, R.P., Eds., Academic Press, San Diego, 1994, 129.
6. Brown-Augsburger, P., Broekelmann, T., Rosenbloom, J., and Mecham, R.P., Functional domains on elastin and microfibril-associated glycoprotein involved in elastic fibre assembly, *Biochem. J.* 318, 149, 1996.
7. Butler, W.T., Ridall, A.I., and McKee, M.D., Osteopontin, in *Principles of Bone Biology,* Bilezikian, J.P., Raisz, L.G., and Rodan, G.A., Eds., Academic Press, San Diego, 1996, Chap. 13.
8. Carpenter, G. and Cohen, S., Epidermal growth factor, *J. Biol. Chem.* 265, 7709, 1990.
9. Cleary, E.G., The microfibrillar component of the elastic fibers, morphology and biochemistry, in *Connective Tissue Disease. Molecular Pathology of the Extracellular Matrix,* Uitto, J. and Perejda, A.J., Eds., Marcel Dekker, New York,1987, 140.
10. Denhardt, D.T. and Xiaojia, G., Osteopontin: a protein with diverse functions, *FASEB J.* 7, 1475, 1993.
11. Ducy, P. and Karsenty, G., Skeletal Gla proteins: gene structure, regulation of expression, and function, in *Principles of Bone Biology,* Bilezikian, J.P., Raisz, L.G., and Rodan, G.A., Eds., Academic Press, San Diego, 1996, Chap. 14.
12. Faraco, J., Bashir, M., Rosenbloom, J., and Francke, U., Characterization of the human gene for microfibril-associated glycoprotein (MFAP2), assignment to chromosome 1p36.1-p35, and linkage to D1S170, *Genomics* 25,630, 1995.
13. Gibson, M.A., Hatzinikolas, G., Davis, E., Baker, E., Sutherland, G.R., and Mecham, R.P., Bovine latent TGF-β1-binding protein-2: molecular cloning, identification of tissue isoforms and immunolocalization to the elastin-associated microfibrils, *Molec. Cell Biol.* 15, 6932,1995.
14. Gibson, M., Hatzinikolas, A., Kumaratilake, J.S., Sandberg, L.B., Nicholl, J.K., Sutherland, G.R., and Cleary, E.G., Further characterization of proteins associated with elastic fiber microfibrils including the molecular cloning of MAGP-2 (MP25), *J. Biol. Chem.* 271, 1096, 1996.
15. Iozzo, R.V. and Murdoch, A.D., Proteoglycans of the extracellular environment: clues from the gene and protein side offer novel perspectives in molecular diversity and function, *FASEB J.* 10, 598, 1996.
16. Kagan, H.M., Characterization and regulation of lysyl oxidase, in *Regulation of Matrix Accumulation,* Mecham, R.P., Ed., Academic Press, Orlando,1986.
17. Kanzaki, T., Olofsson, A., Moren, A., Wernstedt, C., Hellman, U., Miyazono, K., Claesson-Welsh, L., and Heldin, C.-H., TGF-β1 binding protein: a component of the large latent complex of TGFβ-1 with multiple repeat sequences, *Cell* 61, 1051, 1990.
18. Kjellen, L. and Lindahl, U., Proteoglycans: structures and interactions, *Annu. Rev. Biochem.* 60, 443, 1991.
19. Kobayashi, R., Tashima, Y., Masuda, H., Shozawa, T., Numata, Y., Miyauchi, K., and Hayakawa, T., Isolation and characterization of a new 36-kDa microfibril-associated glycoprotein from porcine aorta, *J. Biol. Chem.* 264, 17437, 1989.

20. Kosmehl, H., Berndt, A., and Katenkamp, D., Molecular variants of fibronectin and laminin: structure, physiological occurrence and histopathological aspects, *Virchows Archiv.* 429, 3ll, 1996.
21. Lane, T.F. and Sage, E.H., The biology of SPARC, a protein that modulates cell-matrix interactions, *FASEB J.* 8, 163, 1994.
22. Lansing, A.I., Rosenthal, T.B., Alex, M., and Dempsey, E., The structure and chemical characterization of elastic fibers as revealed by elastase and by electron microscopy, *Anat. Rec.* 555,1952.
23. Maslen, C.L. and Glanville, R.W., The molecular basis of Marfan syndrome, *DNA and Cell Biol.* 7, 5ll, 1993.
24. Mecham, R.P., Hinek, A., Entwistle, R., Wrenn, D.S., Griffin, G.L., and Senior, R.M., Elastin binds to a multifunctional 67-kilodalton peripheral membrane protein, *Biochemistry* 28, 3716, 1989.
25. Olsen, B.R., Collagen Biosynthesis, in *Cell Biology of Extracellular Matrix,* 2nd ed., Hay, E.D., Ed., Plenum, New York, 1991, Chap. 6.
26. Potts, J.R. and Campbell, I.D., Fibronectin structure and assembly, *Curr. Opin. Cell Biol.* 6, 648, 1994.
27. Prockop, D.J. and Kivirikko, K.I., Collagens: molecular biology, diseases, and potentials for therapy, *Annu. Rev. Biochem.* 64, 403, 1995.
28. Ramirez, F., Fibrillin mutations in Marfan syndrome and related phenotypes, *Curr. Opin. Genet. and Devel.* 6, 309, 1996.
29. Reber-Muller, S., Spissinger, T., Schuchert, P., Spring, J., and Schmid, V., An extracellular matrix protein of jellyfish homologous to mammalian fibrillin forms different fibrils depending on the life stage of the animal, *Develop. Biol.* 169, 662, 1995.
30. Roark, E.F., Keene, D.R., Haudenschild, C.C., Godyna, S., Little, C.D., and Argraves, W.S., The association of human fibulin-1 with elastic fibers: and immunohistological, ultrastructural, and RNA study, *J. Histochem. Cytochem.* 43, 401, 1995.
31. Rosenbloom, J., Abrams, W.R., and Mecham, R., The elastic fiber, *FASEB J.* 7, 1208, 1993.
32. Ross, R. and Bornstein, P., The elastic fiber. I. The separation and partial characterization of its macromolecular components. *J. Cell Biol.* 40, 366, 1969.
33. Ryan, M.C., Christiano, A.M., Engval, E., Werwer, U.M., Miner, J.H., Sanes, J.R., and Burgeson, R.E., The functions of laminins: lessons from in vivo studies, *Matrix Biology* 15, 369, 1996.
34. Sakai, L.Y., Keene, D.R., and Engvall, E., Fibrillin, a new 350-kD glycoprotein, is a component of extracellular microfibrils, *J. Cell Biol.* 103, 2499, 1986.
35. Serafini-Fracassini, A., Elastogenesis in embryonic and post-natal development, in *Ultrastructure of the Connective Tissue Matrix*, Ruggeri, A. and Motta, P.M., Eds., Nijhoff, the Hague, 1984, 140.
36. Timpl, R. and Chu, M.L., Microfibrillar collagen type VI, in *Extracellular Matrix Assembly and Structure,* Yurchenco, P.D., Birk, D.E., and Mecham, R.P., Eds., Academic Press, San Diego, 1994, 207.
37. Van der Rest, M., Garrone, R., and Herbage, D., Collagen: a family of proteins with many facets, *Adv. Mol. Cell Biol.: Extracellular Matrix* 6, 1, 1993.
38. Van der Rest, M. and Garrone, R., Collagen family of proteins. *FASEB J.* 5, 2814, 1991.
39. Vuorio, E. and de Crombrugghe, B., The family of collagen genes, *Annu. Rev. Biochem.* 59, 837, 1990.

40. Yeh, H., Chow, M., Abrams, W.R., Fan, J., Foster, J., Mitchell, H., Muenke, M., and Rosenbloom, J., Structure of the human gene encoding the associated microbrillar protein (MFAP1) and localization to chromosome 15q15-q21, *Genomics* 23, 443, 1994.
41. Yurchenco, P.D., Assembly of laminin and type IV collagen into basement membrane networks, in *Extracellular Matrix Assembly and Structure,* Yurchenco, P.D., Birk, D.E., and Mecham, R.P., Eds., Academic Press, San Diego, 1994, 351.

3 Biology of Osteoclasts and Osteoblasts

J. Edward Puzas and Gregory D. Lewis

CONTENTS

3.1 INTRODUCTION

The skeleton functions in mechanical support, protection of vital organs, as a site for hematopoeisis and as a reservoir for key minerals such as calcium, phosphorus and magnesium. The two key cellular activities responsible for these functions are osteoclastic bone resorption and osteoblastic bone formation. The characteristics and regulatory pathways of these cells are described in detail below. As we better understand the factors that control osteoclast and osteoblast activity it should be possible to devise therapeutic protocols that would lead to a closer control of skeletal metabolism.

0-8493-9237-3/99/$0.00+$.50

3.2 OSTEOCLAST

The osteoclast is a giant multinucleated cell that, when resorbing bone, demonstrates a polarity defined by a ruffled border that is composed of extensive interdigitated villi in direct contact with bone. Osteoclasts vary between 40 to 100 microns in diameter and may contain as many as 10 to 20 nuclei per cell. Active osteoclasts contain extensive mitochondria, lysosomes and a well-developed Golgi apparatus. These cells are also mobile cells and frequently migrate across a bony surface during the process of bone resorption.

3.2.1 Osteoclast Lineage and the Role of Regulatory Factors

The osteoclast is derived from the macrophage lineage and, thus, is a member of the hematopoietic stem cell family. The original experiments that defined the origin of the cell showed that osteoclast-deficient sclerotic bone diseases can be cured by transplanting competent myeloid elements from a syngenic animal or human.[1,2]

The regulatory pathway for osteoclastogenesis utilizes many of the early steps found in all macrophagic cell differentiation. Recent reports have shown that the myeloid and B lymphocyte transcription factor, PU.1, plays a critical role in osteoclast formation.[3] In mutant mice that are devoid of this transcription factor no macrophages of any kind develop nor do osteoclasts form. The animals develop osteopetrosis and a skeletal sclerosis characterized by dense bone, small marrow spaces and a lack of remodeling. Thus, disruptions at the earliest stages of macrophage development are an indication that osteoclast formation is dependent on points of regulation that exist in the formative pathways of myeloid cell differentiation. So far the earliest identified step in myeloid development and subsequent osteoclastogenesis is the step that is inhibited as a result of PU.1 deletion.

A second transcription factor, c-fos, has also been implicated in osteoclast formation. A deletion in c-fos causes a form of osteopetrosis that can be reversed by myeloid cell transplantation. However, c-fos deletion does not interfere with the formation of active macrophages, whereas PU.1 deletion prevents macrophage formation everywhere. Interestingly, c-fos deletion is associated with a substantial increase in the number of macrophages.[4] This suggests that c-fos regulates a branch point in the osteoclast differentiation pathway that is downstream from the PU.1 regulated step.

Other animal and human mutations have further delineated the osteoclast pathway. The op/op mouse, known to have a deficiency in the hematopoietic regulatory protein, CSF-1 (colony stimulating factor-1),[5,6] has no osteoclasts and almost no macrophages. This deficiency is curable by injections of CSF-1. Because most phagocytic cells are non-functional in this mutant model, the CSF-1 control point is probably downstream of PU.1 and upstream of c-fos.

Mice which lack c-SRC also have osteopetrosis,[7] but not because of a lack of osteoclastogenesis. Instead, these animals have an abundant number of cells with an osteoclast phenotype, yet are not competent to resorb bone. Similar observations have been made in animals with mutations in carbonic anhydrase[8] and the proton

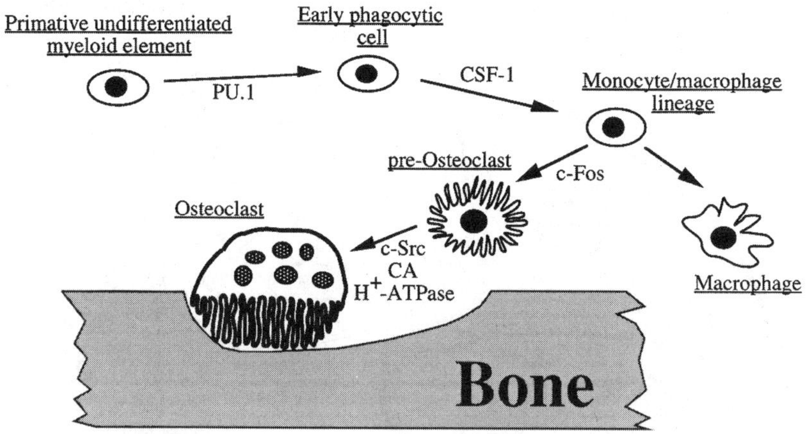

FIGURE 3.1 Osteoclast differentiation pathway. Mature osteoclasts are derived from undifferentiated myeloid elements. These cells progress through a series of steps that are modulated by the action of specific cytokines and regulatory factors. Genetic deletion of the cytokines (CSF-1), regulatory factors (PU.1, c-Fos and c-Src) and the indicated enzymes (carbonic anhydrase, CA and the proton pump, H^+ATPase) allows for the identification of their action at each stage of differentiation.

pump (H^+-ATPase).[9] These enzymes seem to function in the late stages of osteoclastogenesis as they essentially affect the mature cell. Thus, a number of the control points for osteoclast genesis, from the earliest developmental stages to the final functions of the cell, are being uncovered. Figure 3.1 portrays this pathway.

3.2.2 NFκB/Rel/IκB Family of Regulatory Factors

Most recently a new family of transcription factors involved in controlling the genes used by osteoclasts in the process of bone resorption has been discovered. They are the NFκB/Rel/IκB molecules (reviewed in [10]). NFκB was originally characterized as a lymphoid specific transcription factor involved in B lymphocyte maturation. However, subsequent work has shown that a number of immunologic and matrix degradation pathways are under its control. The two key members of the NFκB family are NFκB1 (the gene is termed p50) and NFκB2 (the gene is termed p52). NFκB1 or NFκB2 can dimerize with another pair of factors known as RelA and RelB. The subsequent heterodimer makes up the active transcription factor that can translocate into the nucleus and activate specific gene expression. However, this does not occur until an inhibitory protein (IκB) is dissociated from the heterodimer and degraded. That is, in an inactive cell all three components (NFκB, Rel and IκB) are complexed in the cytosol. Upon activation of specific receptors involved in bone resorption, the IκB subunit is phosphorylated and targeted for proteosome degradation by subsequent ubiquitination. (Ubiquitination is the process by which ubiquitin side chains are added to terminal lysine residues in proteins destined for removal.) This liberates the NFκB/Rel dimer and allows it to enter the nucleus and evoke a response.

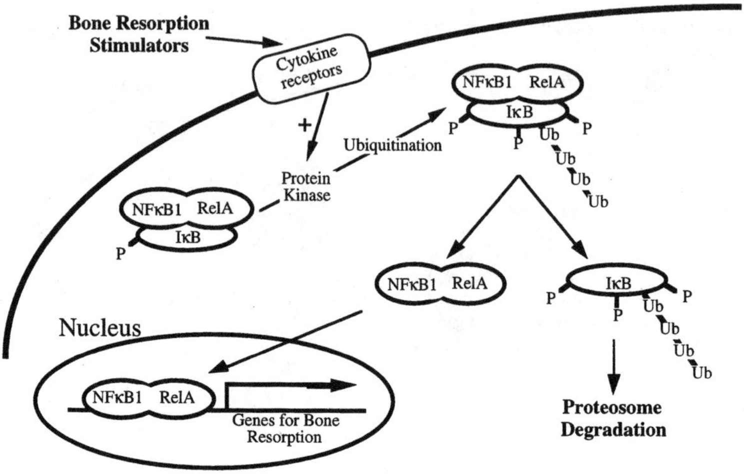

FIGURE 3.2 The NFκB/Rel/IκB pathway. Creation of transgenic mice devoid of NFκB activity demonstrates the importance of this transcription factor in osteoclastogenesis. The NFκB/Rel heterodimer activates a number of genes associated with bone resorption and is under the control of cytokine plasma membrane receptors. Upon activation of a progenitor osteoclast with an appropriate cytokine, an inhibitory factor, IκB becomes phosphorylated and targeted for degradation. The degradation utilizes ubiquitination and proteosome mechanisms. The NFκB/Rel heterodimer is then free to translocate into the nucleus where it initiates the expression of genes needed in osteoclastogenesis.

In animals that have been genetically manipulated to knock out both NFκB1 and NFκB2, a severe osteopetrosis develops because osteoclast-mediated bone resorption does not occur.[11] Deleting either NFκB1 or NFκB2 alone does not lead to the defect. This suggests there is a redundancy in the action of these factors. A summary of these pathways is presented in Figure 3.2.

The most interesting facet of this regulatory pathway is the potentially large number of steps at which it would be possible to intervene and control bone resorption. A number of pharmaceuticals, protease inhibitors and gene therapy protocols could be used to block osteoclastogenesis or osteoclastic activity. For example, sulfasalazine and glucocorticoid hormones modulate IκB metabolism,[12,13] thereby preventing translocation of the NFκB/Rel complex into the nucleus. Although direct experiments using this strategy for the prevention of bone resorption have not yet been attempted, it is conceivable that targeting the proteosome in osteoclasts may be a mechanism to prevent bone loss. The same holds true for genetic alteration of NFκB, Rel or IκB. Any one of a number of strategies may be used to interfere with this pathway. Altering the NFκB or Rel molecules, inactivating the IκB protein kinase, altering the phosphorylation sites on IκB, removing the ubiquitination sites on IκB, and altering the nuclear translocation signals on NFκB, etc., are all potential targets for controlling osteoclast differentiation.

3.3 BONE RESORPTION

Osteoclastogenesis is but the first step in the process of bone resorption. Cell recruitment to a particular site, attachment of cells to bone, demineralization and matrix degradation, motility and apoptosis are all processes that occur as part of the resorptive process.

3.3.1 Recruitment of Osteoclasts

We now know that most prototypic stimulators of bone resorption (such as parathyroid hormone, vitamin D, many interleukins, thyroid hormone, tumor necrosis factor alpha, etc.) stimulate bone resorption indirectly. This means there are no receptors on osteoclasts for these molecules. Rather, auxiliary cells, usually osteoblasts or stromal lining cells, receive the resorption signal and then elaborate a soluble factor or factors that stimulate(s) the final stages of differentiation of a pre-osteoclast.[14] Mounting evidence suggests that the soluble factor activates a TNFα-like receptor on osteoclasts; however, it is likely that more than one factor is associated with the direct activation of osteoclasts.

3.3.2 Attachment of an Osteoclast to a Resorption Site

What signals tell an osteoclast where to resorb bone is not well established. Some investigators have proposed that bone lining cells under the influence of a direct or indirect signal retract partially, thereby exposing the bone mineral to the osteoclast. Once uncovered bone mineral is available, the osteoclast would extend a pseudopod between the cells and onto the bony surface and begin the process of ruffled border formation. Although not yet generally accepted, some histologic evidence for this theory is available.

According to another hypothesis, osteoclasts or stromal lining cells synthesize and secrete enzymes (such as collagenases and other matrix metalloproteinases) that would facilitate osteoclast attachment to the bone surface by removing a protective protein covering. Evidence has been published that systemic stimulators of bone resorption can induce osteoblasts to produce type I collagenase and that osteoclasts can adhere to the surfaces prepared by collagenase action. However, there is only circumstantial proof that these pathways are responsible for directing osteoclast activity.

What is well established is that osteoclasts possess integrin receptors.[15] These plasma membrane receptors are composed of two subunits, alpha (α) and beta (β), with high specificity for bone matrix molecules such as osteopontin and collagen. One widely expressed pair of subunits in the integrin family, $\alpha_v\beta_3$, binds specifically to a tripeptide of arginine-glycine-aspartic acid (RGD) and is present on osteoclasts. Direct experimentation has shown that interference with $\alpha_v\beta_3$ arrests osteoclast attachment to bone and blocks bone resorption. This has been exploited as a therapeutic approach to inhibiting bone resorption. The identification of integrin receptors on osteoclasts does not explain the site-specificity associated with bone resorption, but adds to the understanding of how bone resorption is localized.

3.3.3 Demineralization

Once the osteoclast has established itself on a denuded bone surface it becomes polarized in its orientation. That is, special organellar structures such as the ruffled border and clear zones appear. The ruffled border is a highly interdigitated villar structure that provides for a large surface area through which the osteoclast can interact with bone. Along this border large numbers of protons are secreted through the action of a H^+-ATPase proton pump. This pump is not unlike the one found in renal tubules.[16] As the osteoclast secretes protons into the extracellular space around the ruffled border, its cytosol would become alkaline. To prevent this, osteoclasts have at their plasma membrane border a very active $Cl^-/HCO3^-$ exchanger that allows for the rapid and complete removal of bicarbonate ions. In turn, this allows the osteoclast to decrease the pH to around 5 in the immediate vicinity of the ruffled border and over the bone mineral within that border. At this pH the carbonated hydroxyapatite that comprises the mineral phase of bone becomes soluble and dissolves. As ionic calcium accumulates, some enters the cells and inhibits the proton secretion. Ultimately the cell moves away from its site and the excess calcium in the resorption lacuna diffuses into the extracellular space.

In order to prevent the high concentration of protons from diffusing away from an actively resorbing surface, the osteoclast utilizes another specialized structure not found in any other cell type: the clear zone. This organelle surrounds the osteoclast at the bone-cell interface and acts as a type of sealing gasket. Electron microscopy of this zone reveals an amorphous structure devoid of other cellular structures, hence the name clear zone. Recently some investigators have shown that the clear zone contains proteoglycan-like material and some actin filaments; however, its composition has not been fully elucidated.

3.3.4 Matrix Degradation

Dissolution of the mineral matrix of bone uncovers the collagen and non-collagen proteins of the organic matrix, material that must be removed in the course of bone resorption. Clearly, proteolytic activity must be involved.

Many investigators working in the field of osteoclast biology have likened the space between the ruffled border and bone surface to a lysosomal compartment. This analogy is appropriate, given the low pH, but it is also appropriate because of the large number of hydrolytic enzymes that are secreted into this space. Most lysosomal acid proteases, glycosidases and phosphatases can be found in the space beneath an active osteoclast. Especially important in the degradation of collagen and other proteins are the cathepsins. This family of lysosomal enzymes is known to be present at sites of bone resorption and, under the acidic conditions of the resorption lacunae, can digest native collagen.

All lysosomal enzymes are glycosylated with a complex carbohydrate structure that contains mannose-6-phosphate. The presence of mannose-6-phosphate residues directs the sequestration of the enzymes to the lysosome by virtue of a mannose-6-phosphate receptor that is present on the lysosomal membrane in all types of cells. In the osteoclast, the mannose-6-phosphate receptor also seems to direct the secretion of lysosomal enzymes to the space between the ruffled border and bone. Of interest is the observation that once the osteoclast has completed an episode of bone resorption and moves away from the resorption lacuna, much of the lysosomal secretions remain adsorbed to the bony site.

3.4 OSTEOBLAST

Bone forming cells, by definition, are the cells responsible for the production of authentic bone. For the purposes of this discussion we have defined bone as that tissue which is formed by the deposition of mineral ions within a collagenous framework. The mineral must be in the form of carbonated hydroxyapatite and the collagen must be predominantly type I collagen. Although this definition seems self-evident it does exclude a number of mineralized tissues which, through the years, have been mistakenly grouped with authentic bone. Examples of mineralized tissue that is not bone are dentin and enamel, calcifying cartilage in the growth plate of long bones, renal stones and any organs undergoing pathological calcification (i.e., arterial and aortic walls). Some forms of ectopic or heterotopic bone do fit the criteria of authentic bone. These forms of bone frequently occur after orthopaedic surgery or in rare metabolic disease states.[17,18]

3.4.1 Ultrastructure and Properties

The term "bone forming cell" can be equated with the term "osteoblast". That is, wherever authentic bone is being formed, osteoblasts must be present.

The ultrastructural and histological features of osteoblasts underscore the fact that these cells are very active metabolically. They contain an extensive rough endoplasmic reticulum comprised of polysomal structures that stain intensely basophilic. The predominant genes that are transcribed and translated in these cells deal with the synthesis of an extracellular matrix, i.e., collagenous and non-collagenous matrix proteins. Fully 20% of the total protein produced by osteoblasts is type I collagen. This is extraordinary when one considers the number of genes that need to be expressed for an osteoblast to remain viable. The predominant non-collagen protein secreted by osteoblasts is osteocalcin or bone gla-protein (BGP) which makes up approximately 1% of extracellular matrix protein. Moreover, a host of regulatory factors are produced and deposited in bone by osteoblasts. These include the family of bone morphogenetic proteins (BMPs), the beta transforming growth factors (TGFβs), the insulin-like growth factors (IGFs), platelet derived growth factors (PDGFs), and basic fibroblast growth factor (bFGF) among others. Though these proteins represent a minor component of the extracellular matrix, they play a critical role in bone remodeling (see below).

A well-developed Golgi apparatus is also present in osteoblasts. This structure, usually found near the center of the cell, is responsible for the secretion of collagen and non-collagen proteins.

All osteoblasts are mononuclear with the nucleus positioned eccentrically opposite the rough endoplasmic reticulum. The nuclear material is similar to other eukaryotic cells and remains in a diffuse uncondensed state during interphase. There are usually one to three nucleoli present. A mature functioning osteoblast does not divide.

A characteristic of osteoblasts which can be demonstrated histochemically is the presence of a substantial amount of the enzyme alkaline phosphatase. Bone-specific alkaline phosphatase has been localized to the plasma membrane of osteoblasts and although it is known to be present in large amounts, its true function has not yet been determined. Speculations as to its role in mineralization have been published since 1923[19] and it is clear that alkaline phosphatase activity correlates with bone formation, but its mechanism of action is not yet known. Elevated levels of bone specific alkaline phosphatase in the blood are representative of excessive osteoblast activity, i.e., bone formation. Normal adult levels are 20 to 70 international units/liter of blood (IU/L); in a growing child they are 100 to 150 IU/L, and in pathologic high bone turnover states such as Paget's disease the plasma enzyme levels may rise to 350 to 700 IU/L.

Osteoblasts play a key role in bone resorption. They possess receptors for factors that stimulate bone resorption, i.e., parathyroid hormone, vitamin D, prostaglandins, interleukins, TNFα, etc., and thus constitute the primary target for modulation of osteoclast activity. Most investigators believe that osteoblasts receive and process the systemic signals to resorb bone, and in response, elaborate a molecule or molecules that recruit(s) and stimulate(s) osteoclastic activity.[20-23] Clearly, osteoblasts play a pivotal role in specifying the time and site of bone resorption.

3.4.2 Osteoblast Lineage

Three forms of the osteoblast cell lineage are recognized: progenitor osteoblasts (pre-osteoblasts), mature osteoblasts and osteocytes. Phylogenetically speaking, osteoblasts arise from cells in the condensing mesenchyme and as such are one form of connective tissue. Since mesenchymal cells can give rise to a number of tissue types it is not until a cell is committed to the osteoblast lineage that it can be classified as a bone forming cell.

3.4.2.1 Pre-Osteoblast

A committed progenitor cell destined to become an osteoblast has a number of distinguishing features. First, these cells are located near bone forming surfaces. That is, they are usually present at sites where active, mature osteoblasts are synthesizing bone. Their appearance is that of an elongated cell with an elongated nucleus. Most often they are found in a stratum a few cell layers distant from active osteoblasts. Second, they have the capacity to divide. Frequently mitotic figures can be found in these cells. Third, these cells usually stain less intensely for alkaline phosphatase and there is no evidence of a developed rough endoplasmic reticulum. In other words, they have not yet acquired all of the characteristics of mature osteoblasts.

Pre-osteoblasts give rise to osteoblasts at two distinct sites: the endosteum and the periosteum. Endosteal pre-osteoblasts are cells that are active on trabecular and endocortical bone surfaces. They are derived from the stromal group of cells that, along with the hemopoietic group, populate marrow spaces. These stromal cells are self-renewing and with each cell division have the capacity to create a "determined osteoprogenitor cell (DOPC)" which will ultimately become a mature osteoblast and an "inducible osteoprogenitor stem cell (IOPC)" that will retain stem cell potentiality. The nomenclature of DOPC and IOPC was coined by Friedenstein.[24]

Periosteal pre-osteoblasts are among the cells that form the fibrous periosteum surrounding all bones. They give rise to osteoblasts on bone surfaces and may also provide progenitor cells for fibroblasts. They are derived from a pool of cells that more closely resembles DOPCs.

Differentiation of an osteoprogenitor cell into an osteoblast is not a quantal process. Osteoblasts express all genes necessary for bone formation but do not do so simultaneously.[25] In the early stages of bone development there is extensive proliferation of progenitor cells with expression of growth-related genes (such as c-myc and c-fos). Also, during the proliferative phase, a number of matrix genes begin to be expressed (i.e., type I collagen, fibronectin and some growth factors such as TGFβ). These genes remain active for a number of days and are joined by gene products that are associated with a mature matrix, such as alkaline phosphatase and matrix Gla protein. As the matrix and matrix-maturing proteins are suppressed, new gene products associated with the mineralization phase begin to be expressed (i.e., osteocalcin and osteopontin), thus leading to hydroxyapatite accumulation and complete mineralization.

When viewed as a continuum, the maturation of a pre-osteoblast into a mature osteoblast is a complex process. Gene products are expressed and repressed at specified stages and unless all of the actions are in concert, normal bone matrix will not be formed.

3.4.2.2 Osteoblast

A mature osteoblast is derived from a pre-osteoblast and expresses all of the differentiated functions required to synthesize bone. As discussed above, there is a gradient of differentiation which becomes fully expressed when the mature form of the cell reaches the bone surface. Once the osteoblast has reached the surface its function is to synthesize and secrete collagen, non-collagen matrix proteins and regulatory factors into a structured array and ultimately to mineralize it. Usually, active osteoblasts are found within a matrix that they themselves have synthesized. It is within this matrix at the mineralization front that the process of hydroxyapatite crystal growth occurs. The mineralization front is the advancing edge of calcification and is usually 5 to 50 microns away from the osteoblast surface. The area between the osteoblast and the mineralizing front is often referred to as an "osteoid seam". The depth and character of the osteoid seam can be diagnostic for some forms of bone disease (such as osteomalacia and rickets).

3.4.2.3 Osteocyte

An osteocyte is an osteoblast which has become encased in calcified bone. During the process of bone formation, the osteoblast determines its own fate by calcifying inside a lacunae. Approximately 15% of osteoblasts eventually become osteocytes. Although not all osteoblasts survive as osteocytes, all osteocytes have originated from osteoblasts. As the cell becomes encased in bone, its metabolic activity decreases substantially due to the lack of nutrient diffusion. The only source of nutrients and gas exchange to which the osteocyte has access is through small bone canals known as canaliculi. These channels are the remnants of cellular processes from an osteoblast. The canaliculi form an extensive array of connecting tubules and may serve as a communication as well as a nutrient network.

3.4.3 Regulatory Mechanisms Related to Osteoblasts

This active and important area of current research is one where molecular, biological, immunological, and biochemical techniques have come together in an attempt to understand both normal and disease processes of bone metabolism.

Control of osteoblast function occurs at three levels: endocrine, paracrine and autocrine.

Endocrine control is exerted through the action of hormones such as parathyroid hormone (PTH), 1,25-dihydroxyvitamin D_3, growth hormone, glucocorticoid hormones, gonadal steroids, etc. These agents are secreted into the circulation by endocrine glands and ultimately have a skeletal-wide effect at sites distant from the initial synthesis of the hormone. Of these agents, PTH and 1,25 dihydroxyvitamin D_3 have been the most widely studied with regard to bone formation.

Paracrine control of osteoblast activity occurs when cells adjacent to the osteoblasts produce and release locally acting factors that influence bone formation. There are many examples of this in the skeleton ranging from: i) the initial developmental stages in the embryo; ii) long bone growth and fracture healing; and iii) basal remodeling that occurs throughout life. Specific examples would include the role of basic fibroblast growth factor (bFGF or FGF2) in development and expression of the limb rudiments, the production of the beta transforming growth factors (TGFβs) and bone morphogenetic proteins 2, 6 and 7 by chondrogenic cells in the growth plate and fracture callus, and the production of interleukins by osteoclasts at sites of bone remodeling. All of these examples demonstrate the synthesis of key factors by a non-osteoblast cell type that influences the activity of a nearby osteoblast.

Lastly, in autocrine regulation of osteoblasts factors produced by osteoblasts regulate the cell's own activity. This pathway is best represented in the bone remodeling process wherein the growth factors embedded in bone by osteoblasts are released to influence these cells at a later time. Some of the best-studied of these factors are the insulin-like growth factors IGF-I and IGF-II. These molecules can be extracted from bone and have been shown to stimulate proliferation and differentiation in osteoblasts.

A list of endocrine, paracrine and autocrine factors is presented in Table 3.1.

3.5 BONE FORMATION

3.5.1 Matrix Maturation

One of the major and yet poorly understood areas of collagen metabolism in bone formation is the so-called "maturation of the osteoid matrix". This alteration of

TABLE 3.1
Endocrine, Paracrine and Autocrine Factors Affecting Osteoblasts

Systemic Hormones	Paracrine Factors	Autocrine Factors
Parathyroid hormone	Parathyroid hormone related protein	TGF β 1, 2, and 3
Vitamin D	TGFβ 1, 2, and 3	Fibroblast growth factors (1 and 2)
Glucocorticoid hormones	Fibroblast growth factors (1 and 2)	Insulin-like growth factors
Calcitonin	Insulin-like growth factors	Platelet derived growth factors
Gonadal Steroids (estrogen and testosterone)	Platelet derived growth factors	BMPs 2 to 7
Insulin	BMPs 2 to 7	
	Interleukin-6	

collagen fibers must occur before the matrix is competent to support mineralization. The best way to illustrate this point is to describe the process of bone formation at a remodeling site. From the point of view of collagen synthesis and its mineralization, there are three distinct stages during formation. In the first stage, collagen is deposited at a rapid rate and an ever-thickening osteoid seam is produced. In the second stage, the rate of mineralization increases to match the rate of collagen synthesis and the osteoid seam width remains constant. In the third stage, the rate of collagen synthesis decreases and mineralization continues until the osteoid seam disappears. The maturation of the collagen matrix is expressed as the ratio of the mineralization rate (in microns/day) to the osteoid seam width (in microns). Thus, the maturation of the collagen has as its unit a measure of time, i.e., days. This ratio has become known as the "mineralization lag time" and describes the length of time it takes for the osteoid matrix to acquire the characteristics necessary to support mineralization. The "mineralization lag time" is on the order of 5 to 15 days in adults and its magnitude can sometimes be diagnostic for metabolic bone diseases. Biochemically, the "mineralization lag time" remains undefined. Some theories support a role for crosslinking of collagen in the osteoid, others support the removal of a mineralization inhibitor (see below). Whatever the actual mechanism of osteoid maturation, it is apparent that newly deposited collagen cannot provide a substrate for normal mineralization until it has "matured".

3.5.2 Mineralization

Mineralization of the collagen substructure is another unique function of the osteoblast. Although not all details of this process are known, many significant stages are recognized. The mineral in mature, fully calcified bone is mostly in the form of carbonated hydroxyapatite crystals. These crystals are needle-shaped and rod-like and have a diameter of 30 to 50 angstroms and a length of up to 600 angstroms. They lie linearly along the collagen fibrils and in some instances may penetrate some of the larger fibers. The actual process of mineral precipitation, however, remains obscure. In fact, a number of paradoxical observations have been made in trying to examine the process of calcification. For example, it appears that once hydroxyapatite has been formed, further crystal growth can occur in the absence of

TABLE 3.2
Parameters of Bone Formation Under the Control of Osteoblasts

Bone volume (microscopic area as a percent that is cancellous bone)	22.8%
Osteoid volume (volume of uncalcified osteoid as compared to bone)	4.4 mm^3/cm^3 bone
Osteoid surface (percent of bone surface covered by osteoid)	7.5%
Osteoid seam width	10.0 microns
Mineral apposition rate	0.65 microns/day
Trabecular diameter (mean diameter of trabeculae in cancellous bone)	283.0 microns
Bone-osteoblast interface (% of bone surface in direct contact with osteoblasts)	3.8%

cell activity. In other words, under physiological conditions, the extracellular fluid is supersaturated with regard to calcium and phosphate when in the presence of hydroxyapatite. If crystal growth were not regulated, the extracellular fluid could become depleted of calcium and phosphate. This is the major reason for proposing that there exists an ionic barrier between bone and blood. It is also the reason why devitalized bone will undergo continued mineralization if placed in tissue fluids or bathed in physiological solutions of calcium and phosphate. It appears, therefore, that mineralization is regulated at both the initiation and deposition stages of hydroxyapatite formation.

A quantitative summary of bone formation is presented in Table 3.2.[26] The table presents some histomorphometric parameters that are descriptive of osteoblastic activity. Extreme deviation from these values is often diagnostic of specific bone diseases.

3.6 SKELETAL REMODELING

The integrated activity of osteoclasts and osteoblasts is termed "skeletal remodeling". This process is responsible for a number of key functions. They are: the overall maintenance of skeletal mass, the reformation of fracture callus into normal bone, the adaptation of bone to physical stresses and, in part, the control of mineral homeostasis. In normal remodeling, osteoclast activity precedes osteoblast activity. That is, osteoclasts initiate the resorptive process after which osteoblasts reform the amount of bone resorbed by the osteoclast. As might be expected, breakdown in the lines of communication between these processes can lead to diseases of too little bone or too much bone. Usually, breakdown manifests itself as too little bone formation for a given amount of bone resorption, leading to osteoporosis. However, cases have been documented where more bone is formed than has been resorbed; this can lead to osteopetrosis.

The overall remodeling process is portrayed in Figure 3.3. The figure indicates seven key steps: 1) the recognition of systemic signals by bone lining cells or osteoblasts; 2) the release of regulatory factors for the recruitment of osteoclasts to sites of bone resorption; 3) the resorptive process itself; 4) the release of growth factors and other agents embedded in the bone matrix by the process of bone resorption; 5) the activation of osteoprogenitor cells by these factors; 6) the migration

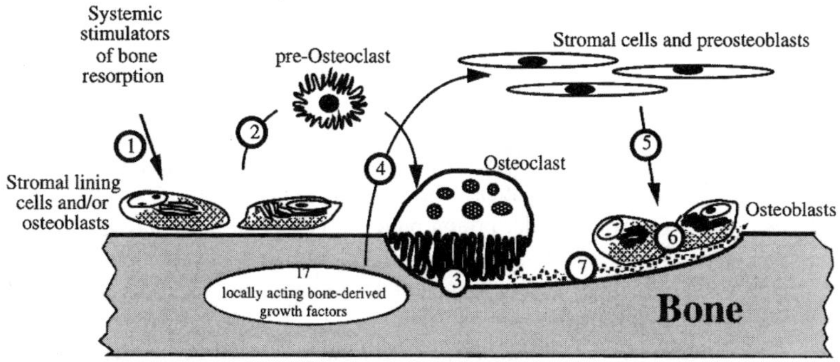

FIGURE 3.3 Diagrammatic representation of bone remodeling. Step 1, stromal lining cells and/or osteoblasts receive a systemic signal to initiate bone resorption. Step 2, soluble factors released from these cells participate in the differentiation of osteoclasts. Step 3, bone resorption proceeds at defined sites. Step 4, release of growth factors stored in bone begins the process of osteoprogenitor differentiation. Step 5, osteoprogenitor cells mature. Steps 6 and 7, mature osteoblasts recognize sites of prior bone resorption and begin the process of bone formation.

and differentiation of osteoblasts at the site of resorption; and 7) the process of formation itself. An excellent histological demonstration of this process is presented in Chapter 1, Figure 1.13, which shows an active osteoclast and active osteoblasts in the remodeling process. Note the fact that osteoblast activity is occurring subsequent to the formation of a resorption lacunae and that the bone is being formed on a prior resorption surface.

As more is learned about the details of these seven steps, it should become possible to manipulate the cells responsible for skeletal remodeling, and thus to alter the course of numerous metabolic and orthopaedic diseases.

REFERENCES

1. Walker, D.G. (1973) Experimental osteopetrosis. *Clin. Orthop. Rel. Res.* 97: 158-174.
2. Walker, D.G. (1973) Osteopetrosis cured by temporary parabiosis. *Science* 180: 275-276.
3. Tondravi, M.M., McKercher, S., Anderson, K., Erdmann, J.J., Quiroz, M., Maki, R., and Teitelbaum, S.L. (1997) Osteopetrosis in mice lacking haematopoietic transcription factor PU.1. *Nature* 386: 81-4.
4. Grigoriadis, A.E., Wang, Z., Cecchini, M.G., Hofstetter, W., Felix, T., Fleisch, H.A., and Wagner, E.F. (1994) c-Fox: A key regulator of osteoclast-macrophage lineage determination and bone remodeling. *Science* 266: 443-448.
5. Kodama, H., Yamasaki, A., Nose, M., Niida, S., Ohgama, Y., Abe, M., Kumegawa, M., and Suda, T. (1991) Congenital osteoclast deficiency in osteopetrotic (op/op) mice is cured by injections of macrophage colony stimulating factor, *J. Exp. Med.* 173: 269-272.
6. Wiktor-Jedrzejczak, W., Bartocci, A., Ferrante, A.W.J., Ahmed-Ansari, A., Sell, K.W., Pollard, J.W., Stanley, E.R. (1990) Total absence of colony stimulating factor 1 in the macrophage deficient osteopetrotic (op/op) mouse. *Proc. Nat. Acad. Sci.* 87: 4828-4832.
7. Soriano, P., Montgomery, C., Geske, R., and Bradley, A. (1991) Targeted disruption of the c-src proto-oncogene leads to osteopetrosis in mice. *Cell* 64: 693-702.

8. Sly, W.S., Hewett-Emmett, D., Whyte, M.P., Yu, Y., and Tashian, R.E. (1983) Carbonic anhydrase II deficiency identified as the primary defect in the autosomal recessive syndrome of osteopetrosis with renal tubular acidosis and cerebral calcification. *Proc. Natl. Acad. Sci.* 80: 2752-2756.
9. Yamamoto, T., Kurihara, N., Yamaoka, K., Ozono, K., Okada, M., Yamamoto, K., Matsumoto, S., Michigami, T., Ono, J., and Okada, S. (1993) Bone marrow-derived osteoclast-like cells from a patient with craniometaphyseal dysplasia lack expression of osteoclast-reactive vacuolar proton pump, *J. Clin. Invest.* 91: 362-367.
10. Verma, I.M., Stevenson, J.K., Schwarz, E.M., Van Antwerp, D., and Miyamoto, S. (1995) Rel/NF-κB/IκB family: intimate tales of association and dissociation, *Genes and Devel.* 9: 2723-2735.
11. Iotsova, V., Caamano, J., Loy, J., Yang, Y., Lewin, A., and Bravo, R. (1997) Osteopetrosis in mice lacking NF-κB1 and NF-κB2. *Nature Medicine* 3:1285-9.
12. Scheinman, R.I., Cogswell, P.C., Lofquist, A.K., and Baldwin, A.S. (1995) Role of transcriptional activation of IκBα in mediation of immunosuppression by glucocorticoids. *Science* 270: 283-286.
13. Wahl, C., Liptay, S., Adler, G., and Schmid, R.M. (1998) Sulfasalazine: a potent and specific inhibitor of nuclear factor κ B. *J. Clin. Invest.* 101:1163-74.
14. McSheehy, P.M.J. and Chambers, T.J. (1986) Osteoblastic cells mediate osteoclastic responsiveness to parathroid hormone, *Endocrinology* 118: 824-828.
15. Ross, F.P., Alvarez, J.I., Chappel, J., Sander, D., Butler, W.T., Farach-Carson, M.C., Mintz, K.A., Robey, P.G., Teitelbaum, S.L., and Cheresh, D.A. (1993) Interactions between the bone matrix proteins osteopontin and bone sialoprotein and the osteoclast integrin $\alpha_v\beta_3$ potentiate bone resorption. *J. Biol. Chem.* 268: 9901-9907.
16. Mattsson, J.P., Schlesinger, P.H., Keeling, D.J., Teitelbaum, S.L., Stone, K.K., and Xie, X. (1994) Isolation and reconstitution of a vacuolar-type proton pump of osteoclast membranes. *J. Biol. Chem.* 269: 24979-24982.
17. Sawyer, J.R., Myers, M.A., Rosier, R.N., and Puzas, J.E. (1991) Heterotopic Ossification: Clinical and Cellular Aspects, *Calcif. Tissue Int.* 49: 208-215.
18. O'Conner, J.M. (1983) *Soft tissue ossification*, Springer-Verlag, New York.
19. Robison, R. (1923) The possible significance of hexosephosphoric esters in ossification. *Biochem. J.* 17: 286-293.
20. Rodan, G.A. and Martin, T.J. (1981) Role of osteoclasts in hormonal control of bone resorption — a hypothesis. *Calcif. Tissue Int.* 33:349-351.
21. Burger, E.H., Van der Meer. J.W.M., and Nijweide, P.J. (1984) Osteoclast formation from mononuclear phagocytes: role of bone forming cells, *J. Cell Biol.* 99:1901-1905.
22. Chambers, T.J., McSheehy, P.M.J., Thomson, B.M., and Fuller, K. (1985) The effect of calcium-regulating hormones and prostaglandins on bone resorption by osteoclasts disaggregated from neonatal rabbit bones, *Endocrin.* 116: 234-239.
23. Martin, T.J. and Ng, K.W. (1994) Mechanism by which cells of the osteoblast lineage control osteoclast formation and activity, *J. Cell. Biochem.* 56: 357-366.
24. Friedenstein, A.Y., Chailakhyan, R.K., Latsinik, N.Y., Panasyuk, A.F., and Keiliss-Borok, I.V. (1974) Stromal cells responsible for transferring the microenvironment of the hemopoietic tissues, *Transplantation* 17: 331-340.
25. Stein, G.S., Lian, J.B., and Own, T.A. (1990) Relationship of cell growth to the regulation of tissue-specific gene expression during osteoblast differentiation, *FASEB J.* 4: 3111-3123.
26. Malluche, H.H. and Faugere, M.-C. (1986) *Atlas of mineralized bone histology,* Karger, New York.

4 Heritable Diseases of Bone and Connective Tissue

Deborah A. Redford-Badwal and
David W. Rowe

CONTENTS

0-8493-9237-3/99/$0.00+$.50

4.1 INTRODUCTION

A rapid expansion in knowledge of the biology of extracellular matrix is having a significant impact on our understanding of the pathophysiological processes that underlie heritable disorders of connective tissue. Much of this progress has come from two parallel avenues: the application of the techniques of molecular biology to the genes that code for the extracellular matrix proteins, and the evolving concept of a common pluripotential stem cell giving rise to a highly differentiated, tissue specific matrix producing cell. The overall objective of this chapter is to provide a basis for clinical orthopedists to understand how these advances in basic science are germane to their practice. This chapter will be divided into three main sections: an overview of extracellular matrix organization with an emphasis of how it meets the needs of various connective tissues; review of the molecular biology of type I collagen as a paradigm for the effect of mutations in other extracellular matrix genes; and an update of the molecular basis of major heritable disorders relevant to orthopedists.

4.2 ORGANIZATION OF THE EXTRACELLULAR MATRIX

Using a relatively limited repertoire of components, the extracellular matrix can meet a diverse set of structural and environmental needs. The same elements are found in connective tissues of all internal organs, dermis, sclera, cornea, and blood vessels in addition to the structural lattices of the bony skeleton and its attachments, such as cartilage, ligaments, tendons, and fasciae. The insoluble fibrils and interstitial polymers evolved to absorb stresses of movement and maintenance of shape, as well as to provide mechanical support and maintain structural integrity. In addition to its structural role, the extracellular matrix must respond to changes in the organism that include growth, remodeling, and repair.

4.2.1 Major Components to the Extracellular Matrix

4.2.1.1 Collagens

The collagen fiber is the major structural element of the extracellular matrix. It consists of a family of structural proteins with the unifying characteristic of three protein chains arranged in a triple helical or braided structure. Collagens are the most ubiquitous and abundant protein in the animal kingdom. Each collagen type (currently 19 identified at the protein and genetic level) is a genetically distinct protein with particular tissue distribution, structural features, and biological properties.

The different collagens can be classified according to their ability to form fibrils. The fibrillar collagens include types I, II, III, V, and XI, and are so named because they can form banded fibers in tissues. The molecules are formed from three polypeptide chains (α chains) arranged in a triple helix approximately 300 nm long. The three α chains may be either a homotrimer (combining three identical α chains), or heterotrimer (combining three dissimilar α chains, two of which may or may not be the same). This group of collagens has a continuous uninterrupted helical domain of approximately 95,000 daltons and is the prototype of all collagen types. The α chains of these collagens consist of a repeating triplet sequence (gly-X-Y)n, where X and Y can be any amino acid but most frequently are proline and hydroxyproline. The presence of glycine, which has no bulky side chain, at every third residue allows the three α chains to wind around a common axis, forming a right-handed superhelix. The three strands are stabilized by regularly occurring interchain hydrogen bonds derived from OH-proline.

Electron microscopic examination of these collagens shows them to have a characteristic cross-striated appearance that results from the highly defined manner in which adjacent collagen molecules self-assemble into a microfibril. They are arranged in a quarter stagger overlap, so that in aggregations approximately 75% of the molecules are in contact with neighbors. This arrangement is fundamental to the strength of the collagen fiber because it permits the proper alignment of crosslinks between adjacent molecules and fibrils. Mutations that disturb the triple helical nature of individual collagen molecules exert their clinical effect by disrupting the formation of the molecular assembly within the microfibril; this in turn compromises the generation of crosslink formation because of improper fiber alignment. See Figure 4.1.

A second group of non-interrupted collagens has a shortened triple helical domain (types VI, VIII, and X). Type X is important to the orthopedist because it is uniquely found in the hypertrophic zone of the growth plate. The other major grouping of collagen types is based on their nonfibrillar nature, with helical domains interrupted by nonhelical segments. Some of these molecules are composed of helical domains that are larger than 95,000 daltons (types IV and VII) and are associated with basement membranes. Others contain three short segments of triple helix (type XI and XII), separated by a nonhelical sequence. These are unusual collagens in that they are crosslinked to the surface of type II or type I collagen fibrils, respectively. Furthermore, they contain a proteoglycan side chain within one of the nonhelical sequences that may be a binding site for fibronectin.

4.2.1.2 Non-Collagenous Proteins

Some of these extracellular matrix components include tenacin, osteopontin, osteonectin, bone sialoprotein, matrix gla protein, osteocalcin, and thrombospondin (COMP). Many of these components are highly specialized and are restricted to specific types of connective tissue. Analysis of patients with mutations within these genes continues to provide insight into their biological function. Gene knockout

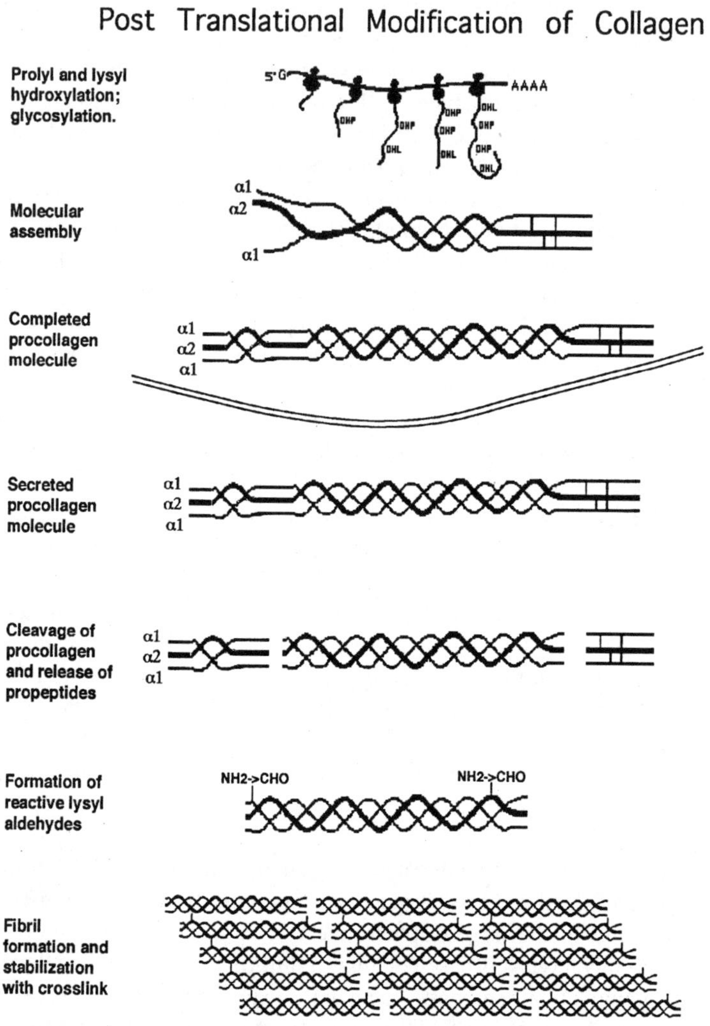

FIGURE 4.1 This diagram highlights selected events of collagen synthesis occurring within the nucleus, endoplasmic reticulum, Golgi apparatus, and extracellular matrix.

experiments in mice involve removing the functional gene product of a particular gene and observing the consequences in the development of the animal. Although relating the results of these experiments to human disease states is often difficult, they have provided valuable insight into the biological role of these extracellular matrix proteins.

4.2.1.3 Proteoglycans

The proteoglycans are a diverse family of large and complex macromolecules that occur in abundance in the extracellular matrix of all connective tissues. These molecules are grouped together because of their glycosaminoglycan (GAG) content. They are sulfated carbohydrate multimeric chains that are covalently linked to a central core protein. They are classified as chondroitin sulfate, dermatan sulfate, heparan sulfate, and hyaluronic acid proteoglycans on the basis of their carbohydrate components. Individual proteoglycan complexes are loosely organized through ionic interactions to hyaluronic acid, the only glycosaminoglycan that is not joined to a core protein. In addition, some of the molecules include multiple chains linked together, e.g., aggrecan, while others have only a single protein chain, e.g., biglycan and decorin. Knock-out experiments with these proteins have shown that each has different tissue related phenotypes that are related to the primary tissue where each is found.

Most, if not all, extracellular matrix proteoglycans bind to other matrix molecules, usually by interaction with the carbohydrate side chain. The binding site in collagen may help regulate the thickness of collagen fibrils in the matrix and may link several extracellular matrix components, as in the interaction between fibronectin and collagen. Proteoglycans also serve as cell adhesion receptors (integrins, see below) and are therefore capable of modulating cellular interaction with the extracellular matrix. Another important function of GAGs is related to their ability to retain a high hydration volume. These proteins have many negatively charged groups (sulfates) which will bind water and occupy a large space relative to their weight. They therefore provide an extracellular carbohydrate-water matrix that may fill most of the intercellular space.

4.2.1.4 Integrins

Integrins are a major family of adhesion receptors produced by most cell types and are a means for the cell to sense and respond to changes in the extracellular matrix composition. The molecule spans the cell membrane with a large extracellular domain and a relatively small cytoplasmic domain. Currently 22 different integrin receptors have been identified. Some of the best-characterized examples of integrins are the fibronectin receptors. Integrins have been loosely subclassified based on their β subunit. β1 integrins affect adhesion between cells and extracellular matrix, the β2 integrins participate in cell-to-cell interactions, and the β3 integrins have a variety of adhesive functions.

4.2.2 Collagen Fibers as a Composite of Individual Components

The interaction of groups of individual collagen types can provide a wide variety of functions for different tissues. When minor collagens are grouped with the corresponding major collagen, it is possible to obtain different physical and biological properties from a rather limited number of individual components. To better understand the molecular interdependence, Figure 4.2 illustrates a hypothetical connective tissue that contains predominantly type I or type II collagen. Once synthesized and secreted into the extracellular matrix, type I or type II collagen fibers begin associating in an ordered manner, forming the microfibril and undergoing crosslinking.

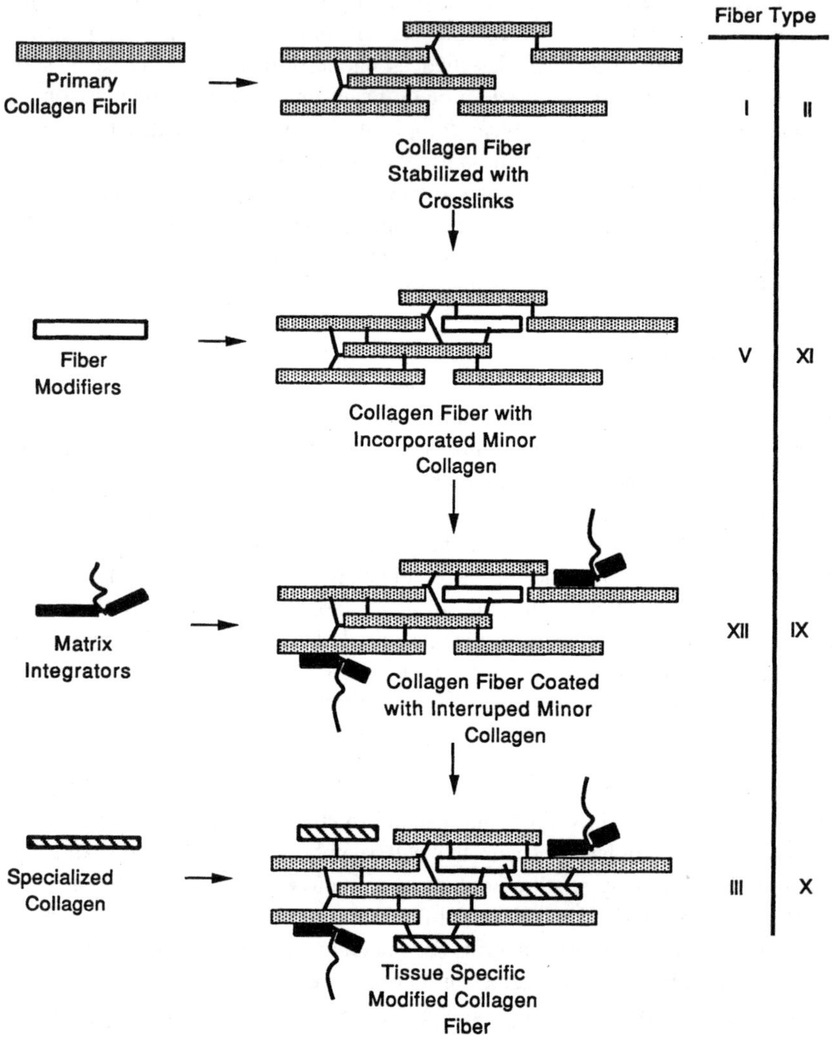

FIGURE 4.2 This diagram demonstrates formation of a collagen fibril. Modifying collagens and specialized collagens join with the major collagen type to form a composite which functions as the primary structural component of extracellular matrix.

The minor collagens become associated with the major collagens and modify their primary function: type I (tensile strength) and II (compressive strength). Within the growing fiber, type V collagen in type I or type XI collagen in type II is incorporated and participates with crosslink formation. The function of the minor intrafiber collagens is unknown, but their relative amount may be thought of as modulating structural properties of the major fiber.

In addition to these minor collagen components, a second collagen can be added to meet special fiber functions. Thus, tissues made up of type I collagen fibers, when located at warmer sites (fetal skin, aorta, viscera, uterus) become enriched in type III collagen, a type that is absent or low in more peripheral tissues (adult skin, bone, tendon, sclera). The denaturing (melting) temperature of type III collagen helix is significantly greater than that of type I collagen. It may therefore allow the tissue to function at a higher ambient temperature than if the tissue were made up exclusively of type I collagen. In cartilage, type X collagen is found in association with type II collagen in the hypertrophic zone of the growth plate. Its unique occurrence in cells undergoing endochondral ossification and the recent identification of mutations within this gene have furthered our understanding in the process of mineralization, and will be discussed below.

4.2.3 Cellular Aspects of the Extracellular Matrix

The emerging concept of a connective tissue stem cell capable of proliferation in the undifferentiated state and subsequently acquiring a differentiated state is helpful in understanding certain diseases of connective tissue. Thus in growing cartilage, there is an area of proliferating immature chondrocytes which subsequently produce a mature cartilage matrix. These same cells then differentiate further to become a hypertrophic chondrocyte and make their own matrix. The initial cartilage matrix supports the linear extension of the growth plate while the hypertrophic matrix provides the environment for bone cell invasion. In an analogous manner, undifferentiated proliferating preosteoblasts expand within the periosteum and subsequently acquire a osteoblast phenotype producing bone osteoid. This matrix provides the scaffold for ordered mineralization of the extracellular matrix necessary for bone strength. The osteoblasts become embedded within the bone matrix and acquire characteristics of the osteocyte. This cell appears to play a role in sensing mechanical forces on bone and initiating early steps of bone remodeling. All of these steps of proliferation and differentiation are controlled by a variety of genes that encode cytokines, growth factors, and transcription factors.

Mutations of these genes have now been associated with human disease. For example, the transcription factor Msx2 stimulates proliferation of preosteoblast and subsequently stimulates genes that initiate the transition to an osteoblast. Boston-type craniosynostosis is associated with a mutation of the Msx2 gene that makes the transcription factor continuously active. Craniosynostosis results when the precursor bone cells within the fontanelles and sutures proliferate excessively and differentiate prematurely. In contrast, another transcription factor Cbfa1 also plays an important role in bone cell differentiation. A mutation which inactivates this gene produces cleidocranial dysostosis, a condition of underdevelopment of the clavicles and failure of fontanelle closure. Analogous mutations in genes controlling the proliferation and maturation of cartilage cells have been identified and are discussed later in the cartilage disease section.

4.3 BIOSYNTHESIS OF TYPE I COLLAGEN: A PARADIGM FOR EXTRACELLULAR MATRIX PROTEINS

Most of the research has been carried out with type I collagen, but the principles learned from studying heritable disorders of this gene are likely to apply to most other collagens and certain non-collagen proteins of the extracellular matrix.

4.3.1 Gene Structure, Transcription, and mRNA Processing

The type I collagen molecule is made up of a trimer of two α 1(I) and one α 2(I) chains. Each of the chains is coded by different genes located on different chromosomes. The genes are composed of exons (regions that code for amino acids) and introns (regions that do not code for amino acids), spanning 18 kb for α 1(I) and 38 kb for α 2(I) gene. There are 51 exons for α 1(I) and 52 exons for the α 2(I) gene. Of the total number, 42 exons code for the amino acids that make up the triple helical region. An additional 4 exons code for the nonhelical C-terminal propeptide, and 5-6 exons code for the N-terminal propeptide.

4.3.1.1 Regulatory Elements of the Collagen Gene

Promoters and enhancers are elements or domains that surround that part of the gene (5′ end) that initiates transcription or modifies the rate of transcription. These domains bind nuclear proteins or transcription factors that alter the structure of the DNA or the interaction of the DNA with other proteins. Mutations in these DNA elements may abolish binding of certain proteins to a promoter element and decrease or eliminate transcription of that gene. The effect of such a change would be a reduction in the level of protein produced by the cell, but the protein would be structurally normal. When a gene is inactivated due to a large deletion or mutation within a promoter element, it is referred to as being “null”.

4.3.1.2 RNA Processing

The excision of the multiple noncoding segments (introns) from the primary RNA transcript is a complex intranuclear process called splicing or post-transcriptional processing. In the case of collagen an 18 or 40 Kb mRNA is reduced to a mature 4.5 to 5.0 kb mRNA molecule. This excision and splicing of the introns and exons must be completed so that subsequent cytoplasmic translation mechanisms can move through the mRNA without encountering a nonsense or stop codon. There is a recognition sequence both at the beginning and end of the intron that is complementary to small nuclear RNA/protein complexes (spliceosomes) which bring the ends of the introns into alignment for the removal and subsequent joining of the adjacent exons. A change in the recognition sequences can result in a retained intron sequence or a skipped exon which can result in a shortened or lengthened protein product. Another example of a processing problem is the recognition of a premature stop or of a defective splicing that occurs where the transcript contains a stop codon.

In cases where a premature stop is encountered, the RNA may not be transported to the cytoplasm. This leads to an underproduction of the α chains. If the segment containing the premature stop is spliced out of the transcript, a shortened protein may be produced, as when exons are missing in type I collagen.

4.3.2 Posttranscriptional Events: Translation and Molecular Assembly

After the mRNA has been processed and exported to the rough endoplasmic reticulum, it undergoes translation to a preprocollagen polypeptide of 1,500 amino acids. The polypeptide chain contains an N-terminal signal peptide which marks the molecule for eventual secretion from the cell. Post-translational hydroxylation and glycosylation steps of prolyl and lysyl residues take place within the endoplasmic reticulum and Golgi apparatus. The sugar moieties may modify the structure of the collagen fiber and participate in collagen/proteoglycan interactions. All posttranslational steps occur prior to the incorporation of the collagen chain into the triple helical structure. Once the α chains are in the fully triple helical state, no further hydroxylation or glycosylation occurs. Genetic defects which delay triple helix formation result in collagen molecules with excessive posttranslational modification.

The individual hydroxylated and glycosylated α chains self-assemble within the endoplasmic reticulum and Golgi apparatus through interactions of amino acids within the noncollagenous C-terminal procollagen domain. Once the trimer is formed, disulfide bonds between interchain cysteine residues stabilize the molecule. Defects in this region of the procollagen chain prevent incorporation of the affected chain into a nascent molecule.

The fully assembled procollagen molecule is secreted by cells into the extracellular space, where the NH_2 and COOH terminal propeptides are enzymatically removed. Failure to remove the N-terminal propeptide results in a rare form of Ehlers-Danlos syndrome (type VII). The collagen fibers in this disease are poorly organized, presumably due to interference of the propeptide with normal fiber aggregation.

4.4 CONCEPTS IMPORTANT TO UNDERSTANDING THE MUTATIONS THAT RESULT IN HERITABLE CONNECTIVE TISSUE DISORDERS

Mutations may be classified by the mode of inheritance. A dominantly inherited trait results from a single gene change that may adversely affect the individual, but does not prevent procreation; consequently, the same trait may be encountered in multiple generations within a pedigree. This form of inheritance pattern is frequently encountered in genes that code for the structural elements of the connective tissues. A recessive mode of inheritance means that both copies of the gene must be mutated for the disease state to occur. In other words, an affected individual has received one copy of the mutated gene from each parent. Connective tissue mutations that are recessive most frequently affect enzymes. This is because half the amount of an enzyme present appears sufficient to carry out the enzyme function. It is only when both alleles become inactive that function is compromised.

With the availability of molecular tools for genetic diagnosis, disorders can now be grouped according to the primary genetic abnormality. Basically four changes that occur within DNA are responsible for all mutations: deletion of genetic material, insertion of material, a change in the sequence of bases, and rearrangement of the genetic material. The results of these genetic alterations can be classified into mutations that alter the structure of the collagen molecule, or mutations that alter the rate at which a normal molecule is produced.

4.4.1 Mutations Which Alter Type I Collagen Structure (Structural Defects)

In defects of structural proteins, transcription, splicing, and translation mechanisms are intact. However, the resulting protein fails to interact properly with component members, thereby jeopardizing the function of the complex.

At present, there is great interest in understanding consequences of mutations in various regions of the collagen molecule. Mutations affecting the α 1(I) chain have a more severe consequence than similar mutations of the α 2(I) chain. The location of the defect within the α chain is also important. Since helix formation begins in the C globular domain and proceeds in a N terminal direction, a mutation in the C terminal region has a more severe consequence than one in the N terminal region because the mutation has disrupted a larger region of the helix.

4.4.2 Mutations Which Alter Type I Collagen Synthesis (Null Mutations)

The second general category of mutations is the result of "null alleles." This means that the mutation that occurred within the gene has either not allowed for the transcription of the gene, or that the nascent RNA chain cannot be spliced properly and therefore is not translated into protein. If the mRNA contains a mutation that produces an early stop codon, a nonfunctional protein is produced. The ultimate result of the null allele is that only half the α chain is produced. This means that the collagen chains that are made into fibers are correct; however the amount of protein that is subsequently produced and secreted into the matrix is greatly reduced.

4.4.3 DNA Linkage

DNA linkage studies identify a molecular marker associated with an inherited disorder. They have the potential for identifying the gene that is responsible for the genetic disease. Linkage is done through the use of restriction fragment length polymorphisms or RFLPs of genomic DNA and through the use of short repetitive sequences within DNA. The process can only be applied to large pedigrees with a positive history for multigeneration individuals afflicted with the disease.

The association of a particular DNA marker with a disease requires the identification of the marker that always segregates with the disease phenotype. This means that the marker is close enough to the diseased gene to always be transmitted to the offspring. The further apart the marker and gene are from each other, the more likely they will not be transmitted together to the offspring. Such a marker therefore is less useful in identifying other individuals with the abnormal gene.

4.5 SPECIFIC DISEASES OF CONNECTIVE TISSUE

The remainder of this chapter will cover the more common diseases of connective tissue that have an impact on the daily practice of the orthopedist. This section is not meant to be exhaustive, but rather to illustrate conditions where the underlying molecular cause can help understand the resulting clinical phenotype. Because extracellular molecules interact with each other in complicated fashion, defects in different molecules can present a similar clinical picture. This section will discuss diseases with primary effects on bone, ligaments, or cartilage.

4.5.1 Heritable Diseases Involving Bone

4.5.1.1 Bone Fracture

Osteogenesis Imperfecta (OI) is one of the best-understood disorders that result from mutations of type I collagen. Historically, the disease was classified into OI congenita (to designate individuals born with multiple fractures) and OI tarda (to designate those who develop fractures later in life). This classification is no longer used because it lacks genetic definition. The classification currently in widest use was developed by Sillence.

Type I OI (Sillence) is the mildest form of the disease. Affected individuals present frequent fractures in childhood, but have normal stature and no major skeletal deformities. In addition to fractures, the only clinical finding is the presence of blue sclera and mild joint laxity. The bone may appear normal by X-ray, but bone mass is decreased. These individuals tend to have fewer fractures after puberty. At menopause, crush fractures become apparent. The orthopedist may be called upon to differentiate these individuals from victims of child abuse. Physical examination, genetic history, and biochemical testing of type I collagen produced by cultured dermal fibroblasts will reveal the presence of OI.

Type I OI is inherited in an autosomal dominant fashion, but also occurs as a new mutation. RFLP studies performed on families with this form of OI have shown linkage to both the α 1(I) and the α 2(I) genes. Studies of cultured fibroblasts have shown decreased production of type I collagen, due either to a premature stop codon, a mutation that alters RNA splicing producing a null allele; or to a frameshift mutation located in the C terminal propeptide, since that part of the chain is not incorporated into the helix. Other mutations resulting in a clinical phenotype of a mild form of the disease will include changes of amino acids within the helix, especially along the N terminal.

Type IV OI, type III OI and type II OI (Sillence) are all distinguished from type I by having greater frequency bone fracture, bone deformity, dentinogenesis imperfecta, significant short stature with scoliosis, and abnormal hearing. A clear autosomal dominant pattern of inheritance or new mutations are usually found within families with these types of OI; most are due to the incorporation of a mutant protein chain, or a dominant negative mutation. It is in these patients that somatic gene therapy offers the greatest hope for a meaningful intervention to supplement the numerous orthopedic procedures that these individuals must endure.

4.5.1.2 Osteoporosis (see also Chapter 5)

Osteoporosis is a major public health problem, affecting more than 25 million people in the United States alone. Unfortunately, the pathogenesis of this common condition is still far from being understood. The influence of environmental factors is significant; however, there is still much to learn about the genetic components. As seen with mild OI, type I collagen has been found to produce osteoporotic conditions, but currently the more routine cases have not been found to have type I collagen mutations. Other genes which are under investigation include the vitamin D receptor gene. Some initial studies have reported that variants in the VDR gene account for a large fraction of the genetic effect on bone density, however, confirmatory studies have not been conclusive. Recent articles have described certain polymorphisms within the collagen gene that are associated with osteoporosis, but these observations will require confirmation.

4.5.1.3 Scoliosis

Marfan syndrome applies to a group of heterogeneous disorders characterized by ocular abnormalities (myopia and lens dislocation); skeletal disproportions (tall stature, dolichostenomelia, arachnodactaly, scoliosis, and pectis deformities); and cardiovascular abnormalities (mitral valve prolapse and aortic aneurysm and dissection). A similar group of conditions, congenital contractural arachnodactyly, is less severe than Marfan syndrome, but the clinical manifestations are primarily confined to the skeleton as well as including additional distinctive features including campodactyly and crumpled ears, while lacking major cardiovascular and ocular manifestations. These are transmitted primarily in an autosomal dominant fashion with full penetrance. Individuals with Marfan syndrome usually die from the cardiovascular complications unless preventive surgery is completed. Mutations within fibrillin 1 (FBN1 on chromosome 15q21) have been shown to cause Marfan syndrome, whereas mutations within fibrillin 2 (FBN2 on chromosome 5q23) have been identified in congenital contractural arachnodactyly. Fibrillins make up microfibrils which are extracellular aggregates that serve to associate elastin with collagen fibers in a manner analogous to a reinforced automobile tire. Fibrillin-1 predominates in microfibrils that are unassociated with elastic fibers and thus, in elastic arteries such as the aorta, fibrillin-1 is found in all three layers of the arterial wall, while fibrillin-2 is concentrated in the media.

4.5.2 Heritable Diseases Affecting Ligaments

Ehlers-Danlos syndrome (EDS) is a group of connective tissue disorders that demonstrate skin hyperextensibility, skin fragility, and joint hypermobility. EDS I-III (Gravis, Mitis, and benign familial hypermobility) are inherited as an autosomal dominant trait. Individuals with these disorders have very soft, velvety hyperextensible skin, impressive joint hypermobility, and easy bruising. Type I EDS can be diagnosed in the newborn period, but usually remains undiagnosed until the evidence of motor delay, which results from joint hypermobility. Distinctions between the three types is based on severity, type I being the most severe, and type III the least. Linkage analysis has shown that some but not all families have linkage to COL5A1. This is another example where linkage studies show an abnormality in different components of the composite system. In fact, some mouse knock-out experiments of decorin have produced a phenotype similar to this type of EDS.

EDS IV, the vascular type, has been shown to result from mutations in the type III collagen molecule. Numerous point mutations and exon skips have thus far been identified. In addition, EDS VIII, the type associated with periodontal disease, has been shown as due to a defect in the COL3A1 gene in some families.

EDS VI, a form that includes extreme ligamentous laxity with severe ocular fragility, retinal detachment, and scleromalacia, is another form that is inherited in an autosomal recessive fashion, the mutations having been found to be within the enzyme lysyl hydroxylase. Young individuals affected with this form of EDS can be suspected of having muscular dystrophy due to motor delay caused by severe muscular hypotonia, but nearly all affected children eventually walk normally.

A rare form of EDS (type VII), also known as arthrochalasis multiplex congenita, which presents with extremely lax joints with congenital hip dislocation and some other findings, has been clinically subdivided into three subgroups, A, B, and C. Within types A and B, specific exon 6 skips or deletions within COL1A1, COL1A2, in the N terminal extensions have been identified to cause this form of EDS. If mutations exist within the helical domain or the C-terminal domains of either COL1A1 or COL1A2, the clinical disease state is OI. Obviously the position of the mutations within the molecule is important in determining the clinical manifestations of the particular mutation. Type C has received much attention because the molecular basis of the disorder has been clarified. This form of EDS is distinguished from others by characteristic congenital hip dislocations that are refractory to surgical correction. Other joints are markedly hypermobile as well. The disease results from defective procollagen cleavage due either to a mutation of the cleavage enzyme or to a deletion or change in the cleavage recognition site within the collagen chain.

4.5.3 Diseases Affecting Cartilage

Cartilage is a heterogeneous tissue, similar to bone, and many mutations in cartilagenous gene products have been identified which result in abnormalities of the cartilage matrix.

4.5.3.1 Type II Collagen Defects

There is a broad range in the spectrum of conditions that have currently been identified as having a mutation within type II collagen. Some of the most severe or lethal phenotypes include achondrogenesis type II and hypochondrogenesis, while the mildest forms have been found in spondyloepiphyseal dysplasia (SED) with precocious osteoarthritis. SED congenita and Kniest dysplasia also have been found to be caused by a mutation within COL2A1. All mutations currently identified have been found within the triple helical domain of the molecule. The most common alteration involves the substitution of an alternative amino acid for glycine which is required in every third position for the integrity of the triple helix, as seen in type I collagen mutations. The mutations are thought to act through a dominant negative mechanism at the molecular level. This means that the product of the mutant allele disrupts the function of the product of the normal allele. All cartilagenous tissues are affected, but those regions that are dependent on filling a space, rather than those responsible for further longitudinal growth, are most severely affected. The condition produces more profound effects on the trunk than on the limbs, leading to a phenotype with a shorter trunk and long limbs.

The mutations that have been identified within COL2A1 causing Stickler syndrome appear to be due to a deficit in the normal amount of protein, or functionally null mutations. In several cases that have been characterized at the molecular level, a splicing error or an inframe premature stop codon sequence has been found. Therefore, similar to the null alleles within mild OI, a null allele within type II collagen has led to the clinical phenotype which includes early osteoarthritic problems, ocular problems, sensorineural hearing loss, and the possibility of an isolated cleft palate associated with Robin sequence.

4.5.3.2 Type X Collagen Defects

Several heterozygous mutations have been found within COL10A1 and have all been associated with Schmid metaphyseal chondrodysplasia, a relatively mild chondrodysplasia. The mutations have thus far mapped to the region of the gene encoding the carboxy collagen triple helix, and appear to involve amino acids playing essential roles in chain association or in termination of the synthesis of the alpha chain prior to the carboxy propeptide. These types of mutations would lead to an insufficient amount of normal protein, because the mutant chains would not be incorporated in the developing collagen fibril. In contrast to the phenotype seen with type II mutations (above), this condition is characterized by more significant effects on tissues responsible for the longitudinal growth, i.e., the growth plates where type X collagen is made. Individuals with mutations in type X collagen show a more normal trunk size with shorter limbs. The hypertrophic zone of the cartilage is disrupted and much smaller than normal. Because the quality of the type II collagen is normal, these patients do not develop degenerative joint disease.

4.5.3.3 Type XI Collagen Defects

Mutations of the COL11A2 gene have recently been described in two families with a Stickler-like syndrome. The affected individuals presented with mild SED, precocious osteoarthritis and sensorineural hearing loss but did not have any eye abnormalities. This lack of ocular involvement is consistent with the finding that the $\alpha2$ chain of type XI collagen forms trimers with the $\alpha1$ and $\alpha3$ chains of type XI collagen in cartilage and the inner ear, but is replaced by the $\alpha2$ chain of type V collagen in ocular tissues.

4.5.3.4 Mutations Affecting the Chondrocyte Lineage: *Achondroplasia*

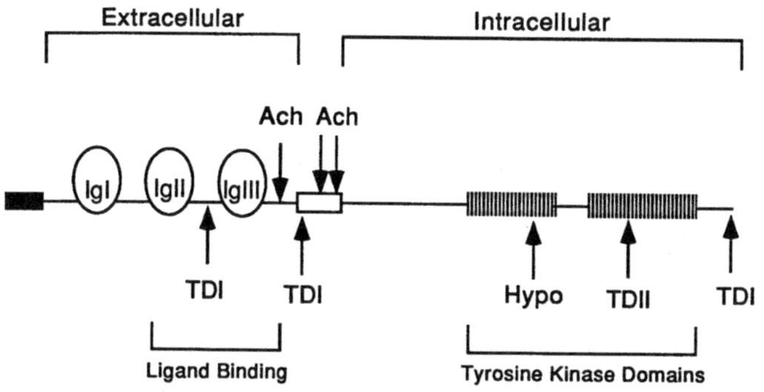

FIGURE 4.3 This scheme summarizes the location of mutations in the FGFR 3 molecule found in various forms of skeletal dysplasias. ■ Signal Peptide; □ Transmembrane Domain; Ig — Immunoglobulin-like domains.

There are four fibroblast growth factor receptors (FGFR). They consist of tyrosine kinase molecules spanning the cell wall and binding and phosphorylating intracellular signal transduction proteins that bind and phosphorylate. Ligand binding induces receptor homo- and heterodimerization which play a role in embryonic development. Several different forms of dwarfism were recently linked to FGFR3 mutations, including achrondoplasia, the most common genetic form of dwarfism; hypochondroplasia, which is similar but less severe; and thanatophoric dysplasia types I and II which are neonatal lethal forms of dwarfism (see Figure 4.3). These syndromes are all characterized by disproportionate short stature, macrocephaly, and, in the case of thanatophoric dysplasia, impaired development of the ribs resulting in early respiratory failure. These dwarfism syndromes are all due to mutations in different structural and functional domains of FGFR3 which is expressed in the resting cartilage of long bones. A single mutation, accounting for >97% of achondroplasia, is a glycine to arginine change at amino acid 380 located within the transmembrane domain of the receptor. It is estimated that ~80% of cases of achondroplasia are new mutations, which is striking when one considers the homogeneity of this mutation at the molecular level.

Hypochondroplasia is due to a substitution of lysine for asparagine at position 540 located in the proximal tyrosine kinase domain of the cytoplasmic domain. The mutations thus far identified within thantophoric dysplasia II have been caused by a lysine to glutamic acid at codon 650 located in the distal tyrosine kinase domain. The underlying molecular defect for TDI is more heterogeneous since two different mutations have thus far been identified.

The ultimate result of these FGFR3 mutations have only recently begun to be understood. It appears that the achondroplasia-class mutations activate FGFR3 signaling in the absence of a ligand (constitutive activation), and that the extent of activation varies according to the mutation and correlates with the severity of the phenotype. The mechanisms by which receptor activation occurs are still speculative, but may involve receptor oligomerization. The mutation in this regulatory element appears to reduce the proliferation of the early chondrocytes, causing a shortening of the growth plate and resulting in short limbs. Further studies are necessary, however, prior to a more complete understanding of the pathophysiology of these FGFR3 mutations.

4.5.3.5 Mutation of Noncollagenous Matrix Proteins of Cartilage

The cartilage oligomeric matrix protein (COMP) is a component of the extracellular matrix of cartilage and is found primarily as a pentomeric molecule. Linkage studies with pseudoachondroplasia first mapped to 19p12-13.1 and later heterozygous mutations in COMP were identified. Pseudoachondroplasia resembles achondroplasia clinically, but is distinguished by a normal appearance and size at birth. COMP is a member of the thrombospondin protein family, but the function of COMP is as yet not well defined. The mutations in COMP causing a disease state are thought to act through a dominant negative fashion on the proliferative capacity of the chondrocyte (thus producing the achrodroplasia like phenotype).

4.5.3.6 Mutation of a Matrix Modifying Enzyme

The diastrophic dysplasia sulfate transporter (DTDST) gene has been found to be responsible for several cases of diastrophic dysplasia, an autosomal recessive disorder, identified at birth by the presence of markedly short extremities and distinctive hands with shortening of the digits and proximal displacement of the thumb (hitchhiker thumb). Linkage studies first localized the gene to chromosome 5q in 1990, but mutations were not identified for another four years. Mutations have been found in one of the affected alleles in three individuals, all creating a premature termination codon, but the mutation in their second allele has yet to be identified.

In addition to causing diastrophic dysplasia, DTDST has also been found to cause two other recessive lethal chondrodysplasias, achondrogenesis type 1B, and atelosteogenesis type II. Mutations in both alleles of DTDST of six individuals affected with achondrogenesis have been found. The pathogenesis of these disorders probably reflects the abundance of sulfated proteoglycans present in cartilage. Observations thus far imply that chondrocytes are unable to transport sufficient sulfate ions to cartilage matrix proteins. The specific clinical phenotype depends on the specific mutations within the DTDST genes.

4.6 FUTURE DIRECTIONS

In this chapter, we have given an overview of the defects that underlie connective tissue disorders frequently treated by orthopedists. For the immediate future, defining the molecular basis of these disorders will provide a better understanding of the heterogeneity of the various traits, will improve our ability to predict the natural course of the disorder, and the response to orthopedic manipulations. It will also provide more accurate data for genetic counseling. A more practical aspect of molecular diagnosis will be new strategies for therapy. These will be based on isolating the connective tissue stem cell from the affected individual, introducing a gene which alters the expression of the mutated gene and then reintroducing the corrected cells back into the affected individual. This type of approach is currently being developed in the murine model of connective tissue diseases, and in some form will eventually be applicable to humans.

ADDITIONAL READINGS

1. Byers, P.H., Disorders of collagen biosynthesis and structure, in *The Metabolic and Molecular Basis of Inherited Disease, Vol III,* 7th ed., C.R. Scriver et al., Eds., McGraw-Hill, p. 4029-4077, 1995.
2. De Moerlooze, L. and Dickson, C., Skeletal disorders associated with fibroblast growth factor receptor mutations, *Cur. Opin. Genet. and Devel.*, 7(3): 378-385, 1997.
3. Dickman, S., No bones about a genetic switch for bone growth, *Science*, 276: 1502, 1997.
4. Horton, W.A., Molecular genetic basis of the human chondrodysplasias, *Endo. and Metab. Clinics of North Amer.*, 25(3): 683-697, 1996.
5. Newham, P. and Humphries, M.J., Integrin adhesion receptors: structure, function and implications for biomedicine, *Mol. Med. Today,* 2(7): 304-313, 1996.
6. Olsen, B.R., Mutations in collagen genes resulting in metaphyseal and epiphyseal dysplasias, *Bone,* 17(2): 45S-49S, 1995.
7. Pope, F.M. and Burrows, N.P., Ehlers-Danlos syndrome has varied molecular mechanisms, *J. Med. Genet.*, 34: 400-410, 1997.
8. Ramirez, F., Fibrillin mutations in Marfan syndrome and related phenotypes, *Cur. Opin. Genet. and Devel.*, 6: 309-315, 1996.
9. Rowe, D.W. and Shapiro, J.R., Diseases associated with abnormalities of structural proteins, in *Textbook of Rheumatology,* 5th edition, Kelly, W.M., Harris, E.O., Ruddy, S., and Sledge, C.B., Eds., W.B. Saunders, Chapter 99, p. 1535-1562, 1997.
10. Rowe, D.W. and Shapiro, J.R., Osteogenesis Imperfecta, in *Metabolic Bone Disease,* 3rd edition, Avioli, L. and Krane, S., Eds., W.B. Saunders, Chapter 23, p. 651-695, 1997.
11. Webster, M.K. and Donoghue, D.J., FGFR activation in skeletal disorders: too much of a good thing, *Trends in Genet.*, 13(5): 178-182, 1997.
12. Wilkie, A.O.M., Craniosynostosis: genes and mechanisms, *Hum. Mol. Genet.*, 6(10): 1647-1656, 1997.

5 Osteoporosis

Felix Bronner

CONTENTS

5.1 INTRODUCTION

With the aging of the American population, osteoporosis, defined as a thinning of bone structure that leads to great susceptibility to bone fracture (Figure 5.1), has become a significant public health problem. This chapter will discuss the epidemiology of osteoporosis, and the biology of the skeleton and of the cells that construct this largely extracellular structure.

Over 90% of the calcium content of the human body, typically 1 to 1.5 kg, is found in the skeleton. In the first two decades of life, skeletal growth and calcium accumulation in bones tend to go in parallel. By the end of the third decade of life, with skeletal growth having come to an end some 10 to 12 years earlier, there occurs a reversal in the relationship between bone calcium deposition and removal. Whereas the bone calcium deposition rate exceeds the bone removal rate, leading to a positive calcium balance during the period of skeletal growth, deposition and resorption after the age of 30 begin to decline, with deposition decreasing faster than resorption. As a result, the mass of bone calcium begins to decrease (Figure 5.2). This decrease is

0-8493-9237-3/99/$0.00+$.50

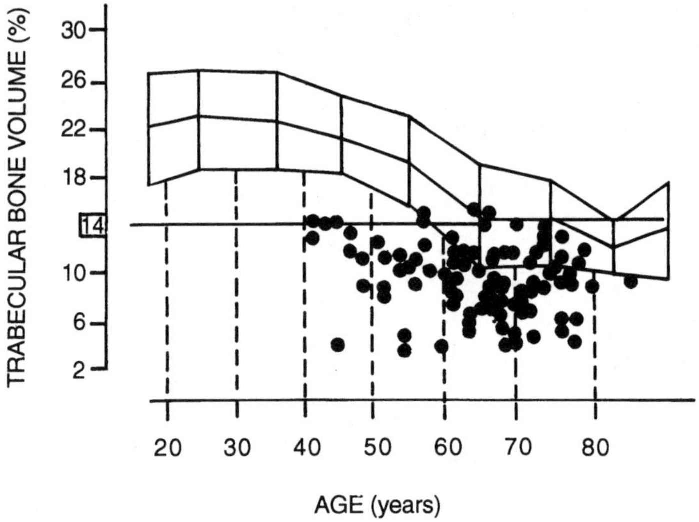

FIGURE 5.1 Trabecular bone volume in women as a function of age. The boxes represent mean values (±SEM) for normal women. The individual data points are from 106 women with primary vertebral osteoporosis, aged 65.9 ± 9.9 years, with a mean trabecular volume of 10.0 ± 28%. A value of 14 is considered the vertebral fracture threshold (vft) in women with osteoporosis. *Note:* The term "fracture threshold" represents a statistical concept, not an absolute value. Actual fracture risk is continuous and progressive over a fairly wide range of bone mineral density. (Reproduced from [21] with permission.)

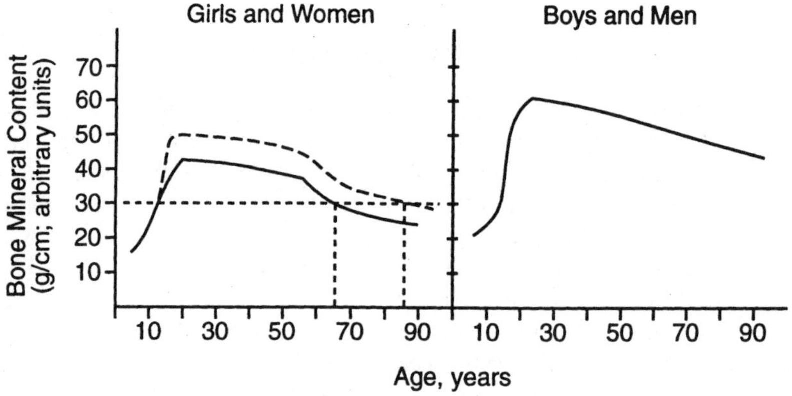

FIGURE 5.2 Bone mineral content as a function of age, determined by photon absorptiometry. The dashed line indicates a theoretical fracture limit. Accordingly, the bone of women 65 years or older would be subject to ready fracture. If, however, bone mineral content of the females had increased as indicated by the stippled curve, the likelihood of ready fracture would be delayed to the age of 86 years and beyond. (From unpublished data, kindly provided by C. Christiansen, Denmark.)

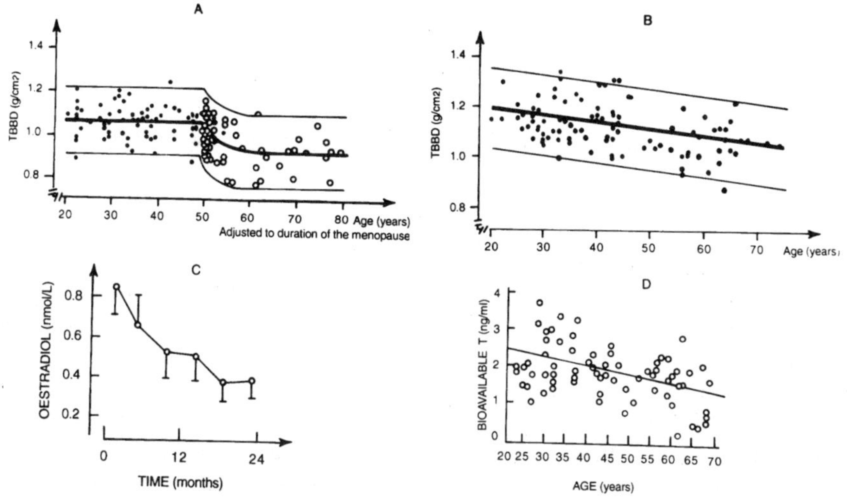

FIGURE 5.3 Total body bone density (TBBD) as a function of age in women (A) and men (B). Plasma estradiol concentration (C) in 31 women, 47 to 54 years old, with irregular menses during a two-year period. Bioavailable testosterone levels in plasma of men (D). TBBD was obtained by measuring total bone mineral content of the body by gadolinium 153 scanning, normalized to skeletal surface areas. (Figures A and B taken from [13]. Figure C taken from [25]. Figure D taken from [24]. All reproduced with permission.)

quite gradual, almost imperceptible, until the age of 50. Thereafter, it accelerates. In women, at the menopause, the loss of bone calcium is sudden and rapid and does not begin to slow until the seventh decade of life (Figure 5.2). In men, the loss of bone mass, beginning at about the age of 50 years, is more gradual. The rate of loss in both sexes becomes about the same after the age of 70 years (Figure 5.3).

5.2 CALCIUM IN BONE

Calcium, along with phosphate, constitutes the principal mineral and structural substance that gives vertebrates their internal support and allows people to stand erect. The skeleton constitutes about 16% of an adult's body weight; 47% of the skeletal weight is dry, fat-free bone and 26% of the latter is calcium.[6]

At least 90% of the crystalline calcium phosphate in bone is hydroxyapatite [$C_{10}(PO_4)_6(OH)_2$]; other calcium phosphates include whitlockite, octacalcium phosphate and brushite, as well as an amorphous calcium phosphate with variable phosphate content.[31]

The precise order in which calcium is precipitated in bone and the path it follows as calcium salts mature and become increasingly less soluble is not yet known. The initial calcium phosphate is deposited on or inside collagen fibrils that have formed extracellularly from collagen molecules that had been extruded by osteoblasts, the bone-forming cells. Additional calcium phosphate is deposited by accretion so that the calcium salt is arranged in a very orderly fashion. The resulting crystals are plate-like, with the surface layers of the bone crystals constituting 50% of the newly formed crystals, but ultimately, in the fully mature crystal, the surface layers constitute only about 25% of the fully mature crystal volume.[31]

5.3 THE EFFECT OF AGING ON THE SKELETON

Figures 5.3A and 5.3B are representative of the available information on how the mineral mass of the skeleton changes with age in women and men. In women (Figure 5.3A), a very modest decline in bone mineral mass between the ages of 30 and menopause is followed by a sharp, exponential decline for the next decade, with a further, more modest, apparently linear decline thereafter. The rapid loss of bone mineral mass that occurs in women in the decade after menopause accounts for some 13% of the total body bone density at menopause and largely affects trabecular bone. In men (Figure 5.3B), on the other hand, bone mineral mass declines linearly, with a rate of approximately 0.2% per year from a peak mass reached in the third decade of life. The Framingham cross-sectional population study[16] showed that elderly men and women well past the menopause have a bone mass that decreases with age in both gender groups in a linear and equivalent fashion.

Loss of trabecular bone volume may involve the loss of whole trabecular plates, rather than their mere thinning, as is the case for cortical bone. As a result, as stated by Parfitt,[28] "…the mainly continuous trabecular network characteristic of a young person [is transformed] into the mainly discontinuous network characteristic of the elderly…" Compressive strength of trabecular bone depends importantly on the connections between these structural elements. Once lost, a trabecular plate cannot be restored.[28] Hence, a major aim of therapy must be prevention of loss of the trabecular elements, as well as slowing of the thinning of cortical bone.

5.4 GONADAL HORMONES AS MAJOR REGULATORS OF BONE CELL FUNCTION

It was Albright who first related osteoporosis in women to the menopause. The incisiveness of this insight is illustrated in Figure 5.3 which shows how the abruptness of loss in gonadal hormone function in women (Figure 5.3C) parallels the abruptness with which their skeleton weakens (Figure 5.3A). The figure also shows how the gradual loss of bone mass in males (Figure 5.3B) is paralleled by a comparably gradual loss in functional testosterone levels (Figure 5.3D). What is more, gonadectomy in both females (Figure 5.4A) and males (Figure 5.4B) is followed by a rapid drop in bone mass, the rate of which is comparable to that in Figure 5.3C. The bone mineral density of men castrated by orchidectomy (whose testosterone levels were at least an order of magnitude lower than those of controls) fell exponentially to stabilize at some 70% of the initial density. This value and the rate of fall ($T_{1/2} \approx 3y$) are comparable to the corresponding values that can be calculated from Figure 5.3A for the rapid phase of bone loss that follows the menopause in women. It has been reported[34] that fractures involving limbs, hips, and ribs occurred

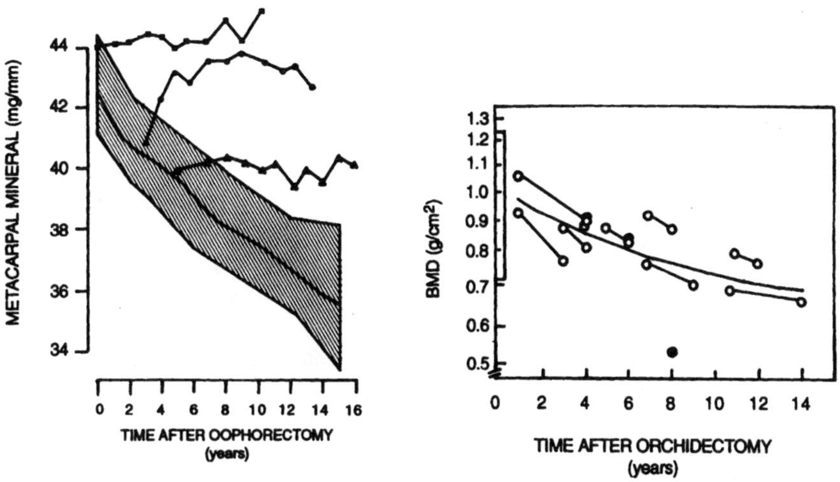

FIGURE 5.4 The effect of gonadectomy on bone. (A) In women. Hatched area is mean ± SD. Single lines represent mean bone loss values in three groups of women given estrogen treatment at 0 (■), 3 (●), and 6 (▲) years after oophorectomy. (B) In men. In 8 of the 12 patients, the measurement was repeated after 1 to 3 years. The line is a second-order regression. (Figure A from [1]. Figure B from [33], with permission.)

twice as frequently in male geriatric patients whose morning levels of serum testosterone were at or below 1040 nmol/L than in those whose testosterone levels were higher. Also, two or more separate incidents of fracture occurred five times more frequently in hypogonadal than eugonadal men.[34] Moreover, in the hips of healthy men, there is a consistently positive relationship between bone mineral density and the logarithm of the ratio of serum testosterone to the serum level of globulin that binds testosterone.[23] This ratio is an index of free testosterone levels.

In a recent review, Riggs et al.[28a] argue that a major factor in the age-dependent thinning of bone in men is due to a low level of bioavailable estrogen. The latter is produced in men by conversion of testosterone. Thus, the decreasing level of testosterone leads to lower estrogen levels in elderly men and it is the low levels of estrogen that are thought to be responsible for the thin bones of men, as also true in women. Only further research can provide support for this hypothesis.

The effects of gonadectomy on bone metabolism are rapid and dramatic. Thus, in oophorectomized women, urinary losses of hydroxyproline and calcium increased within three weeks, and estrogen treatment of only one week was associated with a clear reversal of the effects of oophorectomy.[27] Figure 5.4A shows how promptly metacarpal bone mineral levels stopped dropping when oophorectomized women were treated with estradiol. Similar responses have been reported in men. In situations where puberty is delayed due to gonadal hormone deficiency in boys, or because of anorexia nervosa in young women, normal peak bone density is not reached. Similarly, men who suffer from hypogonadism due to a deficiency of the hypothalamic gonadotropin releasing factor, GnRH, evince a marked decrease in bone density. This can be raised by gonadal hormone replacement, the treatment being more effective in younger men with a less mature bone structure.[16,34] These effects of gonadal hormone deficiencies and replacements in both males and females show that osteoporosis is not a disease confined to women. Rather, its cause must be searched for in how both male and female hormones modulate bone cell metabolism.

5.5 CELLULAR EFFECTS OF GONADAL HORMONES

Osteoblast-like cells possess receptors for both androgens and estrogens and for the insulin-like growth factors. Moreover, these bone cells, whether isolated from men or women, bind male and female hormones.

Osteoclasts also possess gonadal hormone receptors. Cultured avian osteoclasts have been shown to diminish their osteolytic activity in a dose-dependent fashion in response to the addition of estrogens. Cells from human giant cell tumors (an osteoclastoma) contain estrogen receptors and respond to 17β-estradiol *in vitro*.[26]

The discovery of numerous cytokines produced by osteoblasts[17] and of transcripts of several of these (IL-3 and IL-8) in human bone cells[4] suggests that these molecules play an important role as messengers from osteoblasts to osteoclasts or their precursors. These messages may stimulate osteoclastic development and/or activity. On the other hand, when released in reduced amounts (or not at all), as when osteoblasts are under estrogen domination, the repression of the cytokine-induced increase in osteoclastic activity may account for the maintenance of the bone mineral mass in premenopausal women.[18] Osteoblasts respond to testosterone via specific receptors and, when under testosterone domination, also produce less interleukin-6 (IL-6).

There is now evidence that when IL-6 release is stimulated, this in turn acts to enhance the effect of 1,25-dihydroxyvitamin D_3, 1, 25-$(OH)_2D_3$, in stimulating the production of osteoclast progenitors. Estrogen inhibits the IL-6-dependent stimulation by 1,25-$(OH)_2D_3$ and consequently causes less osteoclast precursors to be formed. Thyroid hormone, on the other hand, stimulates the IL-6-dependent enhancement of the action of 1,25-$(OH)_2D_3$; as a result there is increased production of osteoclast-like cells.[30]

Estrogen or androgen, when added to a bone cell culture, causes diminution of the inhibition of bone cell activity that otherwise results from parathyroid hormone addition.[11,12] Estradiol also stimulates osteoblast proliferation, thymidine incorporation *in vivo*, and synthesis of collagen mRNA and of collagen.[9,10]

If, as has become evident from cell culture experiments, gonadal hormones stimulate and maintain osteoblastic metabolism, a decrease in gonadal hormone levels would be accompanied by downregulation of osteoblasts, reduction of collagen synthesis and the diminution or even cessation of the cascade of events that lead to the formation of bone. Contrariwise, osteoclast activity would be enhanced if osteoclasts and/or their progenitor cells were to be relieved from gonadal hormone inhibition, thus being able to spread out over the bone surface and resorb bone at a maximum rate. One interesting consequence, it has recently been shown,[5] is that the nature of mineralization is changed. Under estrogen domination bone has a lower mineral density, on average, than when bone forms under the absence of estrogen.

In the latter case, bone seems more brittle, i.e., its impact resistance is diminished. In addition, whatever inhibition operated on precursor cells would also be relieved.

In the absence of gonadal hormones, osteoblastic activity would be diminished and osteoblast generation would be reduced, whereas osteoclastic activity and osteoclastogenesis would approach a maximum. As a result, those regions of bone where osteoblasts and osteoclasts are most numerous, as on trabecular surfaces, would be subject to the most intense destruction. Predictably, therefore, gonadectomy would lead to the most rapid bone loss; the menopause, with its fairly drastic loss of ovarian function, would lead to rapid bone loss (Figure 5.3A), but to less loss than in the case of oophorectomy. The fairly gradual diminution of testosterone function in men would be — and is — accompanied by the relatively slow bone loss recorded for men (Figure 5.3B).

Notwithstanding the profound effects of gonadal hormones on bone, fracture healing seems unaffected in animals deprived of their gonads.

5.6 MODULATION OF SKELETAL FUNCTION

5.6.1 Genetic

It seems obvious that many genes, mostly as yet unidentified, must be involved in specifying the processes that lead to skeletal assembly, shape, size, and turnover. One gene that has recently been identified as having a potential role in bone density is linked to polymorphism in the vitamin D receptor gene. Morrison and collaborators[22] have shown that "allelic variants in the gene encoding the vitamin D receptor can be used to predict differences in bone density…" Postmenopausal women with a bone density two standard deviations below that of young women were found to exhibit a significantly higher incidence of the genotype associated with low bone density.

Nevertheless, several surveys have failed to find a valid correlation between conditions associated with or characteristic of osteoporosis and a specific state of the vitamin D polymorphism receptor. Clearly the likely complexity of the interaction of the many genes involved in specifying and expressing skeletal characteristics makes it unlikely that only one gene or its expression plays the major role in skeletal health.

5.6.2 Vitamin D

Attempts to overcome osteoporosis, or at least to slow the course of bone mineral decrease, have for many years utilized vitamin D, either by itself or together with calcium supplementation. Results with vitamin D alone have been variable, some investigators reporting significant reductions in the fracture rate, others failing to find any effect. One review[8] of the effect of 1,25-dihydroxyvitamin D_3 on the course of bone loss concluded that the more favorable outcomes, such as reducing fracture rates, were associated with higher doses of the metabolite. Conceivably, individuals who responded to vitamin D supplementation had a vitamin D receptor allele that required a higher than normal amount of vitamin D for bone density to come nearer to normal. Typically, vitamin D supplementation of women with osteoporosis will increase calcium absorption and urinary calcium output, with no effect on the overall retention of calcium. Indeed, in a study of two postmenopausal women who were treated with 3.75 mg vitamin D (150,000 international units) for six weeks, the rate of bone calcium deposition and removal went down, not up.[15] It is of course possible that the two postmenopausal subjects did not have an allelic defect and increased vitamin D intake therefore was without effect. A positive effect of adding 1,25-dihydroxyvitamin D to calcium supplementation has been reported, but the patients in that study received corticosteroid therapy.[29] The latter influences bone loss more from the spine than from other sites which do not show a vitamin D response. Conceivably, administration of vitamin D is less effective than administration of 1,25-$(OH)_2D_3$, as the conversion of vitamin D to the dihydroxylated metabolite is regulated. Further study is needed, but the overall results reported for vitamin D and its congeners do not seem encouraging.

Pharmaceutical companies have synthesized various vitamin D analogs in an attempt to emphasize desirable characteristics, such as longer half-life, and minimize undesirable effects, such as hypercalcemia. Some of these compounds have been subjected to clinical trials in patients with osteoporosis and modest gains or diminished rates of loss of bone mass have been reported. It seems likely that vitamin D or appropriate analogs may be of benefit when added as a supplement to the diet of the elderly, but vitamin D or its analogs are not likely to constitute major therapy for osteoporosis in the near future.

5.6.3 Parathyroid Hormone (PTH) and Calcitonin (CT)

From the role PTH plays in the developing and growing organism, it is clear the action of PTH can be classified as anabolic and it is in this sense that PTH, especially when administered intermittently, has been used in osteoporosis. While the anabolic effects of PTH have been fairly clear in animal experiments, especially in ovariectomized or castrated rats, therapeutic effects in human patients have been less clear-cut. Combining PTH with 1,25-$(OH)_2D_3$ or antiresorptive agents such as calcitonin, bisphosphonates, or estrogen has generally led to more promising results, but the number of patients studied for any one treatment has been small.

Based on the hypocalcemic effect when CT is administered acutely, therapeutic use of CT in osteoporosis was proposed and experimented with early. Calcitonin has been shown to inhibit osteoclast metabolism transiently by causing the cell to stop its rhythmic pseudopodal activity, causing the osteoclast to round up and become quiescent, although the ultimate viability of the cell seems relatively unaffected. Treatment with CT has been reported to reduce the incidence and rate of new fractures in patients with osteoporosis. Calcitonin also has analgesic effects of unknown mechanism and the difficulty of enteric administration has been partially overcome by a nasal preparation that the patient can self-administer. The most potent CT preparation is a synthetic salmon preparation, many times more potent than human CT. One reason for this appears to be a longer biological half-life of the salmon CT, partly due to greater resistance to enzyme degradation and higher affinity for the CT receptor.

5.6.4 Other Hormones

In addition to the specific calcitropic hormones, parathyroid hormone, and calcitonin, a number of other hormones (gonadal hormones, thyroxin, growth hormone, insulin-like growth factors, glucocorticoids, insulin, glucagon) play a role in modulating bone metabolism and, therefore, may also change the course of osteoporosis.

Gonadal hormone effects on bone cells have been discussed in Sections 5.4 and 5.5, above. Estrogens may be given daily or in a cycle that includes progesterone. A major advantage of estrogen treatment over other treatments that combat loss of bone is that estrogen treatment also lowers the incidence of cardiovascular disease that occurs in untreated postmenopausal women. Estrogen treatment also appears to diminish the incidence of Alzheimer's disease.

There is as yet no consensus on treating elderly men with testosterone or hormones that act at an earlier point in the biochemical cascade that leads to male hormone production.

Although thyroid hormones modulate or interact with many steps in the pathways that determine the status of the skeleton, they have not been used to treat osteoporosis as such. This is also true for insulin and glucagon.

Glucocorticoids modify the expression of a variety of genes in osteoblastic cells and act permissively for other hormones. Large doses of glucocorticoids inhibit osteoprogenitor proliferation and bone formation, specifically decreasing the mRNA levels of $\alpha 1$ (I) collagen. These actions are responsible for the development of Cushing's disease and the bone loss associated with prolonged treatment of patients with asthma, inflammatory bowel disease, granuloma, and collagen-vascular disease. Thus, glucocorticoids have anabolic effects on bone under certain conditions; the overall effect, however, is catabolic, inducing rather than overcoming osteoporosis.

The insulin-like growth factors (IGF-I and IGF-II) are synthesized in the liver in response to growth hormone from the pituitary gland. Upon release from the hepatocyte, the IGFs become bound to binding proteins (IGFBBs) both in the liver and also in the skeleton, the second richest depot for IGFs, next to the liver. IGFs are also synthesized by osteoblasts. The availability of recombinant human IGF-I (rhIGF-I) has facilitated clinical studies intended to determine whether bone formation rates increase as a result of treatment with IGF-I. Low doses of rhIGF-I, administered on a continuing basis, seem to have stimulated bone formation in osteoporotic males,[19] but more and larger studies are needed before treatment with IGF-I can become a modality.

5.6.5 Exercise

Vigorous exercise is well-known to lead to increased muscle and bone mass. Contrariwise, life under conditions of hypogravity is associated with loss of muscle and weight-bearing bone (see Section 5.6.6, below). Given an adequate intake of calcium and appropriate levels of gonadal hormones, physical exercise will increase peak adult skeletal mass.[14] However, when gonadal hormone levels are depressed, as in postmenopausal osteoporosis, exercise alone will not arrest the decline in bone mass; exercise combined with estrogen therapy is more effective than estrogen alone. The mechanism by which weight-bearing exercise enhances bone mass is not known. The effect of exercise appears mediated by bone cells — osteocytes in particular have been implicated — which respond by increased metabolic activity.

5.6.6 Spaceflight

From data obtained in the course of the Skylab experiments in 1973, it appears that the bones stressed most by gravity, e.g., the calcaneus, are most affected by weightlessness. Bone mineral loss under these conditions appears progressive for several months or more. Recovery after return to earth is slow and may not be complete for some years.

Changes in calcium metabolism as a result of spaceflight include increases in plasma calcium, a decrease in plasma parathyroid hormone levels, and an initial increase followed by a subsequent decrease in plasma 1,25-dihydroxyvitamin D_3 levels. These changes probably contribute to the negative calcium balance observed in space fight, as they would lead to a diminution of active calcium absorption in the intestine and diminished renal calcium reabsorption.

5.6.7 Caffeine

The 12th Framingham study examination identified caffeine intake as a risk factor, especially for women under 65 years of age,[20] but other studies have failed to find such an effect. In men under 75 years of age, the Framingham study found no effect of caffeine intake; the risk of hip fractures was, however, nearly doubled in men 75 years and older who drank two or more cups of coffee per day. How caffeine might act, whether directly on bone cells or indirectly, is not known.

5.6.8 Tobacco

Daniell[7] was the first to observe that smokers 60 to 69 years of age had lost cortical bone at an average rate of 1.02% per year, whereas nonsmokers lost only 0.69% per year, a statistically significant difference. Nonobese smokers lost significantly more bone than nonobese nonsmokers. There was, however, no statistically significant difference between obese smokers and obese nonsmokers; moreover, as also observed by others, the obese population lost significantly less bone than nonobese.

While some investigators have failed to find that smoking affects the incidence of osteoporosis, most have shown that smoking does constitute a risk factor for osteoporosis.

5.6.9 Alcohol

A variety of studies have confirmed that alcoholism is associated with diminished bone mass and density in both men and women. In men, chronic alcoholism has been found[32] to lead to osteoporosis in half of the population of alcoholics under the age of 50 years, whereas this percentage is negligibly small in normal males (Figure 5.3B). Increasingly, evidence in human and animal studies points to a direct effect of alcohol on bone cells themselves, with severe impairment of bone remodeling having been observed in chronic alcoholics who have normal biochemical parameters of calcium metabolism.[2]

5.7 THERAPY CONSIDERATIONS

It seems obvious that adequate calcium intake is necessary to permit full expression of the genetic program that leads to skeletal shape, size, and mass. It is equally evident that skeletal development is a complicated, multifactorial process that involves many hormones, with gonadal hormones, growth hormone, and insulin-like growth factors playing a principal role. Bone mass begins to decrease after the third decade of life. The question therefore arises whether this can be arrested or slowed. Moreover, inasmuch as the decrease in bone mass implies that the formation rate is now smaller than the rate at which bone is being destroyed, one needs to consider whether therapy should consist of stimulating formation or inhibiting destruction, or both.

The data depicted in Figure 5.4A suggest that estrogen treatment can markedly slow the loss of bone in oophorectomized women, but from available information it seems unlikely that bone loss can be totally arrested. However, with hormone replacement therapy and appropriate calcium intake, loss of bone mass can be slowed to a minimum. The effect of this slowing, illustrated in Figure 5.2, is to delay significantly the age at which fracture of a given bone becomes probable under what until that time had been a harmless impact. In light of what is now known about the biology of bone cells, gonadal hormone replacement will stimulate osteoblast function and number. This in turn will reduce the production of cytokines such as interleukin 6, which stimulate osteoclastogenesis.

An alternative approach is to attempt to influence osteoclast function directly. This has been done by administering *calcitonin*, *fluorides*, or *bisphosphonates*.

Calcitonin inhibits the osteoclast, causing it to round up and cease its metabolic activity, at least transiently. As discussed above, Section 5.6.3, calcitonin has been reported to reduce the incidence and rate of new fracture formation in osteoporotic patients and to decrease the pain associated with collapsed vertebrae. Administration of calcitonin that is not isogenous may lead to immune resistance.

Attempts at using *fluoride* to combat osteoporosis date back many years. Results have been variable, with enough encouraging results for trials to continue and for new trials to be initiated. Fluorides become deposited in bone, with the fluoride ion substituting for the hydroxyl ion in carbanatohydroxyapatite. Fluoroapatite is less soluble than hydroxyapatite so that resorption of bone mineral is slowed significantly. Fluoride treatment seems to result in enhancement of the cancellous bone mass, but without a concurrent decrease in the fracture rate. Moreover, there are indications that fluoride therapy leads to a higher hip fracture rate.

Bisphosphonates, at relatively high concentrations, alter the bone mineral to make it less soluble, thereby reducing osteoclastic activity. More recently formulated bisphosphonates act at relatively low concentrations, probably by directly inhibiting the osteoclast. The long-term effects of inhibiting osteoclastic activity are not known. Over the short term, the reduction in osteolysis has caused bone mass loss to slow, even to disappear, and to reduce the incidence of fractures and the loss of height.

Treatment of osteoporosis in recent years has benefited greatly from the wider availability of multiple treatments — hormonal, bisphosphonate, combinations of the two, plus nutritional support. For example, bisphosphonate treatment can supplement replacement hormone therapy in cases where the latter has not adequately slowed the decrease in bone mass. Moreover, it is becoming possible to evaluate bone quality beyond bone mass. As a result, individualization of treatment is both possible and recommended, and patients that do not tolerate one type of treatment can still be treated.

REFERENCES

1. Aitken, J.M., D.M. Hart, J.B. Anderson, R. Lindsay, and D.A. Smith. Osteoporosis after oophorectomy for non-malignant disease. *Brit. Med. J.* 1: 325-328, 1973.
2. Bikle, D.D., H.K. Genant, C. Cann, R.R. Recker, B.P. Halloran, and G.J. Strewler. Bone disease in alcohol abuse. *Ann. Int. Med.* 103: 42-48, 1985.
3. Bikle, D.D., B.R. Halloran, and E. Morey-Holton. Spaceflight and the skeleton: lessons for the earthbound. *Gravitational and Space Biol. Bull.* 10: 119-135, 1997.
4. Birch, M.A., A.F. Ginty, C.A. Walsh, W.D. Fraser, J.A. Gallagher, and G. Bilbe. PCR detection of cytokines in normal human pagetic osteoblast-like cells. *J. Bone Miner. Res.* 8: 1155-1171, 1993.
5. Boyde, A., J.E. Compston, J. Reeve, K.L. Bell, B.S. Noble, S.J. Jones, and N. Loveridge. Effect of estrogen suppression on the mineralization density of iliac crest biopsies in young women as assessed by backscattered electron imaging. *Bone* 22: 241-250, 1998.
6. Bronner, F. and R. Lemaire. Comparison of calcium kinetics in man and the rat. *Calcif. Tiss. Res.* 3: 128-248, 1969.
7. Daniell, H.W. Osteoporosis and the slender smoker. Vertebral compression fractures and loss of metacarpal cortex in relation to postmenopausal cigarette smoking and lack of obesity. *Arch. Intern. Med.* 136: 298-304, 1976.
8. Dawson-Hughes, B., S. Harris, C. Kramich, G. Dallal, and H.M. Rasmussen. Calcium retention and hormone levels in black and white women on high- and low-calcium diets. *J. Bone Miner. Res.* 8: 779-788, 1993.
9. Ernst, M., C.H. Schmid, and E.R. Froesch. Enhanced osteoblast proliferation and collagen gene expression by estradiol. *Proc. Nat. Acad. Sci. (U.S.A.)* 85: 2307-2310, 1988.
10. Ernst, M., J.K. Heath, and G.A. Rodan. Estradiol effects on proliferation, messenger ribonucleic acid for collagen and insulin-like growth factor-I, and parathyroid hormone-stimulated adenylate cyclase activity in osteoblastic cells from calvariae and long bones. *Endocrinology* 125: 825-833, 1989.
11. Fukayama, S. and A.H. Tashjian, Jr. Direct modulation by estradiol of the response of human bone cells (SaOS-2) to human parathyroid hormone (PTH) and PTH-related protein. *Endocrinology* 124: 397-401, 1989.
12. Fukayama, S. and A.H. Tashjian, Jr. Direct modulation by androgens of the response of human bone cells (SaOS-2) to human parathyroid hormone (PTH) and PTH-related protein, *Endocrinology* 125: 1789-1794, 1989.
13. Gotfredsen, A., A. Hadberg, L. Nilas, and C. Christiansen. Total body mineral in healthy adults. *J. Lab. Clin. Med.* 110: 362-368, 1987.

14. Halioua, L. and J.J. Anderson. Lifetime calcium intake and physical activity habits: independent and combined effects on the radial bone of healthy premenopausal Caucasian women. *Amer. J. Clin. Nutr.* 49: 534-541, 1989.
15. Hall, B.D., D.R. Macmillan, and F. Bronner. Vitamin D-resistant rickets associated with high fecal endogenous calcium output. A report of two cases. *Amer. J. Clin. Nutr.* 22: 448-457, 1969.
16. Hannan, M.T., D.T. Felson, and J.J. Anderson. Bone mineral density in elderly men and women: results from the Framingham osteoporosis study. *J. Bone Miner. Res.* 7: 547-553, 1992.
17. Horowitz, M.C. Cytokines and estrogen in bone: antiosteoporotic effect. *Science* 260: 626-627, 1993.
18. Jilka, R.L., G. Hangoc, G. Girasole, G. Passeri, D.C. Williams, J.S. Abrams, B. Boyce, H. Broxmeyer, and S.C. Manolagas. Increased osteoclast development after estrogen loss; mediation by interleukin-6. *Science* 257: 88-91, 1992.
19. Johansson, A.G., E. Lindh, G. Kollerap, and S. Ljunghall. Dose-dependent effects of IGF-I on metabolism of collagen type I in male osteoporosis. *J. Bone Miner. Res.* 10: S393, 1995.
20. Kiel, D.P., D.T. Felson, M.T. Hannan, J.J. Anderson, and P.W.F. Wilson. Caffeine and the risk of hip fracture: the Framingham study. *Amer. J. Epidemiol.* 132: 675-684, 1990.
21. Meunier, P.J. Bone quantity versus bone quality. In: *Osteoporosis. Contributions to Modern Management.* BEC Nordin, Ed. Parthenon: Park Ridge, NJ. 31-37, 1990.
22. Morrison, N.A., J.C. Qi, A. Tokita, P.J. Kelly, L. Crofts, T.V. Nguyen, P.N. Sambrook, and J.A. Eisman. Prediction of bone density from vitamin D receptor alleles. *Nature* 367: 284-287, 1994.
23. Murphy, S., K.T. Khaw, A. Cassidy, and J.E. Compston. Sex hormones and bone mineral density in elderly men. *Bone Miner.* 20: 133-140, 1993.
24. Nahoul, K. and M. Roger. Age-related decline of plasma bioavailable testosterone in adult men. *J. Steroid. Biochem.* 35: 293-299, 1990.
25. Nilas, L. and C. Christiansen. The pathophysiology of pre- and postmenopausal bone loss. *Brit. J. Obstet. Gynecol.* 96: 580-587, 1989.
26. Oursler, M.J., L. Pederson, L. Fitzpatrick, B.L. Riggs, and T.C. Spelsberg. Human gliant cell tumors of the bone (osteoclastomas) are estrogen target cells. *Proc. Nat. Acad. Sci. (U.S.A.)* 91: 5227-5231, 1994.
27. Pacifici, R., C. Brown, E. Puscheck, E. Friedrich, E. Slatopolsky, D. Maggio, R. McCracken, and L.V. Avioli. Effect of surgical menopause and estrogen replacement on cytokine release from human blood mononuclear cells. *Proc. Nat. Acad. Sci. (U.S.A.)* 88: 5134-5138, 1991.
28. Parfitt, A.M. The physiologic and histomorphometric significance of bone histomorphometric data. In: *Bone Histomorphometry: Techniques and Interpretation,* Recker, R.R., Ed. CRC Press, Boca Raton, FL, 53-87, 1983.
28a. Riggs, B.L., S. Khosla, and L.J. Melton III. A unitary model for involutional osteoporosis: estrogen deficiency causes both type I and type II osteoporosis in postmenopausal women and contributes to bone loss in aging men. *J. Bone Miner. Res.* 13: 763-773, 1998.
29. Sambrook, P., J. Birmingham, P. Kelly, S. Kempler, T. Nguyen, N. Pocock, and J. Eisman. Prevention of corticosteroid osteoporosis. A comparison of calcium, calcitriol and calcitonin. *New Eng. J. Med.* 328: 1747-1752, 1993.

30. Schiller, C., R. Gruber, G.-M. Ho, K. Redlich, H.-J. Gober, F. Katzgraber, M. Willheim, O. Hoffmann, P. Pietschmann, and M. Peterlik. Interaction of triiodothyronine with 1α, 25-dihydroxyvitamin D_3 on interleukin-6-dependent osteoclast-like cell formation in mouse bone marrow cell cultures. *Bone* 22: 341-346, 1998.
31. Simmons, D.J. and M.D. Grynpas. Mechanisms of bone formation *in vivo*. In: *Bone: Vol 1. The Osteoblast and Osteocyte*. B.K. Hall, Ed. Caldwell, NJ. Telford Press, 193-302, 1990.
32. Spencer, H., N. Rubio, E. Rubio, M. Indreika, and A. Seitam. Chronic alcoholism. Frequently overlooked cause of osteoporosis in men. *Am. J. Med.* 80: 393-397, 1986.
33. Stepan, J.J., M. Lachman, J. Zverina, V. Pacovsky, and D.J. Baylink. Castrated men exhibit bone loss: effect of calcitonin treatment on biomechanical indices of bone remodeling. *J. Clin. Endocrin. Metab.* 69: 523-527, 1989.
34. Swartz, C.M. and M.A. Young. Male hypogonadism and bone fracture (Letter to the editor). *New Engl. J. Med.* 318: 996, 1988.

Section II

Mineral Metabolism of Bone

6 Calcium Metabolism and Homeostasis

Felix Bronner

CONTENTS

6.1 INTRODUCTION

6.1.1 Distribution of Calcium in Nature

Calcium is the fifth most-abundant element of the globe. It is found in a variety of rocks and throughout most waters. The average calcium concentration of the crust of the Earth is almost 1 mol/kg (40 mg/kg), with more than 80% occurring in the form of limestone ($CaCO_3$) deposits.

As cells evolved, they learned to get rid of excess calcium, adapting calcium extrusion to a variety of cellular processes — protein secretion, intracellular signaling, and the many calcium-dependent processes that have come to light in recent years. When organisms began to leave the ocean to conquer the land, they required mechanisms of support and developed external and, ultimately, internal skeletons which contained calcium as the principal cation. In turn, those calcium deposits also served as storage depots, i.e., for the accumulation and release of calcium, thereby maintaining the plasma calcium concentration constant, typically 2.5 mM.

0-8493-9237-3/99/$0.00+$.50

6.1.2 Distribution of Calcium in the Body

The adult human body contains about 1 kg of Ca, with less than 1% of that amount found outside the skeleton. The body's calcium traffic involves multiple gradients of calcium concentration and changes in state from solid to liquid and back. Calcium ingested in a meal may require solubilization before it can be absorbed. Because the calcium concentration in the luminal fluid of the intestine following a meal generally exceeds the free calcium concentration of lymph and blood (0.5 and ~1 mM, respectively) the ion, in moving across the intestinal epithelium, moves down a chemical gradient. Calcium enters bone from blood and is precipitated in the form of various calcium phosphate phases, e.g., whitlockite, carbonate, phosphate, and hydroxyapatite.

When calcium is mobilized from bone, it changes its state from solid to liquid and returns to the circulation. Excretion in the urine involves a change in concentration, from 0.5 to 3 mM. Excretion in sweat and in the stool as endogenous fecal calcium probably involves no change in concentration as the calcium passes through the skin or into the intestinal lumen, but evaporation of sweat and water reabsorption in the intestine markedly change the calcium concentrations of the final products.

Total cellular calcium varies between 1 and 5 mmol/kg, but the free intracellular calcium concentration is only about 100 nmol/L in most cells. Thus, there is a very large gradient between free and bound intracellular calcium, the latter accounting for nearly the entire cellular calcium. It is undoubtedly this huge gradient that has made it possible for calcium to be such an effective intracellular signal.

6.1.3 Calcium Movement in the Body

The principal tissues that participate in extracellular calcium movement are the intestine, the blood, the kidney, and the skeleton, as well as some endocrine organs. Sensing of calcium levels by some of these tissue cells is via a calcium receptor located on the plasmalemma.[6]

Figure 6.1 summarizes in schematic form the pathways that calcium follows as it is ingested, absorbed, transported to and from the skeleton, and excreted from the body. Details of the processes involved are presented below.

6.2 CALCIUM IN FOOD AND DIET

Foods that contain more than 2.0 mmol calcium per portion include milk, cheese, ice cream, broccoli, cheese pizza, custard, Cream of Wheat, and a whole orange (but not orange juice). A detailed study of the dietary sources of calcium in the second U.S. National Health and Nutrition Examination Survey (1976-1980) found[1] that dairy products contributed about 55% of dietary calcium. In 1984, U.S. women 35 to 50 years old consumed on average 13.3 mmol of calcium, a value that is significantly lower, however, than the daily recommended dietary allowance (RDA) for women of 20 mmol. Men aged 19 to 50 years consumed 125% of their RDA for calcium when surveyed for one summer day in 1985.

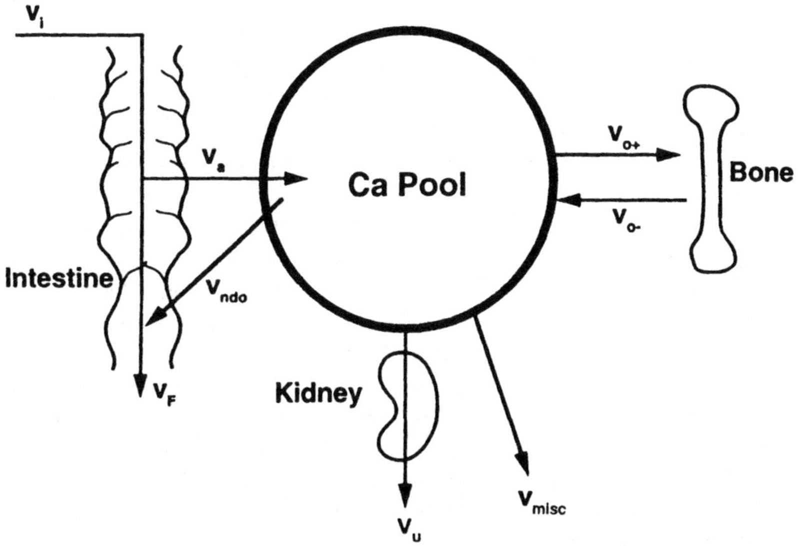

FIGURE 6.1 Schematic diagram of the flow of calcium through the body. The Ca pool includes calcium in solution in blood plasma, in the extracellular fluid, and in or associated with bone, described in units of mass, e.g., mmol. v_i = Ca ingested in food: v_a = Ca absorbed in food: v_{ndo} = endogenous Ca lost in stool: v_u = Ca excreted in urine: v_F = total Ca excreted in stool: v_{misc} = Ca lost from the body via sweat, semen, menstrual fluid, milk: v_{o+} = Ca deposited in bone: v_{o-} = Ca resorbed from bone. v's represent rates in units of mass per unit time, e.g., mmol/day. v_T = rate at which Ca enters or leaves the pool, i.e., $v_a + v_{o-} = v_{o+} + v_u + v_{ndo} + v_{misc}$. In a nonlactating organism, v_{misc} is generally negligibly small. For illustrative numbers of the various parameters, see Table 6.3. (Reproduced from [4], with permission.)

The diet of people in industrialized countries is increasingly made up of foods that have undergone substantial processing. While processing of foods may alter some nutrient content, the calcium content of these foods is less likely to be affected. Moreover, processing may render a given food more digestible, and fortification with nonfat dry milk powder enriches the food's calcium content.

6.3 CALCIUM ABSORPTION

For calcium to be absorbed, it must move across the intestinal epithelium. Only calcium in solution in the intestinal lumen can undergo absorption. Food calcium may already be in solution as in milk, or it may become solubilized as the result of the combined actions of gastric acid and intestinal enzymes and of intestinal contractions and peristalsis, all of which act to bring about digestion and solubilization.

Bioavailability of food calcium depends to a considerable extent on how well it is solubilized following digestion. The more completely a food is digested, the greater the proportion of calcium that can be solubilized and become available for absorption.

Calcium moves across the intestinal epithelium by two routes: through the cell, i.e., transcellularly; and between cells, i.e., paracellularly.[5] The transcellular movement is saturable, regulated largely by vitamin D, and takes place in the proximal intestine, mostly the duodenum. Paracellular transport occurs throughout the intestine and is not subject to acute regulation.

Transcellular movement of calcium is a metabolically active process, requiring oxygen, and against a chemical gradient. It is a saturable process that involves three sequential steps: entry across the brush border membrane; intracellular movement from one to the other pole of the cell; and extrusion at the basolateral cell membrane.

Calcium enters intestinal cells through the brush border membrane, down an electrochemical gradient, with the intracellular fluid negative with respect to the lumen and its free calcium content 100 nM, compared with the lumen content in the millimolar range. Calcium entry into the cell is mediated by calcium channels which also restrict calcium entry severely. If that were not the case, extracellular calcium, moving down its electrochemical gradient, would flood the cell. There is evidence that duodenal cells — where most of the transcellular calcium movement takes place — contain a vitamin D-dependent element in the brush border that permits increased cell entry.

Once calcium has entered the cell, it must diffuse through the cell interior to the basolateral membrane where extrusion takes place. The rate at which a calcium ion can diffuse through the interior of an intestinal cell is only about 1/70 of the rate of transcellular calcium transport in the duodenum. This means that, in the duodenal cell, calcium moves transcellularly at a rate some 70 times greater than the rate at which the ion alone can diffuse. This implies that there must exist in the duodenal cell a mechanism that significantly and markedly enhances the self-diffusion of the calcium ion. This is accomplished by an intracellular calcium-binding protein, calbindin D_{9k} ($M_r \approx 9$ kDa[5,9,15]).

This molecule was discovered by Wasserman and colleagues.[15] Its biosynthesis is totally dependent on vitamin D, it contains two calcium-binding sites, has a quaternary structure resembling an E-F hand, a pI of 4.3, and K_d for calcium of about 0.3 μM. Under conditions of maximum transport, V_m, the calbindin D_{9k} (CaBP) concentration in the cell is about 0.2 mM, sufficient to augment the diffusion rate of calcium to the required value. Figure 6.2 shows that calcium transport, as measured by an in vivo loop technique or an in vitro everted sac technique, is directly proportional to the tissue calbindin D_{9k} content.

The action of calbindin D_{9k} may be compared to that of an intracellular ferry. It should be pointed out that this process is equivalent to what is postulated to occur in the muscle cell where myoglobin is thought to ferry oxygen across the cell, thus speeding up the loading and unloading of oxygen to and from the tissue.[13,17]

Because the cell interior is electronegative with respect to the outside of the cell and because the intracellular calcium content is about two orders of magnitude below that outside the cell, calcium extrusion from the cell is necessarily against an electrochemical gradient. It is effected by a Ca-ATPase, a large, membrane-spanning molecule ($M_r \approx 123$ kDa) that couples the hydrolysis of ATP to the transport of Ca^{2+}. Available information, based on the primary structure of the pump molecule from a cDNA isolated from a human teratoma library,[7] indicates that on the cytoplasmic side of the

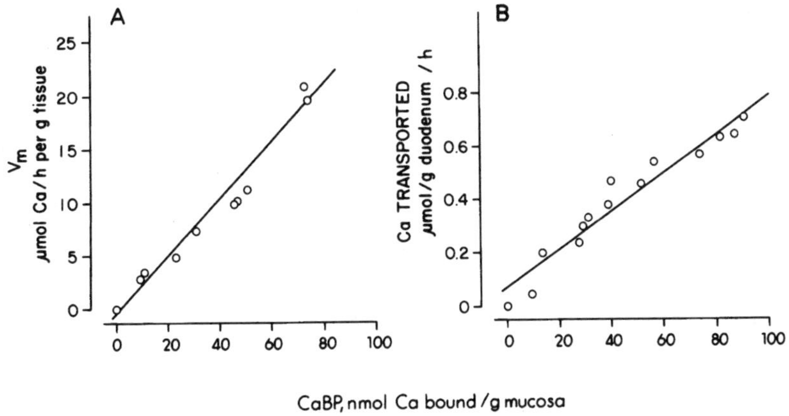

FIGURE 6.2 Relation between intestinal calcium transport and calbindin D_{9K} (CaBP) content. (A) V_m, calculated from in situ duodenal, jejunal, and ileal loop experiments, shown as a function of calbindin D_{9k} content. (B) Calcium transport, as evaluated from everted duodenal sac experiments, shown as a function of calbindin D_{9k} content. (Reproduced from [5] with permission).

membrane there is a calmodulin-binding domain and a cAMP-dependent phosphorylation site. The latter is located near the carboxyl terminus. Also on the cytoplasmic side is a putative calcium-binding domain somewhat nearer the N terminus, and a "hinge region" thought to bring about the conformational change in the transmembrane elements. This change would then propel the calcium through the channel-like transmembrane elements to the outside of the cell. The conformational change is thought to be the sequel to a phosphorylation step, and the site on the molecule that is thought to undergo phosphorylation has been identified. Vitamin D has been found to increase the pumping capacity of the intestinal cell, presumably by increasing the number of pumps per cell.[16]

Many cells contain a Na/Ca exchanger. However, Na/Ca exchange does not appear to play a significant role in calcium extrusion in the intestine, where the Ca-ATPase is the major mechanism for Ca extrusion.

The nonsaturable component of transepithelial calcium transport, i.e., paracellular movement, occurs throughout the length of the small intestine, with the rate of calcium movement out of the lumen approximating 16%/h in the rat.[4] As evident from Figures 6.2 and 6.3, calbindin D_{9k} and active (saturable) calcium transport vary inversely with calcium intake, whereas net and non-saturable absorption vary linearly with intake.

Substances whose effect on calcium absorption is mediated by their effect on paracellular transport are sugars like mannitol or lactose, amino acids such as L-lysine, or medium-chain triglycerides. Some detergents and bile salts similarly enhance calcium absorption by acting on the paracellular pathway.

The most efficient way of increasing the amount of calcium that is absorbed is to increase intake of calcium in a form that is readily digested and solubilized. Increased intake will, with time, lead to diminished absorption by the active route.

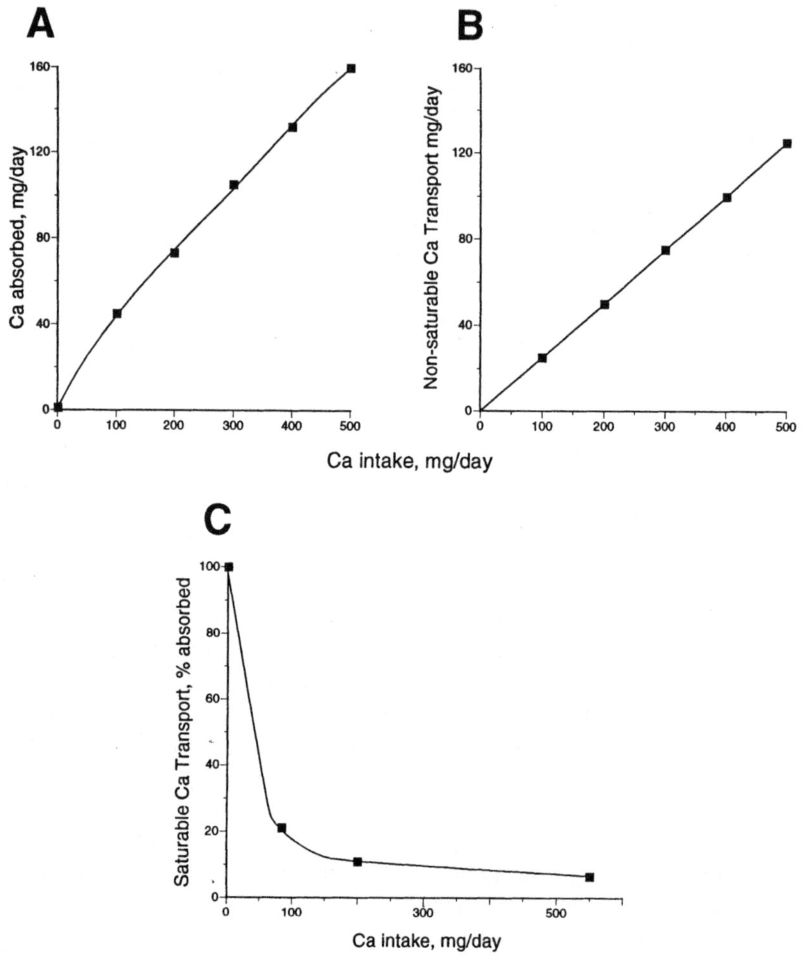

FIGURE 6.3 Diagram of total calcium absorption (A), non-saturable calcium transport (B), and saturable calcium transport (C) as a function of calcium intake. Total calcium absorbed is the sum of non-saturable and saturable calcium transport, the latter the product of the percent absorbed multiplied by the intake. Graphs adapted from data in references [4,8].

The amount transported by the passive route, on the other hand, increases with increased intake. Because of the down-regulation of the active transport route with increased calcium intake, the relative role played by the active transport route also decreases as calcium intake increases.[5] Dietary manipulation leads to relatively rapid changes in the serum levels of 1,25-$(OH)_2$-D_3. Therefore, up- and down-regulation of the active transport component will happen relatively quickly — within 24 h in the rat — so that dietary manipulation of calcium intake is an effective and safe procedure. Administration of vitamin D will, to be sure, enhance the active component of calcium transport, but it needs medical supervision and may lead to other complications, such as hypercalcemia, hypercalciuria, and depressed bone turnover.

TABLE 6.1
Distribution of Calcium in Normal Human Plasma

Form	mM	Percent of total
Ionized	1.18	47.5
Protein-bound	1.14	46.0
Phosphate	0.04	1.6
Citrate	0.04	1.7
Other complexes	0.08	3.2
Total	2.48	100.0

Adapted from [14]

6.4 CALCIUM IN BLOOD

Virtually all blood calcium is found in the plasma, so the plasma calcium content, 2.5 mM, is the parameter dealt with in biology and medicine. The plasma calcium concentration is closely regulated in vertebrates. It has about the same value in all species and varies relatively little with age and physiological status.

Table 6.1 lists the compounds and forms of calcium in human blood, typical of mammalian blood. As shown in Table 6.1, somewhat less than half of the total plasma calcium is bound to protein, albumin being the major component. Somewhat more than half of the plasma calcium is not bound to protein, mostly in the form of the free ion, and a small portion, ~6%, is bound to citrate, phosphate, and other complexes. Although dissociation constants between calcium and its ligands in the plasma vary, the rate at which equilibrium is established with albumin is so rapid (<5 s) that total and ionized calcium concentrations will give equivalent functional information under nearly all circumstances, even though it is the ionized calcium concentration that is the relevant functional variable.

Plasma calcium levels tend to be higher in men than in women; they decrease with age in both women and men.[10] The age-dependent decrease in plasma calcium is related to the increasing proportion of hydroxyapatite as bone mineral matures. This in turn leads to an increase in the calcium affinity of the average calcium binding sites in the bone mineral, thereby causing the plasma calcium to drop.

The plasma calcium is in extremely rapid, dynamic equilibrium with calcium in the extracellular fluid, plasma constituting about 17% of the extracellular fluid volume. As a result, the plasma calcium concentration resulting from an intravenous calcium load will be reduced within less than 1 min. to about one sixth of what it would have been if none of the injected calcium had left the plasma compartment. Following this initial expansion, the calcium load is disposed of in a strictly exponential manner, the plasma calcium concentration returning to the pretreatment (baseline) value with a $t_{1/2}$ that approximates the time it would take for the plasma to be cleared of half of its load in about 27 circulations.[3]

In addition to the bone, the other major gateways for calcium entry to and exit from the circulation are the gut and the kidney. The latter in particular has often been implicated as a significant regulator of blood calcium. If, however, one calculates the time required for a load to be cleared by the kidney or the gut, it is apparent that neither of these organs can compete effectively with bone.[3]

The initial pool of calcium distribution, i.e., the extracellular water, seems to be largely independent of the functional state of the organism. In other words, a calcium load will be diluted approximately six-fold, whatever the state of the organism. On the other hand, the rate at which the blood is cleared of its calcium load by the skeleton is very much dependent on the endocrine status and age of the individual. Thus, the rate of clearance — i.e., the rate at which the plasma calcium returns to the preinjection level — is faster in young than in old individuals, and faster in euparathyroid than in parathyroidectomized animals.[3]

To explain how bone can overcome a calcium load, the nature of the interaction of plasma calcium with bone needs analysis. Each time the blood plasma courses over bone, half of the positive or negative difference between the concentration of the plasma calcium as it enters and leaves the bone is abolished. Consequently, the plasma calcium seems to be in rapid, dynamic equilibrium with calcium-binding sites in bone.

Such a dynamic equilibrium is generally considered in terms of the solubility product of ionic calcium and phosphate in the blood. However, the equilibrium for bone calcium-binding sites can be equally well described in terms of an apparent half-concentration constant, K_m. When there is no net gain or loss of calcium from the plasma, the free energy of calcium binding must be zero. Consequently, the plasma calcium level $[Ca_s]$ must equal the mean K_m of the bone calcium-binding sites. In other words, $K_m = [Ca_s]$. Calculations of the permeability of bone for calcium make it unlikely that calcium enters bone by fluxing through bone cells. Rather, calcium must move between bone cells, with the calcium-binding sites therefore located on (or in) the bone mineral itself.

The nature and type of calcium-binding sites in bone mineral have not been described as such. However, at least five phases of calcium phosphate are likely to occur in bone (Table 6.2). Inasmuch as calcium-binding affinity varies inversely with solubility, then the K_m must also follow suit. Because the calcium phosphate phases with the highest calcium-to-phosphorus ratio are least soluble, they must have the lowest K_m. Moreover, the average K_m of a given section of bone will depend on the bone salts it contains. Mature bone, having a high content of hydroxyapatite, would therefore be associated with a low K_m and a relatively depressed plasma calcium level, whereas in newly forming bone the bone salt would be less mature, and its average K_m and the associated plasma calcium level would be relatively high. Shifts in the mean K_m and associated plasma calcium level would then be brought about by shifts in the proportions of calcium-binding sites in bone.

The question then arises how those rapid shifts in the proportion of calcium-binding sites, leading to a change in the K_m, can be brought about. The model of regulation that has been proposed[3] is based on the rapid changes in shape that bone cells have been observed to undergo. Osteoblasts and osteoclasts, together with the

TABLE 6.2
Solid Phases of Calcium Phosphate Linked to Biological Calcification[a]

Name	Formula	Molar ratio of Ca to P
Hydroxyapatite	$Ca_{10}(PO_4)_6(OH)_2$	1.66
Whitlockite	$(Ca,Mg)_3(PO_4)_2$	1.50
Amorphous $CaXPO_4$	$Ca_9(PO_4)_6$(variable)	1.30-1.50
Octacalcium phosphate	$Ca_8H_2(PO_4)_6.5H_2O$	1.33
Brushite	$CaHPO_4.(2H_2O)$	1.00

Note: At least 90% of the cystalline solid is hydroxyapatite, based on X-ray diffraction analysis.

[a] Listed in order of increasing acidity, solubility, and, by inference, increasing K_m, i.e., decreasing calcium-binding affinity.

Adapted from [12].

bone-lining cells and osteocytes, constitute the cell population of the mammalian skeleton, but only osteoblasts and osteoclasts are metabolically active, and are the cells that primarily regulate bone growth and turnover.

Osteoblasts possess receptors for parathyroid hormone, PTH, and 1,25-dihydroxyvitamin D_3, 1,25-$(OH)_2$-D_3, whereas only osteoclasts possess receptors for calcitonin, CT, the third of the three major calcitropic hormones. A very early response of osteoblasts to PTH or 1,25-$(OH)_2$-D_3 is to round up, followed by a cascade of events such as inhibition of collagen synthesis, characteristic either of an arrest or a marked slowing of metabolic activity. Calcitonin, on the other hand, induces a rounding up of osteoclasts and transient inhibition (or slowing) of their metabolic activity.

Shape changes of bone cells may be thought to be associated with changes in the average calcium-binding affinity of bones by causing a change in the relative proportion of high- and low-affinity calcium-binding sites. Osteoblasts, when extended and apposed to bone, are hypothesized to block the low-affinity extremes of the population of calcium-binding sites (Figure 6.4A). But when osteoblasts retract under the action of PTH or 1,25-$(OH)_2$-D_3, they expose these low affinity sites (Figure 6.4B). As a result, plasma calcium goes up.

Conversely, osteoclasts may be thought to be associated with binding sites that have high affinity for calcium. Thus, when osteoclasts are caused to contract, as under the action of calcitonin (Figure 6.4C), high-affinity calcium-binding sites are exposed and the plasma calcium level falls.

Plasma calcium regulation therefore involves a cell-mediated modulation of the available calcium-binding sites on bone mineral. The shape changes of osteoblasts or osteoclasts in turn represent the initial steps in the cascade of events that lead to bone formation and resorption, but plasma calcium regulation depends only indirectly on those latter events.

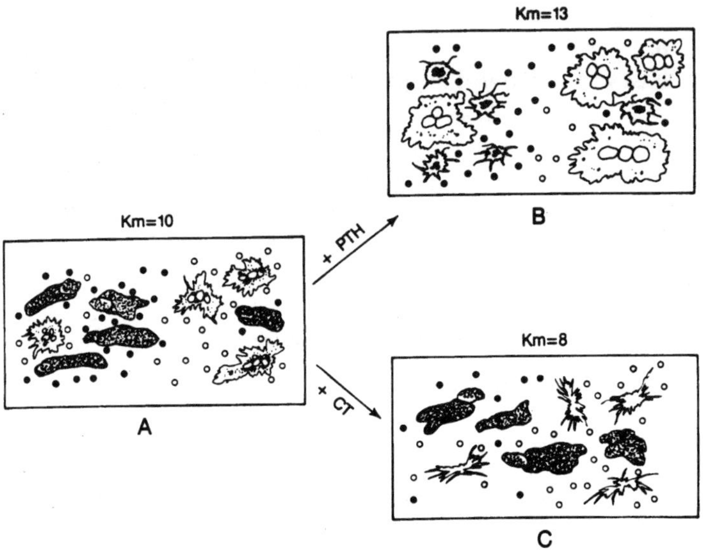

FIGURE 6.4 Diagram representing the effect of the acute administration of parathyroid hormone (PTH) or calcitonin (CT) on the spatial relationships of osteoblasts and osteoclasts on a bone surface. The open and closed circles represent, respectively, the K_m values of high-affinity and low-affinity bone calcium-binding sites. Diagram (A) represents a normocalcemic situation, with an equal number of high- and low-affinity sites. Diagram (B) represents the result of PTH administration, where the shrinkage of osteoblasts has exposed low-affinity sites, leading to an average K_m of 13 and hypercalcemia. Diagram (C) represents the results of CT administration, where the shrinkage of osteoclasts has exposed high-affinity sites, leading to an average K_m of 8 and hypocalcemia. *Note:* High-affinity sites are considered to have an apparent Km of 5 mg Ca/dL, and low-affinity sites an apparent K_m of 15 mg Ca/dL. For the sake of convenience, the K_ms refer to total plasma calcium, rather than the theoretically correct ionic calcium concentration, approximately half of the plasma total (Table 6.1). Bone mineral with a high Ca/P ratio is considered to have a relatively higher affinity for calcium binding than bone mineral with a low Ca/P ratio (see text and Table 6.2). (Reproduced from [3], with permission.)

6.5 CALCIUM IN BONE

Calcium, with phosphate, constitutes the principal structural substance of the skeleton that gives vertebrates their internal support and, in the case of people, allows them to be erect. The skeleton constitutes about 16% of an adult's body weight. Approximately 47% of the skeletal weight is dry, fat-free bone, and 26% of the latter is calcium. Table 6.2 lists the various phases in which calcium phosphate occurs in bone. The precise order in which calcium is precipitated and the path it follows as calcium salts mature and become increasingly less soluble are not yet known. The final calcium salt is a carbanatohydroxyapatite, i.e., an apatitic type of calcium phosphate that also contains, at least on the surface, calcium carbonate.

The mechanism of calcification, many years of study notwithstanding, is not fully known. The initial calcium phosphate is deposited on or inside collagen fibrils that have formed extracellularly from collagen molecules that had been extruded by osteoblasts, the bone-forming cells. Once the calcium phosphate molecule is in place, additional calcium phosphate is deposited by accretion so that the calcium salt is arranged in a very orderly fashion. The crystals are platelike, with a long axis of 30 to 70 nm and a short axis of 10 to 25 nm. The surface layers of the bone crystals constitute 50% of the newly formed crystals, but ultimately they constitute only about 25% of the fully mature crystal volume.[12]

Calcium exists in bone in two forms: in solution, as part of the fluid that surrounds and exists in bone; and in a solid state, as the phases of calcium phosphate described above and listed in Table 6.2. The bone calcium pool contains five to six times more calcium than is found in the extracellular fluid, but constitutes only a small fraction of the total body calcium. For example, in a 220-g male rat, the extracellular calcium amounts to 0.67 mmol of Ca and the bone calcium pool contains about 3.45 mmol of Ca, whereas the total skeletal calcium amounts to about 120 mmol.[11]

The bone calcium pool serves two functions: as the source of calcium that becomes deposited as bone salt, and as the source of the exchangeable calcium, i.e., the calcium that leaves and reenters blood, with the concentration of blood plasma calcium determined by the average calcium-binding capacity of the bone salt.

Bone calcium resorption, i.e., the phase transformation of solid to solution and the return of that calcium into the circulation, also decreases with age, but somewhat less rapidly than does the bone calcium deposition rate. As a result, the individual goes into negative bone calcium balance, i.e., the bone mass decreases. This is illustrated in Table 6.3. Note in particular in Table 6.3 how the bone calcium deposition rate decreases with age, with corresponding decreases in the calcium balance.

Modeling and remodeling of bone also involve structural changes, i.e., osteoclast-mediated dissolution of calcium and partial or total degradation of the extracellular matrix from which the bone salt has been removed. These structural changes necessarily proceed more slowly than the initial steps which involve calcium binding and release by the bone salt.

When bones are immobilized in casts, there is an initial loss of bone as a result of the relative acceleration of resorptive processes. With time, there is also an effect on modeling and remodeling. Modeling is diminished and remodeling accelerated. Inasmuch as bone mass is always lost when bone is remodeled, bones in casts become thinner. Moreover, casts also cause muscles to weaken, so that loss from bones in casts is the result of inherent changes in bone modeling and remodeling, as well as the result of progressive muscle weakening. If there is a choice between internal fixation and cast application, the former is preferable, because it would lead to lesser bone loss.

Thus, bone formation and bone resorption are terms which designate a cascade of events, with calcium constituting the principal cation of bone salt, which in turn is the major product of the osteoblasts.

TABLE 6.3
Components of Calcium Metabolism

	Young Male	Young Female	Postmenopausal Female
Body wt, kg	76	40	62
Age, y	17	14	55
Plasma Ca, mg/dL	10.3	10.1	9.8
Ca Pool, mg	6100	4000	3080
Pool turnover, mg/day	1500	1400	640
Ca intake, v_i, mg/day	1160	1200	640
Urinary Ca output, v_u, mg/day	250	200	100
Fecal endogenous Ca output, v_{ndo}, mg/day	150	200	76
Total fecal Ca output v_F, mg/day	860	900	564
Calcium balance, Δ, mg/day	+50	+100	–24
Ca absorbed, v_a, mg/day	450	500	152
Percent Ca absorption	39	42	24
Bone Ca deposition rate, v_{o+}, mg/day	1100	1000	476
Bone Ca removal rate, v_{o-}, mg/day	1050	900	500
Fraction to bone, v_{o+}/v_T	0.73	0.71	0.74
Fraction excreted, $v_u + v_{ndo}/v_T$	0.27	0.29	0.26

Notes: Plasma calcium is part of the calcium pool which includes all extracellular calcium and the calcium in solution in bone.

Pool turnover, $v_T = v_a + v_{o-} = v_{o+} + v_u + v_{ndo}$

Data adapted from [2,4].

6.6 CALCIUM EXCRETION

6.6.1 Urine

In an adult who weighs 70 kg, the nephron filters approximately 1700 mmol Ca/day. The urinary calcium output of this person might be 5 mmol/day, or 0.3% of the filtered load. Actual calcium excretion in the urine is a complicated function of an individual's prior calcium intake, vitamin D and nutritional status, sex, reproductive status (if female), as well as age and therefore skeletal maturity.

Calcium in the lumen of the nephron is subject to two transport processes: a paracellular, concentration-dependent transepithelial movement, which accounts for most of the calcium reabsorption in the kidney, and a transcellular movement that constitutes active transport against an electrochemical gradient. Calcium is reabsorbed, i.e., moves transepithelially, in the proximal tubule (straight and convoluted), mostly by a passive mechanism, although some movement may be transcellular and involve entry via calcium channels and extrusion via a Ca-ATPase. Very little calcium is reabsorbed as the luminal fluid passes through the thin limbs of Henle. As the fluid enters the thick ascending limb of the nephron, calcium reabsorption is resumed, largely by a passive process. Active transepithelial calcium transport occurs principally in the distal convoluted tubule (DCT). Once the luminal fluid has passed the region of the DCT, it enters those regions of the nephron designated as connecting and collecting ducts, where transport is essentially by a paracellular route.

In addition to vitamin D, the major regulator of urinary calcium excretion is parathyroid hormone (PTH), causing increased reabsorption of calcium from the renal tubule, while phosphate excretion is simultaneously increased.

6.6.2 Stool

Calcium in the stool has two sources: unabsorbed food calcium and endogenous calcium, i.e., calcium that entered the intestinal lumen with the various body fluids such as bile, *succus entericus*, etc., and has not been reabsorbed.

In humans, the amount of endogenous calcium found in the stool approximates the amount of calcium excreted in the urine. In the rat, on the other hand, the amount of endogenous calcium is ten times greater than the urinary calcium output. There is a tendency for the endogenous fecal calcium to go up as calcium intake goes up, but there is no indication that the endogenous calcium secreted into the intestine along with the various fluids constitutes a regulatory route.

6.7 CALCIUM REQUIREMENT

Skeletal calcium is the immediate and most direct source of calcium for the body. To minimize depletion of skeletal calcium stores, net calcium absorption, i.e., the difference between intake and fecal output, must equal or exceed urinary calcium excretion. The minimum dietary calcium requirement can therefore be estimated from the sum of endogenous fecal calcium output and urinary calcium excretion, divided by the fractional calcium absorption. Endogenous fecal calcium output tends to equal the amount excreted in the urine. Therefore, an approximate estimate of the minimum calcium requirement is twice the daily urinary calcium output divided by the fractional calcium absorption. For example, according to Table 6.3, a postmenopausal woman excretes in the urine 100 mg Ca/day (2.5 mmol/day), her endogenous fecal output is 76 mg/day (1.9 mmol/day) and her fractional absorption averages 24%. The amount of calcium she would have to consume to remain in zero balance therefore is 100 + 76/0.24 or 733 mg Ca/day. If her excretion had been estimated at 200 mg/day, because her endogenous fecal calcium output had not been measured, her minimum requirement would be 833 mg/day. In either case, her intake was insufficient to keep her in balance.

REFERENCES

1. Block, G.M., Dresser, C.M., Hartman, A.M., and Carroll, M.D. Nutrient sources in the American diet. Quantitative data from the NHANES II Survey. I. Vitamins and minerals. *Am. J. Epidemiol.* 122: 13-26, 1985.
2. Bronner, F., Richelle, L.J., Saville, P.D., Nicholas, J.A., and Cobb, J.R. Quantitation of calcium metabolism in postmenopausal osteoporosis and in scoliosis. *J. Clin. Invest.* 42: 898-905, 1963.

3. Bronner, F. and Stein, W.D. Modulation of bone calcium-binding sites regulates plasma calcium: an hypothesis. *Calcif. Tissue Int.* 50: 483-489, 1992.
4. Bronner, F. Calcium. In: *Handbook of Nutritionally Essential Mineral Elements,* B.L. O'Dell and R.A. Sunde, Eds. Marcel Dekker: New York, pp. 13-61, 1997.
5. Bronner, F., Pansu, D., and Stein, W.D. An analysis of intestinal calcium transport across the rat ntestine. *Am. J. Physiol.* 250 (Gastrointest. Liver Physiol.: 13): G562-G569, 1986.
6. Brown, E.M., Pollak, M., Chu, Y.-H.W., Seidman, C.E., Seidman, J.G., and Hebert, S.C. The cloning of extracellular Ca^{2+}-sensing receptors from parathyroid and kidney: molecular mechanisms of extracellular Ca^{2+}-sensing. *J. Nutr.* 125: 1965S-1970S, 1995.
7. Carafoli, E. Biogenesis: Plasma membrane calcium ATPase: 15 years of work on the purified enzyme. *FASEB J.* 8: 993-1002, 1994.
8. Duflos, C., Bellaton, C., Pansu, D., and Bronner, F. Calcium solubility, intestinal sojourn time and paracellular permeability codetermine passive calcium absorption in rats. *J. Nutr.* 125: 2348-2355, 1995.
9. Feher, J.J., Fullmer, C.S., and Wasserman, R.H. Role of facilitated diffusion of calcium by calbindin in intestinal calcium absorption. *Am. J. Physiol.* 262: (Cell Physiol 31): C517-C526, 1992.
10. Roof, B.S., Piel, C.F., Hansen, J.J., and Fudenberg, H.H. Serum parathyroid hormone levels and serum calcium levels from birth to senescence. *Mech. Aging Develop.* 5: 289-304, 1976.
11. Sammon, P.J., Stacey, R.E., and Bronner, F. Role of parathyroid hormone in calcium homeostasis and metabolism. *Am. J. Physiol.* 218: 479-485, 1970.
12. Simmons, D.J. and Grynpas, M.D. Mechanisms of Bone Formation *in vivo*. In: *Bone* Vol. 1 *The Osteoblast and Osteocyte.* Telford Press: Caldwell, NJ, pp. 193-302, 1990.
13. Stein, W.D. and Hoshen, M.B. The role of ligand-binding proteins in increasing the transcellular flux of metabolites, in particular that of calcium, bilirubin and fatty acids. *Comp. Biochem. Physiol.* 115B: 307-312, 1996.
14. Walser, M. Ion association VI. Interaction between calcium, magnesium, inorganic phosphate, citrate and protein in normal human plasma. *J. Clin. Invest.* 40: 723-730, 1961.
15. Wasserman, R.H., Corradino, R.A., and Taylor, A.N. Vitamin D-dependent calcium binding protein: purification and some properties. *J. Biol. Chem.* 243: 3978-3986, 1968.
16. Wasserman, R.H., Smith, C.A., Brindak, M.E., De Talamoni, N., Fullmer, C.S., Penniston, J.T., and Kumar, R. Vitamin D and mineral deficiencies increase the plasma membrane calcium pump of chicken intestine. *Gastroenterology* 102: 868-894, 1992.
17. Wyman, J. Facilitated diffusion and the possible role of myoglobin as a transport molecule. *J. Biol. Chem.* 241: 115-121, 1966.

7 Metabolism of Phosphate and Metals

Felix Bronner

CONTENTS

7.1 PHOSPHATE METABOLISM

Phosphate is the principal anion of bone mineral and therefore plays a major role in skeletal metabolism. Phosphate also plays an important role in energy metabolism through the high energy bond and the many phosphorylation reactions central to cellular metabolism. This chapter will only discuss events involving the inorganic phosphate ion, P_i. The terms phosphorus and inorganic phosphate will be used interchangeably, with cited phosphate concentrations referring to the quantity of inorganic phosphorus, even though it is in the form of phosphate that phosphorus fluxes through the body.

7.1.1 Phosphate in Body, Blood, and Food

The human body's phosphorus content rises from 0.6% fat-free body weight at birth to 1.2% in the adult. About five sixths of this resides in the skeleton. The remainder is found in the soft tissues, largely the musculature. The total phosphorus content

0-8493-9237-3/99/$0.00+$.50

of human plasma is 12 mg/dL, and the inorganic plasma phosphate content is about 4 mg/dL or 1.3 mM. This is the parameter tested for and reported when the examining physician orders a blood phosphate analysis.

In contrast with the homeostatically maintained plasma calcium level, the plasma P_i (inorganic phosphate) level is subject to variation. Marked changes in dietary phosphate can bring about significant changes in the plasma P_i level in experimental animals. In humans, hypophosphatemia can result from phosphate leaks in the kidney. Dietary phosphate insufficiency, on the other hand, is virtually never encountered in humans, as the typical Western diet contains abundant amounts of phosphate. Soft drinks are but one example of rich phosphate sources; meat and fish, while modest sources of calcium, are significant dietary sources of phosphate.

Phosphate intakes by people are typically twice as great as calcium intakes. A 70 kg person on the usual Western diet is likely to consume 1.4 g of phosphate. This individual, if in phosphate balance, would absorb about 70% (1g) and excrete about 1 g in the urine.

7.1.2 Intestinal Absorption

Phosphorus is absorbed in the intestine by two mechanisms: an active, transcellular transport mechanism that is sodium-dependent and is largely localized in the jejunum; and a passive, purely concentration-dependent mechanism that functions throughout the length of the intestine and is paracellular. Phosphate absorption is essentially a straight-line function of phosphorus intake. This means that the saturable, active component contributes little to total absorption.

Active phosphate transport in the jejunum is vitamin D-dependent, but the mechanism is not understood. Phosphate entry across the brush border is against a gradient and therefore requires metabolic energy. Phosphate exit from the cell is down an electrochemical gradient. A sodium/phosphate cotransporter molecule has been tentatively identified in intestinal brush border. Whether or not intracellular diffusion of phosphate is enhanced is not known.

7.1.3 Renal Excretion

Urinary phosphate excretion, like intestinal absorption, involves active and passive transport routes. A very substantial fraction, perhaps as much as half of the phosphate filtered at the glomerulus, is reabsorbed in the proximal nephron, mostly in the first few convolutions of the proximal tubule.

An additional 15 to 20% of the filtered phosphate is reabsorbed in the straight portion (pars recta) of the proximal nephron. Very little phosphate gets reabsorbed in the thin portions of the nephron, with the remainder reabsorbed in the distal nephron. There is some uncertainty about how much phosphate is handled by the various components of the distal nephron, but most is likely to be transported in the distal convoluted tubule, with the quantitative role played by the connecting and collecting duct segments uncertain.

The major regulator molecule of renal phosphate transport is parathyroid hormone (PTH), which induces an increase in urinary phosphate excretion by diminishing phosphate reabsorption. Receptors for PTH are found on the basolateral membrane of segments of the nephron involved in phosphate transport. The mechanism by which PTH induces phosphaturia probably parallels or utilizes the PTH-sensitive adenyl cyclase, but how this enzyme in turn functions in the cascade of events that leads to diminished phosphate reabsorption is not known. Other regulators of renal phosphate handling are calcitonin which appears to diminish phosphate reabsorption, possibly vitamin D, and noncalcitropic hormones such as insulin, glucocorticoid, thyroid hormone, and growth hormone. None of these, however, has been shown to act directly.

7.1.4 Phosphate Deficiency and Rickets

Alimentary phosphate depletion and deficiency have been studied principally in farm and experimental animals, as the condition is rarely encountered in human beings. Symptoms, however, appear to be similar in all mammalian species. The principal interest in this condition stems from the fact that true phosphate deficiency leads to frank and full-blown rickets and osteomalacia. Pure alimentary calcium deficiency, on the other hands, does not lead to rickets, and pure vitamin D deficiency will lead to rickets in some species but not others, depending on the relative importance of vitamin D to phosphate absorption and reabsorption in a given species. Inasmuch as plasma phosphate is only moderately regulated, there is no clear correlation between hypophosphaturia and rickets.

Phosphate deficiency is associated with a marked increase in bone resorption. Indeed, one may think of the resorption of bone as the body's attempt to mine its phosphate stores in order to provide phosphate for other functions whose importance to survival is greater than an intact skeleton. In the phosphate-depleted organism, plasma calcium will tend to be elevated, and calciuria is a prominent sign of that condition. Rats made severely phosphate-deficient will excrete in the urine up to 10 mg of calcium per day, whereas control animals typically excrete less than 1 mg of calcium per day. This situation may be explained by recognizing that the molar calcium: inorganic phosphate ratio of bone is 1.6. As a result, the organism is confronted with the need to dispose of 1.6 moles calcium for every mole of P_i resorbed from bone. It does so largely via the urinary route, but it is not surprising that plasma calcium is high normal or elevated in phosphate deficiency.

Alimentary phosphate deficiency is aggravated by vitamin D deficiency. Acute vitamin D deficiency lowers the general turnover rate of calcium in the body and, high PTH levels notwithstanding, leads to hypocalcemia, but to only modest decreases in bone mineral. If vitamin D deficiency is superimposed on phosphate deficiency, the absence of vitamin D depresses calcium metabolism. As a result, phosphate-deficient and vitamin D-deficient animals have smaller skeletons and absorb less calcium. However, their urinary calcium output is even higher than that of the phosphate-deficient controls (supplied with vitamin D), because they are still mining their skeletons for phosphate and can absorb even less phosphate than controls.

Vitamin D promotes jejunal phosphate absorption and renal phosphate reabsorption. Therefore, vitamin D deficiency superimposed on phosphate deficiency aggravates the latter. At the same time, parameters of calcium metabolism are depressed and the organism becomes severely rachitic.

Disorders exist in which both phosphate absorption in the intestine and/or reabsorption in the kidney are depressed. These include the initial stages of severe burns, diabetic ketoacidosis, cases of severe vomiting, certain malabsorption states, and conditions in which large amounts of phosphate-binding antacids have been administered. Unless permitted to continue, these conditions will not normally lead to significant skeletal defects.

7.1.5 Phosphate Excess

Because plasma phosphate is rather poorly regulated in the body, hyperphosphatemia is most often an indication of renal disease, usually due to a reduction in the glomerular filtration rate encountered in hospitalized patients. Hyperphosphatemia may lead to secondary hyperparathyroidism and renal osteodystrophy. It can also result from vitamin D intoxication. Rhabdomyolysis, whether resulting from contusions, pressure necrosis, some viral infections, or other causes, can lead to severe hyperphosphatemia, often associated also with renal failure. Soft tissue effects of these conditions, frequently leading to extraskeletal or metastatic calcification, are more significant than direct changes in the skeleton, which are small and not well documented.

7.2 METALS IN BONE

The mineral phase of bone, made up principally of calcium and phosphate, in the course of mineral deposition takes up from the circulation a variety of metals that may be present in the bloodstream as the blood plasma courses over the skeletal tissue. Uptake by the bone mineral will be a function of the affinity of a given metal for the bone mineral and the extracellular matrix, and of the metal's concentration in the plasma. If, in addition, the metal interacts with bone cells, their metabolism may be affected and this in turn may alter osteoblast and osteoclast function. Fluoride and bisphosphonates are examples of compounds that become part of the bone mineral, but also have an inhibitory effect on osteoclasts.

Once a metal becomes incorporated in the bone mineral, its return into the circulation will depend on when the bone mineral that contains the metal will be resorbed. Metals deposited or exchanged with other metals on the surface of the bone mineral tend to be exchanged off rapidly. As new bone mineral is deposited, the opportunity for isoionic or heteroionic exchange diminishes and osteoclastic resorption becomes the dominant process responsible for the metal's re-entry into the circulation. There it is subject to the stochastic processes of loss from the circulation via excretion (urine and stool), redeposition in bone, or soft tissue uptake. The latter usually accounts for only a minute fraction of the loss out of the circulation, but, from a toxicological viewpoint, may constitute the most significant event for the organism. Because the turnover of bone mineral varies in trabecular and cortical bone and in various regions of the skeleton, accumulation of a given metal in the skeleton will be in those regions with the lowest turnover rate. For this reason, one can think of bone not only as a reservoir for a variety of elements, including metals, but as an organ that provides storage for the unexcreted fraction of a body burden.

7.2.1 Aluminum

Interest in the interaction between aluminum and bone was stimulated as a result of the observation that patients with renal dystrophy accumulated aluminum in their skeleton in quantities that tended to exceed those accumulated by patients with comparable rates of bone turnover, as in hyperparathyroidism. Moreover, all accumulation was markedly enhanced as a result of long-term dialysis, leading to bone disease characterized by impaired mineralization and diminished bone cell activity. Bone disease of this type has also been described in individuals with chronic renal disease who are not on dialysis, and in persons receiving total parenteral nutrition and in aluminum welders.

The usual plasma level of 2 μg/L can be exceeded by high intakes of aluminum. As plasma concentrations of aluminum increase or when renal aluminum excretion decreases, bone uptake of aluminum goes up. Bone accumulation is also increased in diabetes mellitus, a risk factor for aluminum bone disease. Aluminum appears to enter skeletal tissue along with calcium, competing with it, inhibiting hydroxyapatite formation *in vitro*, and probably also *in vivo*, even though the Al concentrations that interfere with calcification *in vivo* are likely to be higher.

The amount of surface-stainable aluminum appears to be the best available indicator of aluminum toxicity. When surface levels of aluminum exceed 30%, bone formation and/or mineralization are adversely affected.

7.2.2 Boron

Boron has been found to modify vitamin D deficiency in chicks and rats, but the effects are minor and have not been explored in humans. A study limited to six postmenopausal women failed to find convincing effects of boron supplementation. At present, boron does not appear to play a functionally important role in bone or calcium metabolism.

7.2.3 Cadmium

Cadmium poisoning, acute or chronic, typically results from exposure as a result of mining or environmental contamination resulting from mining. The three organ systems that are principally affected by cadmium poisoning are the kidney, the skeleton, and the respiratory system. The latter is implicated particularly in acute poisoning due to cadmium contamination by dust. Principal renal symptoms are proteinuria, glycosuria, and micoglobulinuria. Osteomalacia and osteoporosis are the skeletal symptoms that have been identified in patients who have had a chronic low-dose exposure for a long time. In individuals with skeletal symptoms, calcium deficiency aggravated the disease. High doses of vitamin D, leading to increased calcium absorption, have been reported to overcome or minimize the symptoms.

Cadmium causes desquamation of intestinal epithelial cells and changes in cell-to-cell binding in renal cells. As a result, the hydroxylation of 25-hydroxyvitamin D_3 in the kidney is interfered with, diminishing the synthesis of intestinal and renal calbindins. This in turn diminishes active intestinal calcium transport in the duodenum and active calcium reabsorption in the kidney tubule. In addition, cadmium binds to calbindin competitively with calcium. All told, cadmium intoxication induces increased renal calcium loss and reduced intestinal calcium absorption.

The effect of cadmium on bone is a double one. It interacts directly with bone cells, diminishing their ability to mineralize, inhibiting procollagen C-proteinases. This prevents collagen self-assembly in the extracellular matrix and decreases collagen production. A second, indirect effect is to accelerate bone turnover, particularly bone resorption. The increase in bone resorption may be due to stimulation of parathyroid hormone release resulting from the cadmium-induced tendency toward hypocalcemia.

7.2.4 Chromium

This transition element is thought to be an essential micronutrient, as it seems to be essential for optimal glucose utilization and its deficiency may aggravate glucose intolerance in infants. As yet, its skeletal role has remained largely unexplored. Chromium deficiency or chromium excess may lead to bone changes. Deficiency is difficult to produce in the laboratory and unlikely to be encountered in humans, even though low intakes in the elderly have been associated with glucose intolerance. The association of high local metal concentrations including chromium from failed joint prostheses has been reported, but the specifics of the effects of chromium excess on bone cells and tissues are not known.

7.2.5 Lead

Lead contamination of the environment, largely due to the widespread use of lead compounds in paints and in gasoline, has become a major public health problem. Although the use of lead-containing gasoline has been severely restricted in the United States, and exterior and interior paints are now formulated without lead in many countries, lead contamination continues to remain an important problem throughout the world. As is true for many trace elements, the body lead burden is located largely in the skeleton, which serves as the major site of lead deposit. Even when there is little or no further lead ingestion or inhalation, lead is liberated from bone as bone turns over. Consequently, the skeleton is not only the major site of lead deposit, but can become the major source of endogenous lead. It is lead that is released into the circulation and enters soft tissues that constitutes the major health hazard.

When lead is ingested, it largely follows the routes of calcium. It binds to calbindin in the duodenum, therefore vitamin D enhances lead absorption. In situations of calcium deficiency, when intestinal calbindin levels are high, lead absorption is enhanced. On high calcium intakes, most of the calcium and therefore, presumably, most of the lead is absorbed in the ileum. Lead that has entered the body fluids leaves these via the urine, via the intestine, and by entry into bone. Lead behaves like calcium in movements into, within, and out of bone and one can calculate that when lead leaves the body pool, it has a 60 to 70% chance of entering bone. Nearly two thirds of the lead flow would be to cortical bone and a little over one third to trabecular bone. However, trabecular bone turns over faster than cortical bone. Therefore, when lead originating in bone enters the circulation, more than a third would be of trabecular origin.

The overall effect of lead poisoning on bone is unclear. Toxic lead levels may distort the normal macrodistribution of lead in bone, but this is not established. In children of adequate nutritional status who had been chronically exposed to low to moderate lead levels, no significant changes were observed as far as their vitamin metabolism or bone mineral content were concerned. There also were no significant changes in plasma calcium and phosphate levels.

7.2.6 Silicon

Silicon is classified chemically as part of the carbon family which includes germanium, tin, and lead. Typical plasma and tissue concentrations of silicon in humans are 10 to 20 μg/g wet weight. In connective tissues, silicon concentrations are higher, mainly because silicon is an integral component of glycosaminoglycans and their protein complexes.

Because animal experiments had suggested that silicon supplementation hastened or increased mineralization, silicon, often in organic rather than in inorganic form, has been proposed as a dietary supplement in or as treatment for osteoporosis. Published data are, however, insufficient to support this approach.

One reason for interest in possible silicon effects on bone is that granules of special glasses have been used for repair of bone defects in the dental field. These vitreous materials contain silicon, as do materials to complete suturectomy for the treatment of craniosynostosis. In the case of the granules, analyses of the material embedded in the jaws showed that silicon had diffused into the surrounding tissue, but it is not clear whether the presence of silicon caused the observed failure of osteoinduction. In the light of the increasing use of metal implants, study of the effect of silicon on bone seems desirable.

7.2.7 Strontium

Strontium is not an essential element and interest in strontium metabolism stems from the fact that ^{90}Sr is an abundant and potentially hazardous by-product of nuclear fission. Although above-ground tests of nuclear explosions have largely ceased, the fact that strontium behaves in the body much like calcium has helped maintain interest in this element.

Fed in large amounts, strontium has long been known to cause rickets in experimental animals. It interferes with intestinal calcium absorption and the synthesis of 1,25-$(OH)_2D_3$. It also interferes with mineralization, apparently via direct action on bone cells, although the nature of this action is as yet unclear. One way in which bone formation may be interfered with by strontium is to delay the natural progression of osteoid to bone, i.e., at the stage of conversion of cartilage to bone.

Nontoxic amounts of strontium have been reported to be beneficial in osteoporosis. In rats, 0.19% $SrCl_2$ in the diet stimulated bone formation and raised the trabecular calcified bone volume by 10%. More recently, Marie et al. (1993) have reported that an organic distrontium salt, S12911, inhibited the increase in bone resorption in ovariectomized rats, without reducing bone formation. It is unclear, however, how much of this effect is due to strontium.

In conclusion, as strontium replaces calcium, the metabolism of calcium is depressed, with high strontium intakes leading to rickets and poor bone formation and mineralization. As yet, beneficial effects of small quantities of strontium remain uncertain.

SUGGESTED READINGS

Phosphate

Gmaj, P. and Murer, H. Cellular mechanisms of inorganic phosphate transport in kidney. *Physiol. Rev.* 1986; 66:36-70.

Lee, D.B.N., Brautbar, N., and Kleeman, C.R. Disorders of Phosphorus Metabolism. In: *Disorders of Mineral Metabolism.* Vol. III. *Pathophysiology of calcium phosphorus and magnesium.* Bronner, F. and Coburn, J.W., Eds. New York: Academic Press, 1981: 282-423.

Hruska, K.A. and Connolly, J. Hyperphosphatemia and Hypophosphatemia. In: *Primer on the Metabolic Bone Diseases and Disorders of Mineral Metabolism.* 3rd ed., Fawn, M.J., Ed. Philadelphia: Lippincott-Raven, 1996: 238-245.

Other Metals

Bronner, F. Metals in Bone: Aluminum, Boron, Cadmium, Chromium, Lead, Silicon and Strontium. In: *Principles of Bone Biology.* Bilezikian, J.O., Raisz, L.G., and Rodan, G.A., Eds. San Diego: Academic Press, 1996: 295-303.

Marie, P.J., Gabra, M.T., Hott, M., and Miravet, L. Effect of low doses of stable strontium on bone metabolism in rats. *Miner. Electrol. Metab.* 1985; 11: 5-13.

8 The Calcitropic Hormones: Parathyroid Hormone, Calcitonin, and Vitamin D

Felix Bronner

CONTENTS

8.1 INTRODUCTION

Three systemic hormones are involved in the regulation of calcium metabolism: parathyroid hormone (PTH), vitamin D, and calcitonin (CT). PTH and CT are both peptides; vitamin D is a secosterol whose hormone-like action was recognized about 40 years ago. PTH and CT interact with plasma membrane receptors of their target cells, whereas vitamin D, after a two-step transformation in liver and kidney to 1,25-dihydroxyvitamin D, acts on target cells via a gene-mediated mechanism. As a result, PTH and CT have quite rapid effects, whereas the vitamin D-mediated responses tend to be somewhat slower. One target of vitamin D is the parathyroid cell; consequently, there exists some interaction between vitamin D and PTH, but most responses associated with one hormone occur independently of the action of the other.

0-8493-9237-3/99/$0.00+$.50

8.2 PARATHYROID HORMONE

8.2.1 Chemistry, Biosynthesis, and Metabolism

PTH is a protein of 84 amino acids (Figure 8.1). It is synthesized in the form of a precursor, termed "prepro PTH," a protein of 115 amino acids. The "pre" sequence of 25 amino acids is thought to be a signal sequence that permits establishing a polyribosomal/membrane junction in the rough endoplasmic reticulum. The second cleavage, i.e., the removal at the amino terminal of the six amino acid sequence that constitutes the "pro" segment, occurs in the Golgi complex about 15 min after the signal sequence has been cleaved off. The hormone molecule, i.e., the 84-amino acid polypeptide, is then extruded, probably by means of exocytosis. It is thought the hormone is located inside a vesicle or granule whose limiting membrane fuses with the plasma membrane. This step is followed by lysis of the membrane and eventual extrusion or release of the hormone molecule into the circulation.[8]

Parathyroid cells are equipped with a cell surface calcium receptor that is coupled to a G-protein which then initiates the intracellular signaling that leads to PTH release and to increased hormone synthesis. The receptor is a protein made up of 1,085 amino acids ($M_r \approx 110$ kDa) with seven membrane-spanning elements, an extracellular domain of some 600 amino acids, and a 222-amino acid residue that constitutes the cytoplasmic tail. The receptor is a member of the super-family of G-protein-coupled receptors.[5]

PTH, upon release from the gland cells into the circulation, is transported to its target tissues, bone and kidney, as well as to the liver. The half-life of the intact hormone in the circulation is under 5 min. In the liver, the molecule undergoes cleavage, either between residues 33 and 34 or at several other sites that are near the 33/34 site; it is also cleaved near its middle. Most fragments, except the 1 to 34 amino-terminal sequence, have no or only limited biological activity. The 1 to 34 fragment has biological activity that appears to be identical, both qualitatively and quantitatively, to that of the intact hormone. The functional significance of the 35 to 84 sequence of the intact hormone is not known.

The genes of murine, bovine, and human PTH have been cloned. The human and bovine gene, like their hormone products, are more alike, while the rat gene (and hormone) exhibits fewer homologies with the human gene (and hormone). The human gene is located near the end of the short arm of chromosome 11, close to the genes encoding the hormones calcitonin and insulin.

When PTH interacts with the receptor site on the plasma membrane of kidney or bone cells, there results a stimulation of the adenyl cyclase system leading to increased production of 3′,5′-cAMP. This is a specific test for PTH, inasmuch as only target cells respond to PTH by an increase in the adenyl cyclase activity and their cAMP content.

One of the earliest responses of the osteoblast, the bone cell that is equipped with PTH receptors, is a shape change, i.e., a retraction of peripheral lamellipodia, probably modulated via cAMP.[12] The change in shape would then be the first step in the cascade of steps that ultimately leads to increased bone resorption, mediated by the osteoclast.

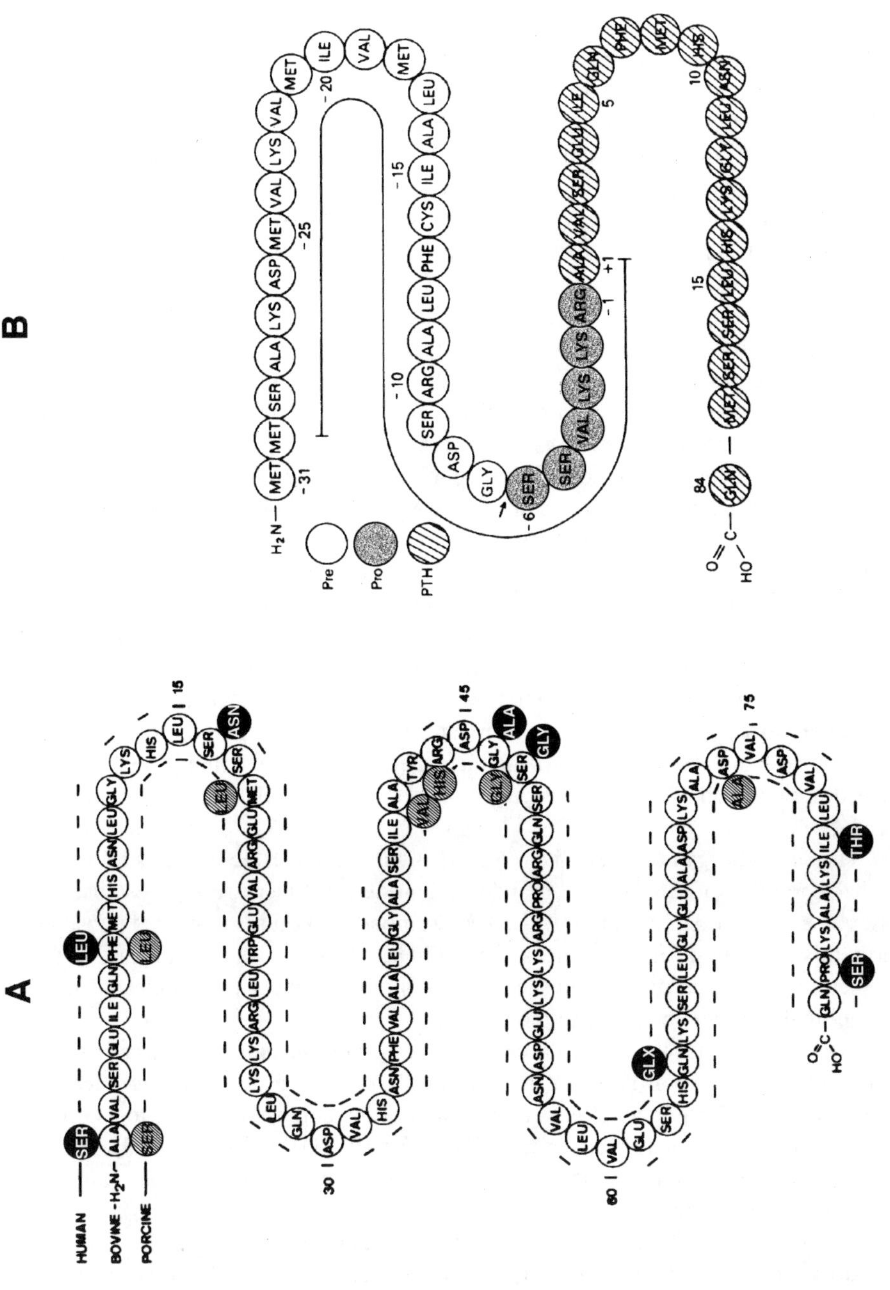

FIGURE 8.1 Amino acid sequence of parathyroid hormone (A), and the prepro- and pro-hormone (B).

8.2.2 Function

The principal function of PTH is to regulate the calcium concentration of extracellular fluid. This is accomplished by altering the transfer of calcium from and into bone, by changes in renal calcium reabsorption, and by indirectly inducing changes in intestinal calcium absorption.

In the normal mammalian organism, major regulation of the bone calcium balance is effected by modulation of bone calcium resorption. In the parathyroidectomized animal, the relationship between bone calcium deposition and resorption rates is altered both quantitatively and qualitatively. In the normal organism, the rate of bone calcium deposition is virtually constant, regardless of how much calcium enters the body via the gut. Instead, the increase in the bone calcium balance is brought about by a drop in bone resorption. This drop is in direct proportion to the amount of calcium absorbed. In the organism without functioning parathyroid glands, on the other hand, the intensity of both parameters is reduced to nearly one half. Moreover, as calcium comes in from the gut, bone resorption goes down, but at a lesser rate than in the normal animal. At the same time, the rate of bone calcium deposition goes up, at a rate that is almost twice as fast as in the normal animal. In other words, in the presence of PTH, regulation of calcium flow to the skeleton is exerted almost exclusively by means of the resorptive processes, whereas in the absence of PTH, the regulatory action of bone calcium resorption, although still dominant, is lessened.[11]

These effects may be explained as having resulted from the complementary behavior of osteoblasts and osteoclasts. When PTH is released from the parathyroid glands in response to a drop in the plasma calcium, osteoblasts assume their contracted state and their metabolic activities such as collagen synthesis and secretion are largely arrested. Osteoclasts in turn spread out, occupying some of the space freed up by osteoblastic retraction, and their metabolic action is intensified, leading to resorption of bone mineral and degradation of the extracellular matrix and collagen fibers.[4]

The second organ that responds to PTH is the kidney. PTH causes an increase in the proportion of renal cAMP found in the urine. This increase has been used to assess the amount of circulating PTH. The hormone also causes a marked phosphaturia; this is the best-known clinical effect. Finally, PTH leads to an increase in the glomerular clearance of calcium, i.e., the amount of calcium that is cleared from the luminal fluid and returned to the plasma.

The mechanisms by which PTH causes increased phosphate excretion and diminished calcium excretion have not been fully clarified. The phosphaturic effect of PTH may be due to a direct effect of PTH on phosphate transport and/or to its effect on sodium or bicarbonate reabsorption. The effect of PTH on calcium reabsorption may involve a modulation by the hormone of the intercellular space and a resultant increase in paracellular calcium flux.

The indirect effect of PTH on intestinal calcium absorption is mediated by 1,25-dihydroxyvitamin D_3, 1,25-$(OH)_2$-D_3, the active metabolite of vitamin D, the renal hydroxylation of which is stimulated by PTH. The increase in $1,25\text{-(OH)}_2\text{-D}_3$ leads to increased synthesis of intestinal calbindin D_{9K}, the molecule responsible for transcellular calcium transport (Chapter 6).

The normal plasma calcium level is quite invariant at 2.5 mM. Following parathyroidectomy, plasma calcium drops to about 1.5 mM and remains much less constant. The ability to maintain the plasma calcium steady is markedly impaired in the parathyroidectomized or parathyroprivic state.[11] In the euparathyroid animal, the presence of the hormone permits inflow of calcium from bone during periods when inflow from the gut is nil or low, as in nonfeeding periods. This compensatory mechanism is largely absent in the parathyroidectomized animal. This absence also accounts in part for the greater diurnal variation in the plasma calcium that characterizes the parathyroprivic animal. In addition, as calcium turnover in bone is slower in animals without parathyroids, the calcium pool expands more when calcium enters it from the gut.

PTH is released from the gland when the extracellular calcium level drops, and its release is inhibited when extracellular calcium rises. The extracellular changes in calcium concentration, mediated by the calcium receptor,[15] are paralleled by changes in intracellular calcium, but the mechanism by which intracellular calcium alters hormone release and thereby affects hormone synthesis is not known.

8.3 PARATHYROID HORMONE-RELATED PEPTIDE (PTHrP)

This sister molecule of parathyroid hormone functions as a paracrine regulator of the growth and development of various tissues, including bone. It is widely expressed in the developing embryo, especially in epithelial cells, and also in adult skin. PTH receptors are also PTHrP receptors and therefore are referred to as PTH/PTHrP receptors. PTHrP may play an endocrine role in fetal bone development and in the metabolic response of maternal bone during lactation; it may also be involved in regulating placental calcium transport. It had been suggested that in the fetus PTHrP plays a role in the regulation of calcium metabolism that is similar to that assumed by PTH after birth. PTHrP contributes to the regulation of smooth muscle tone and seems to play a role, as yet unclarified, in brain.[9]

Recent studies have suggested that PTHrP plays a major role in modulating proliferation, differentiation and apoptosis of chondrocytes, and from haploinsufficiency studies — i.e., studies on progeny from one normal parent and one totally deficient in the PTHrP gene — it appears the hormone influences bone formation postnatally, trabecular architecture in particular.[13]

PTHrP was cloned from tumor tissue isolated from patients with malignant hypercalcemia and cancer is the disease most frequently associated with PTHrP. Its action on bone is a dual one: the amino terminal fragments, like those of PTH, interact with the receptor on osteoblasts, inducing both anabolic and catabolic events. The carboxy terminus of PTHrP, on the other hand, shares no homology with that of PTH and seems to inhibit bone resorption in culture. *In vitro* results cannot as yet be reconciled with *in vivo* events.

Human Calcitonin

1 5 10 15
Cys-Gly-Asn-Leu-Ser-Thr-Cys-Met-Leu-Gly-Thr-Tyr-Thr-Gln-Asp-

20 25 30
-Ph-Asn-Lys-Phe-His-Thr-Phe-Pro-Gln-Thr-Ala-Ile-Gly-Val-Gly-

-Ala-Pro-NH_2

Human CGRP

S
1 10 15
Ser-Cys-Asn-Thr-Ala-Thr-Cys-Val-Thr-His-Arg-Leu-Ala-Gly-Leu-

20 25 30
-Leu-Ser-Arg-Ser-Gly-Gly-Val-Val-Lys-Asp-Asn-Phe-Val-Pro-Thr-

35
-Asn-Val-Gly-Ser-Glu-Ala-Phe-amide

FIGURE 8.2 Amino acid sequence of calcitonin and calcitonin gene-related protein (CGRP).

8.4 CALCITONIN

8.4.1 Chemistry and Biosynthesis[1]

Calcitonin is a 32-amino acid polypeptide (Figure 8.2) that is synthesized in the parafollicular cells, also known as "C" or "clear" cells of the thyroid gland. These cells arise embryologically from the fifth branchial pouch and migrate into the thyroid gland in mammals; in fish they form the ultimobranchial body, a distinct entity. Remarkably, there is considerable similarity between calcitonin from fish and mammals, and the bovine and human molecules differ more from each other than do human and salmon calcitonin. The latter exists in three forms, one of which is the most potent, biologically speaking, of all calcitonins that have been sequenced.

Calcitonin was one of the first hormones to be sequenced, but its function has remained unclear. It has a pronounced, transient hypocalcemic effect; it is this effect that was utilized to purify and determine its structure. However, its role in calcium metabolism is unclear.

Studies of the calcitonin gene have shown that it gives rise by differential splicing (Figure 8.2B) to two products, calcitonin and another protein called the calcitonin gene-related peptide (CGRP; Figure 8.2B). Whereas calcitonin is expressed in the C cells of the thyroid, CGRP is expressed largely in the central nervous system. As is true for many gene products, the messenger RNA for calcitonin is translated into a precursor molecule of 136 amino acids (in the rat), which is then cleaved into three fragments, one of which is the hormone. In the case of the messenger RNA for CGRP, the precursor is again split into three peptides, one of which is CGRP.

The function of CGRP is unknown. Systemic and local administration of CGRP increase the rate and force of contraction of the isolated atrium of the heart. Administration of CGRP to normal human subjects leads to vasodilatation and to flushing of the face. Some of these effects can also be induced by calcitonin, but require much greater doses. This can be explained by cross-reaction of receptor binding, plus the existing homology of these two products of a single gene. CGRP is a 37-amino acid polypeptide.

8.4.2 Function

Calcitonin interacts with a receptor located on the plasma membrane of osteoclasts. This interaction leads to a stimulation of the adenyl cyclase system, with increased accumulation of cAMP. The interaction of calcitonin with the osteoclast causes the latter to stop its searching action, expressed by the movement of pseudopod-like extensions that move over the extracellular bone surface and presumably precede the release of lysosomes and dissolution of bone. Thus, the action of calcitonin inhibits osteoclast metabolism. Osteoblasts do not have receptors for calcitonin.

At the level of the whole organism, the function of calcitonin is not understood. When calcitonin was first discovered, it was thought to function in a push-pull fashion with PTH, PTH causing bone resorption to be enhanced, while calcitonin inhibited bone resorption. However, extensive studies of animals deprived of endogenous calcitonin have failed to reveal major changes in bone metabolism.[10] Animals that have been deprived of their C cells exhibit virtually no change in their steady-state plasma calcium level and the rates of bone calcium deposition and resorption are unchanged, as are their urinary calcium and endogenous fecal calcium outputs. Calcium absorption is also unchanged.[10] Patients with medullary thyroid carcinoma and excess amounts of circulating calcitonin also seem to have no obvious disturbance of calcium metabolism. Intravenous administration of calcitonin to men has been reported to have led to diuresis and to increased fractional excretion of sodium and chloride.

The major effect of a deficiency in calcitonin is the inability to overcome a hypercalcemic challenge as readily as when calcitonin can be released normally. When a large amount of calcium is given so as to expand the calcium pool, the rate at which the expanded pool returns to the preinjection value in a calcitonin-deficient organism is about half what it would be normally.[4]

8.5 VITAMIN D

In contrast with the peptides, PTH, and calcitonin, vitamin D is a secosteroid, a cyclopentanoperhydrophenanthrene-related structure. The amount of the vitamin that the body can produce from precursors in the absence of sunlight is insufficient to meet the need for this compound. This is especially true for growing infants and children who live in northern climates and for the elderly, many of whom have very little exposure to ultraviolet light during northern winter months. When vitamin D was identified in the early 1920s, the compound was classified as a vitamin, i.e., as an essential micronutrient. About 40 years after its identification, as the metabolism of vitamin D became known, it became clear that the mode of action of the biologically active metabolite derived from vitamin D was close to that of steroid hormones, that is, the genomic induction of specific proteins.

8.5.1 Chemistry and Metabolism[6]

Cholesterol is the precursor compound that, in a series of steps, becomes converted to 7-dehydrocholesterol, the provitamin D. The latter accumulates in the skin and, under the action of ultraviolet light, is converted to vitamin D in two steps. In the first step, one of the rings (B) is opened up, yielding the secosteroid structure typical of the vitamin. The second step involves a rearrangement of the "previtamin D" to vitamin D. Neither of these will take place in the absence of sunlight (or ultraviolet light), hence the need for ingesting preformed vitamin D in the absence of sunlight.

Vitamin D undergoes two sequential hydroxylations, one in the liver, the other in the kidney. In the liver cell, vitamin D undergoes hydroxylation at carbon 25. In the kidney cell, 25-hydroxyvitamin D_3 is further hydroxylated to 1,25-dihydroxyvitamin D_3, 1,25-$(OH)_2$-D_3, biologically the most active vitamin D metabolite. Alternatively, 25-hydroxyvitamin D_3 can be hydroxylated at the 24-carbon, to form 24,25-$(OH)_2$-D_3.

From the regulatory viewpoint, the relative amount of 1,25-$(OH)_2$-D_3 or 24,25-$(OH)_2D_3$ plays a key role, as the major functions of vitamin D in kidney, intestine, and bone are associated with the effects due to 1,25-$(OH)_2$-D_3. Under conditions of calcium deficiency, production of 1,25-$(OH)_2$-D_3 is increased. This in turn leads to an increase in the active step of intestinal calcium absorption, enhanced renal reabsorption, and stimulation of bone metabolism. Under conditions of calcium excess, the production of 1,25-$(OH)_2$-D is downregulated and larger amounts of 24,25-$(OH)_2D$ are produced.

8.5.2 Function

The major functions of vitamin D are to enhance active calcium transport in intestine and kidney and to enable bone cells to function at a suitably high level of intensity. In addition, vitamin D appears to have a series of pleiotropic functions related to development and cell differentiation.

Once calcium enters the cell, it encounters a series of calcium-binding sites associated with either mobile or fixed molecules or organelles. Vitamin D seems to increase the number of these calcium-binding sites in the Golgi apparatus and endoplasmic reticulum. The synthesis of the intestinal calbindin (calbindin D_{9K}, CaBP) is totally dependent on vitamin D. As explained in Chapter 6, active calcium transport varies directly and proportionately with the cellular content of calbindin D_{9K}. The calbindin molecule acts as a ferry, effectively shuttling calcium from the luminal to the serosal pole of the intestinal cell at a rate directly proportional to the cellular content of calbindin D_{9K}.

Calcium extrusion is also enhanced by vitamin D, as vitamin D repletion leads to an increase in the number of pump molecules.[14]

Quantitatively speaking, the major effect of vitamin D is on the intestinal calbindin D_{9k}. It has been estimated[2] that neither entry, nor extrusion, nor binding of calcium to fixed intracellular sites is the limiting rate; rather, it is the intracellular diffusion of the calcium ion that is severely limiting in the absence of the cellular calbindin D_{9k}.

Kidney — Vitamin D acts in the kidney to increase calcium reabsorption. It regulates transcellular calcium movement in the distal convoluted tubule (DCT) in a manner analogous with what it does in the intestine. The biosynthesis of the renal calcium-binding protein (calbindin D_{28K}; Mr: 28 kDa) is totally dependent on vitamin D. The protein is thought to function in the DCT by amplifying transcellular transport of calcium.[3]

Bone — The effect of vitamin D on bone is to increase the rates of bone formation and resorption. Receptors for 1,25-$(OH)_2$-D_3 have been found only in osteoblasts, so the effect of vitamin D on bone resorption is likely to be indirect, i.e., via the osteoblast. The principal molecular effect of 1,25-$(OH)_2$-D_3 on osteoblasts is to increase their production of the extracellular matrix molecule, the Gla protein (also known as osteocalcin). Treatment of osteoblasts in culture leads to a state equivalent to enhanced differentiation — that is, a higher level of alkaline phosphatase and shape changes — but the relationship of these observations to the *in vivo* effect of vitamin D has not been clarified.

The role of vitamin D in mineralization is problematic from the viewpoint of mechanisms. Soft bones and the clinical signs associated with rickets are well known, but many of these can be attributed to a phosphate deficiency that is aggravated by the lack of vitamin D.

Experimental vitamin D deficiency leads to minor bone changes in rats. Hypocalcemia due to vitamin D deficiency is not generally associated with obvious skeletal changes visible on radiographic examination. Moreover, it has been reported that in some animals the provision of abundant minerals, either in the diet or systemically, can overcome the skeletal defects associated with vitamin D deficiency. While it seems probable that vitamin D plays a hormone-like role in bone cells, as it does in cells of the duodenum and the DCT of the kidney, the nature of this role and its relationship to mineralization are not yet clarified. There is little doubt, however, that bone turnover of calcium is diminished in vitamin D deficiency.[7]

REFERENCES

1. Becker, K.L., E.S. Nylén, R. Cohen, and R.H.Snider, Jr. Calcitonin: Structure, Molecular Biology, and Actions. In: *Principles of Bone Biology,* J.P. Bilezikian, L.G. Raisz, and G.A.Rodan, Eds. Academic Press: San Diego. pp. 471-494, 1996.
2. Bronner, F., D. Pansu, and W.D. Stein. An analysis of intestinal calcium transport across the rat intestine. *Am. J. Physiol.* 250 (Gastrointest. Liver Physiol. 13): G561-G569, 1986.

3. Bronner, F. and W.D. Stein. $CaBP_r$ facilitates intracellular diffusion from Ca pumping in distal convoluted tubule. *Am. J. Physiol.* 225 (Renal Fluid and Electrolyte Physiol. 24): F558-F562, 1988.
4. Bronner, F. and W.D. Stein. Calcium homeostasis — an old problem revisited. *J. Nutr.* 125: 1987S-1995S, 1995.
5. Brown, E.M., M. Pollak, Y.-H.W. Chen, C.E. Seidman, J.G. Seidman, and S.C. Hebert. The cloning of extracellular Ca^{2+}-sensing receptors from parathyroid and kidney: molecular mechanisms of extracellular Ca^{2+} sensing. *J. Nutr.* 125: 1965S-1970S, 1995.
6. Collins, E.D. and A.W. Norman. Vitamin D. In: *Handbook of Vitamins*. 2nd ed., L.J. Machlin, Ed. Dekker: New York, pp. 59-98, 1991.
7. Hurwitz, S., R.E. Stacey, and F. Bronner. Role of vitamin D in plasma calcium regulation. *Am. J. Physiol.* 216: 254-262, 1969.
8. Kronenberg, H.M., T. Igarashi, M.W. Freeman, T. Okazaki, S.J. Brand, K.M. Wiren, and J.T. Potts, Jr. Structure and expression of the human parathyroid gene. *Recent Progr. Horm. Res.* 42: 641-663, 1986.
9. Mosley, J.M. and T.J. Martin. Parathyroid-Hormone Related Protein: Physiological Actions. In: *Principles of Bone Biology,* J.P. Bilezikian, L.G. Raisz, and G.A. Rodan, Eds. Academic Press: San Diego, pp. 363-376, 1996.
10. Sammon, P.J., R.E. Stacey, and F. Bronner. Further studies on the role of thyrocalcitonin in calcium homeostasis and metabolism. *Biochem. Med.* 3: 252-270, 1969.
11. Sammon, P.J., R.E. Stacey, and F. Bronner, Role of parathyroid hormone in calcium homeostasis and metabolism. *Am. J. Physiol.* 218: 479-485, 1970.
12. Sato, M. and G.A. Rodan. Bone Cell Shape and Function. In: *Cell Shape Determinants, Regulation and Regulatory Role*. W.D. Stein and F. Bronner, Eds. Academic Press: New York, pp. 329-362, 1989.
13. Vortkamp, A., L. Kaechoong, B. Lanske, G.V. Segre, H.M. Kronenberg, and C.J. Tabin. Regulation of rate of cartilage differentiation of Indian hedgehog and PTH-related protein. *Science* 273: 613-621, 1996.
14. Wasserman, R.H. and C.S. Fullmer. Vitamin D and intestinal calcium transport: facts, speculations and hypotheses. *J. Nutr.* 125: 1971S-1979S, 1995.

9 Systemic and Local Modifiers of Bone Metabolism Other Than the Calcitropic Hormones

Felix Bronner

CONTENTS

9.1 INTRODUCTION

Parathyroid hormone, calcitonin, and vitamin D are considered the primary hormones that regulate calcium and bone metabolism. Other hormones that act directly or indirectly on bone include the gonadal steroids, the adrenal glucocorticoids, the thyroid hormones, growth hormone and somatomedin, and insulin and glucagon.

9.2 GONADAL STEROIDS

Mineral metabolism and bones and cartilage are profoundly affected in conditions of excess or deficiency of the gonadal steroids. Osteoblasts and osteoclasts have receptors that respond to estrogens[4] or testosterone.[2] Estrogens, probably acting on precursor cells via cytokines, inhibit osteoclast differentiation. Moreover (cf. Chapter 8), the inhibitory effect exerted by parathyroid hormone on osteoblasts is diminished when estrogen or androgen is added to an osteoblast culture. Estrogen

0-8493-9237-3/99/$0.00+$.50

therapy, often combined with supplementary calcium, is the treatment of choice in postmenopausal osteoporosis (Chapter 5).

Estrogen administration leads to diminished urinary calcium output and a resulting improvement in the body's calcium balance. Although estrogens do not appear to affect intestinal calcium absorption directly, there is controversy in the literature as to whether estrogen therapy improves calcium absorption.

Testosterone seems to have mechanisms of action similar to those of estrogen. At one time, testosterone was used to treat women with postmenopausal osteoporosis, partly because testosterone administration leads to significant improvement in the nitrogen balance. However, because of the undesirable masculinizing effect, it is rarely used today.

9.3 CORTICOSTEROIDS

Cortisol, corticosterone, and deoxycorticosterone are the major products of the zona fasciculata of the human adrenal gland and represent the chemical response of the body to stress. They have a pronounced effect on bone metabolism, inhibiting cartilage growth and development, impairing synthesis of the bone matrix, and inhibiting bone formation. These antianabolic actions of the corticosteroids may in part result from their inhibition of protein synthesis. As a result, bone resorption is stimulated.

Glucocorticoids seem to have no acute effect on urinary calcium excretion,[7] but chronic administration causes calcium excretion to rise. Long-term administration of glucocorticoids or glucocorticoid excess may induce excess calcium mobilization from the skeleton and thus lead to hypercalciuria. The major metabolic effect of glucocorticoids is on bone. An excess of these hormones, as in Cushing's disease, or when administered exogenously, is associated with decreased bone growth in children, loss of bone volume in adults, and the impairment of fracture healing. Glucocorticoids inhibit incorporation of sulfate into cartilage[10] and of amino acids into cartilage collagen;[3] thus, they have an antianabolic effect. Glucocorticoid insufficiency, if untreated, is life-threatening. It is associated with hypercalcemia, which may be the result of excessive osteoclastic activity that would normally be modulated by glucocorticoids.

9.4 THYROID HORMONES[6]

The two principal thyroid hormones are triiodothyronine and thyroxine, the latter containing four atoms of iodine. Even though they are peptides and not steroids, the most probable mechanism of action of the thyroid hormones involves nuclear localization and genomic activation by a ligand-receptor complex. This in turn leads to selective synthesis of specific proteins. Consequently, the action of the thyroid hormones can be likened to that of steroid hormones.

Both thyroid hormone excess and hypothyroidism have significant effects on bone metabolism. Hyperthyroidism is associated with a marked increase in bone resorption, particularly in cortical bone, caused mainly by increased osteoclastic activity due in part to the action of prostaglandins and transforming growth factor-β(TGF-β). At the same time, bone turnover is increased. However, the stimulation of bone calcium resorption seems greater than that of bone calcium deposition. As a result, the bone calcium balance, especially in cortical bone, is diminished. Hyperthyroidism is often associated with an increase in hydroxyproline excretion in urine and sometimes with increased hydroxyproline levels in serum, indications of heightened collagen turnover. Alkaline phosphatase levels are increased in hyperthyroidism.

In hypothyroidism, the effects on calcium metabolism are the obverse of what occurs in the case of thyroid hormone excess. Bone turnover is slowed, hydroxyproline excretion is diminished, and there is a tendency to mild hypocalcemia and diminished serum phosphate levels. Hence, urinary calcium and phosphate excretion are also lower than normal. The bone calcium pool is diminished.

Thyroid hormone promotes skeletal growth in prepubertal children by acting on cartilage growth directly and by stimulating the growth hormone-insulin growth factor pathway. Therefore, hypothyroidism in children is associated with diminished skeletal growth and an increase in density in the zone of provisional calcification and delayed appearance of the centers of epiphyseal ossification.

9.5 GROWTH HORMONE AND SOMATOMEDINS (INSULIN GROWTH FACTORS)

The growth hormone molecule is a large protein consisting of 191 amino acids, the active core of which involves the N-terminal two thirds of the sequence, while the remainder, the C-terminal one third, is thought to stabilize the molecular structure. Growth hormone is the major hormonal growth factor, acting on bone and cartilage. The hormone promotes growth through the insulin growth factors (IGFs), low molecular weight (~7000 Da) peptides synthesized in the liver. IGF receptors have been found in adipocytes, hepatocytes, lymphocytes, and bone cells.

Growth hormone is essential for normal growth and development. One form of human dwarfism is caused by defective production of growth hormone, an autosomal recessive characteristic. Growth hormone is essential for IGF synthesis. Patients with acromegaly, i.e., enlarged stature due to excess growth hormone production, exhibit increased rates of calcium uptake and release by the skeleton, with formation stimulated more than resorption. Acromegaly is associated with hypercalciuria, and in some patients, with increased calcium absorption from the intestine. The mechanism(s) by which growth hormone and/or IGFs act on these processes is unknown; direct action on transcellular calcium transport seems unlikely.

9.6 INSULIN AND GLUCAGON[12]

It seems probable that bone cells are also a direct target of the action of insulin, although other tissues — adipose, muscle, and liver — are generally considered the major targets.

Insulin deficiency leads to a diminution of bone turnover, with bone calcium removal markedly enhanced in insulin-deprived animals.[13] Insulin-deprived rats in the growth phase are only slightly hypocalcemic, but have stopped adding calcium to their skeletons. In other words, their bone balance, instead of being positive, is zero or slightly negative. Insulin deficiency is associated with a drop in active calcium absorption in the intestine and a rise in urinary calcium output; this suggests a diminution of the calcium-conserving capacity of the kidney.

Glucagon administration produces transient hypocalcemia in several mammalian species, including humans, presumably by direct interaction with the skeleton. There is evidence that glucagon inhibits parathyroid-stimulated osteoclastic action, but it probably has no effect in unstimulated bone cells.

9.7 PROSTAGLANDINS AND CYTOKINES

Prostaglandins, particularly prostaglandin E_2, and cytokines (e.g., transforming growth factors, insulin-like growth factors, interleukins) are messenger or signaling molecules that act on neighboring cells or on the cell by which the factor is released. They thus constitute local modifiers, as opposed to systemic modifiers like hormones that travel through the general circulation to reach their intended target.

9.7.1 PROSTAGLANDINS

These compounds, all related to prostanoic acid, are products of arachidonic acid metabolism. They can be divided into three major classes, A,E, and F, with PGE_2 of particular importance in bone metabolism. Prostaglandins are potent multifunctional regulators of bone formation and bone resorption, being produced by bone cells as well as cells adjacent to bone cells. Prostaglandins thus participate actively in the cellular cross-talk that results from systemic hormone stimulation of bone cell formation or resorption.

Prostaglandin E_2 has long been known to stimulate bone resorption and many factors that enhance bone resorption also stimulate prostaglandin production. Glucocorticoids and interleukin-4, which inhibit bone resorption, also inhibit prostaglandin synthesis.

Prostaglandins have a biphasic effect on bone formation. In bone organ culture, prostaglandins, in the presence of cortisol, stimulate the differentiation of osteoblast precursors and cell replication. This may be mediated by cAMP. *In vivo* prostaglandins have been implicated as involved in fracture repair and heterotopic ossification.

It has been suggested that the anabolic action of prostaglandins depends on the presence of osteoblastic lineage cells and on mechanical loading. Indeed, the mechanosensory response of bone cells appears to involve increased release of prostaglandins. However, vibrational forces acting on osteoblasts have been shown to bring about up-regulation in the mRNA expression of two growth-related protoncogenes (c-fos and c-myc) without intervention by prostaglandins.[11]

Yet prostaglandins also inhibit collagen synthesis in cell and organ culture. Differences in action are probably brought about by differences in ligand specificity and resulting differences in cellular signaling. Moreover, cytokines, like interleukins or tumor necrosis factor, contribute to the various effects ascribed to prostaglandins in cell culture.[8]

Although parathyroid hormone, PTHrP, 1,25-dihydroxyvitamin D_3, and thyroid hormone all stimulate prostaglandin production, only thyroid hormone seems to require the presence of prostaglandin in the culture to exert its resorbing effect. Both estrogen and androgen inhibit prostaglandin production. For example, estrogen administration to an oophorectomized rat suppresses the increase in prostaglandin production that resulted from oophorectomy.

9.7.2 Cytokines

Human osteoblast-like cells produce several cytokines, i.e., granulocyte-colony stimulating factor (G-SCF), granulocyte-macrophages stimulating factor (GM-SCF), interleukin (IL)-1β, interleukin-6, leukemia inhibitory factor (LIF), transforming growth factor (TGF)-β, and tumor necrosis factor (TNF)-α. These cellular products are not unique to bone cells, but are also associated with other cells, as they are part of what constitutes cellular cross-talk, i.e., chemical messengers or signals that evoke various responses. A specific example is IL-6 which plays a role in osteoclastogenesis. IL-6 production by osteoblasts is diminished under estrogen domination and enhanced when estrogen production is reduced, as in the menopause.

The knowledge concerning the above factors is constantly expanding, yet it is difficult to summarize their multiple roles other than to say that as messenger molecules they react in a variety of developmental and metabolic events and sequences, many of which play important roles in bone metabolism.

For example, TFG-β, a potent stimulator of matrix formation,[1] also stimulates a variety of other factors (e.g., fibronectin, osteonectin, osteopontin, among others) and inhibits osteocalcin and the plasminogen activator. The quantitative importance of these effects remains to be evaluated. Systemic injection of TFG-β has been shown[9] to stimulate cancellous bone formation in young and adult rats, but whether this observation has therapeutic significance has not been established.

Colony-stimulating factors, also known as macrophage colony-stimulating factors because they play a role in cell and tissue development and differentiation, also have these functions for bone cells, notably in osteoclastogenesis,[5] inducing osteoclast fusion, spreading, and cell survival. Again, a role in therapy needs is yet to be determined.

REFERENCES

1. Bonewald, L.F. Transforming Growth Factor-β. In: *Principles of Bone Biology.* J.P. Bilezikian, L.G. Raisz, and G.A. Rodan, Eds. Academic Press: San Diego, pp. 647-660, 1996.
2. Colvard, D.S., E.F. Eriksen, P.E. Keeting, E.M. Wilson, D.B. Lubahn, F.S. French, B.L. Riggs, and T.C. Spelsberg. Identification of androgen receptors in normal human osteoblast-like cells. *Proc. Nat. Acad. Sci. (U.S.A.)* 86: 854-857, 1989.
3. Daughaday, W.H. and I.K. Mariz. Conversion of proline-U-C^{14} to labeled hydroxyproline by rat cartilage in vitro: Effects of hypophysectomy, growth hormone, and cortisol. *J. Lab. Clin. Med.* 59: 741-751, 1962.

4. Ernst, M., C.H. Schmid, and E.R. Froesch. Enhanced osteoblast proliferation and collagen gene expression by estradiol. *Proc. Nat. Acad. Sci. (U.S.A.)* 85: 2307-2310, 1988.
5. Hofstetter, W., R. Felix, and M.G. Cecchini. Colony-Stimulating Factors. In: *Principles of Bone Biology.* J.P. Bilezikian, L.G. Raisz, and G.A. Rodan, Eds. Academic Press: San Diego, pp. 673-686, 1996.
6. Klaushofer, K., F. Varga, H. Glantschnig, N. Fratzl-Zelman, E. Czerwenka, H.J. Leis, W.-M. Jong, and M. Peterlik. The regulatory role of thyroid hormones in bone cell growth and differentiation. *J. Nutr.* 125: 1996S-2003S, 1995.
7. Massry, S.G. and J.W. Coburn. The hormonal and non-hormonal control of renal excretion of calcium and magnesium. *Nephron* 10: 66-112, 1973.
8. Raisz, L.G. Physiologic and pathologic roles of prostaglandins and other eicosanoids in bone metabolism. *J. Nutr.* 125: 2024S-2027S, 1997.
9. Rosen, D., S.C. Miller, E. DeLeon, A.Y. Thompson, H. Bentz, M. Mathews, and S. Adams. Systemic administration of recombinant transforming growth factor beta 2 (rTGF-β2) stimulates parameters of cancellous bone formation in juvenile and adult rats. *Bone* 15: 355-359, 1994.
10. Schryver, H.F. The effect of hydrocortisone on chondroitin sulfate production and loss by embryonic chick tibiotarsi in organ culture. *Exp. Cell Res.* 40: 610-618, 1965.
11. Tjanchawinata, R.R., V.L. Vincent, and M. Hughes-Fulford. Vibrational force alters mRNA expression in osteoblasts. *FASEB J.* 11: 493-497, 1997.
12. Verhaeghe, J. and R. Bouillon. Effects of Diabetes and Insulin on Bone Metabolism. In: *Principles of Bone Biology.* J.P. Bilezikian, L.G. Raisz, and G.A. Rodan, Eds. Academic Press: San Diego, pp. 549-561, 1996.
13. Wood, R.J., L.H. Allen, and F. Bronner. Regulation of calcium metabolism in streptozotocin-induced diabetes. *Am. J. Physiol.* 247 (Regulatory Integrative Comp. Physiol. 16): R120-R123, 1984.

10 Metabolic Bone Disease

Michael Kleerekoper

CONTENTS

10.1 INTRODUCTION

As our understanding of metabolic bone diseases has increased over the years, so too has our diagnostic capability and our therapeutic options. For the three most common metabolic bone diseases — osteoporosis, Paget's disease of bone, and hyperparathyroidism — these advances have resulted in the diagnosis being established in the asymptomatic, pre-clinical stage. In many respects, this has removed the orthopedist from the clinical picture except for very late stage complicated disease. Nonetheless, since the orthopedic surgeon is often the first entry into the medical system for musculoskeletal symptoms, or the first site of referral by primary care physicians for patients in whom they diagnose potential metabolic bone disease, it is important that the orthopedic surgeon remain current with pathophysiology, diagnostic technology, and therapies.

10.2 OSTEOPOROSIS

Case Report *— A 63-year-old woman presented to her primary care physician with complaints of moderate exacerbation of chronic low back pain. The physical examination was unremarkable, but the physician ordered X-rays of the lumbosacral spine. The radiologist reported that there was generalized demineralization, but no other abnormalities. The conclusion from the radiologist was "possible osteoporosis."*

With this information, the patient was referred back to the radiologist for measurement of bone mineral density by dual energy X-ray absorptiometry (DXA). Bone mineral density of the lumbar spine (L2 to L4) was reported to be 815 mg/cm^2,

0-8493-9237-3/99/$0.00+$.50

corresponding to a T-score of –2.9. The radiologist concluded that the patient had osteoporosis. The patient was referred to you for further evaluation and management of symptomatic osteoporosis.

The definition of osteoporosis has changed from a disease of fractures to a disease of fracture risk, such that the fractures now become the complications of the disease rather than the disease itself. Patients with these complications of fragility fracture (mainly wrist, vertebra, or proximal femur) will still be referred to the orthopedic surgeon, but this group now represents the minority of patients with diagnosed osteoporosis. The patient described above is much more typical in that the diagnosis is based purely on the documentation of a diminished bone mineral density (BMD). Bone mineral density is a surrogate for bone strength and there is ample documentation from cross-sectional and prospective studies that the lower the BMD, the greater the likelihood of fracture. Additionally, in those who have sustained a fracture, the mean BMD is generally lower than those who have not yet fractured. Bone mineral density can be measured at multiple skeletal sites — finger, forearm, spine, proximal femur, and heel — using a variety of techniques. These include single and dual energy X-ray absorptiometry, quantitative computed tomography, radiographic absorptiometry, and broadband ultrasound attenuation.

In general, fracture risk doubles for every standard deviation decrement in measured BMD. The population of healthy, young, premenopausal women, aged 20 to 40, is taken as the reference population with a relative lifetime risk of fracture of 1.0. Every standard deviation below the mean for this reference population is designated as a T-score. This patient in whom the T-score was –2.9 has an almost sixfold increased risk of fracture than healthy women aged 20 to 40.

This patient was referred for evaluation and management of "symptomatic osteoporosis" because she did have osteoporosis, she did have low BMD in the spine, and she had backache. This is, unfortunately, an all too common misconception. Low BMD per se is not associated with any symptoms whatsoever. The symptoms only occur as a result of the fracture and long-term sequelae of the fracture. Since the radiographs in this patient did not detect any vertebral fracture, it can be stated with confidence that her back pain was not due to osteoporosis. The aim of therapy for osteoporosis in this case is to minimize her risk of fracture, not to alleviate her symptoms. The symptoms are due to disease other than osteoporosis and therefore, while needing attention and therapy, will not respond to specific therapy for osteoporosis.

The new definition did not alter the demographics of osteoporosis or osteoporotic fractures in that older postmenopausal white women are those most affected, while men are affected less often. The bone loss that is the hallmark of osteoporosis results from changes in bone remodeling induced by the marked reduction in estrogen production at the time of the menopause. These lower estrogen levels stimulate osteoclast-mediated bone resorption which in turn stimulates osteoblast-mediated bone formation. However, the increase in bone resorption exceeds that of bone formation and bone loss ensues. Available therapies for osteoporosis act by inhibiting bone resorption, thereby minimizing further bone loss. In some patients, there is even a modest increase in BMD, mainly resulting from filling in of pre-existing resorption cavities. The available drugs are estrogen, calcitonin, and alendronate sodium. Alendronate sodium is the first of a new class of compounds, the bisphosphonates, to receive FDA approval for the prevention and treatment of postmenopausal osteoporosis. These bisphosphonates are analogs of naturally occurring pyrophosphate and they bind avidly to the skeleton to inhibit bone resorption. They appear not to have any direct effect on bone formation. Extensive clinical trials have clearly documented that therapy with alendronate sodium significantly reduces the incidence of osteoporotic fractures. The same has been documented, albeit to a lesser extent, with estrogen and calcitonin. Nonetheless, fractures can still occur in patients treated with alendronate sodium and the orthopedic surgeon is often asked what impact, if any, this might have on the recovery from fracture. It has been well demonstrated in animal models that fractures occurring in test animals who have been treated for a long time with alendronate sodium have no abnormality in fracture healing. Likewise, it has been demonstrated that if alendronate sodium is administered for the first time after the fracture has occurred, that too is not associated with any abnormality in fracture healing. There is also no evidence that estrogen or calcitonin has any effect on fracture healing.

Much has been written about the role of calcium and vitamin D in the prevention and treatment of osteoporosis. The evidence that this is of benefit once skeletal maturity is obtained is small. Nonetheless, calcium supplementation, or dietary calcium, is an inexpensive measure with little real or potential adverse effect. Accordingly, it is recommended that a daily intake of calcium (diet and supplement) be maintained at 1,000 to 1,500 mg. When more specific therapy for osteoporosis is given it is important to maintain an adequate calcium intake since bone accretion cannot occur properly in a calcium-deficient state.

Increasingly, studies have demonstrated that a substantial portion of the elderly in the United States, even the well elderly, are deficient in vitamin D. This is not only of importance for skeletal health, but also of importance for maintenance of striated muscle integrity. Studies in the community of vitamin D-deficient elderly French nursing home residents demonstrated that 1,000 mg of calcium plus 800 units of vitamin D daily significantly reduced the prospectively measured incidence of hip fractures, compared to placebo. While this finding is not directly applicable to the elderly population in the United States, it seems reasonable and cost-effective to ensure that all persons over the age of 75 in the United States consume 800 units of vitamin D daily in their diet. This can be provided as two multi-vitamin capsules per day. It is likely, but as yet unproven, that this may also have a beneficial effect on recovery following hip fracture.

10.3 PRIMARY HYPERPARATHYROIDISM

Case Report *— A 41-year-old male executive presented for routine physical examination, following which a screening biochemical profile was obtained. This revealed a serum calcium of 10.9 mg/dl (reference interval 8.8 to 10.2). With this information, the treating physician obtained a more detailed history looking for potential clinical evidence of primary hyperparathyroidism. None was found. Serum intact PTH was*

73 pg/ml (normal 10 to 65) confirming the diagnosis of primary hyperparathyroidism. The patient was well and symptom-free. However, because of the known deleterious effects of primary hyperparathyroidism on the skeleton, BMD was measured and a T-score in the radial midshaft was –3.1. In the lumbar spine, the T-score was –1.6, and in the femoral neck the T-score was –1.3.

This patient is very typical of the current presentation of primary hyperparathyroidism as the serendipitous finding of hypercalcemia in an otherwise asymptomatic patient. Rarely do patients have such severe primary hyperparathyroidism that there is overt skeletal involvement. However, subclinical skeletal disease, detected by direct measurement of BMD, is a very frequent occurrence. It is presumed that, if left untreated, such patients will have progressive bone loss ultimately leading to clinically manifest bone disease. Surprisingly, prospective studies have confirmed the presence of low BMD in many patients with primary hyperparathyroidism, but have failed to show progressive bone loss in those patients. Even more surprisingly, following successful parathyroidectomy, there is a progressive increase in BMD.

While fractures are an infrequent complication of primary hyperparathyroidism, a number of patients with fractures will be found to have mild primary hyperparathyroidism. In general, this should not affect the operative management of the fracture, but might prove to be an important factor should there be a delay in fracture healing. Similarly, any patients scheduled for elective orthopedic procedures, such as joint replacement surgery, should be free of primary hyperparathyroidism prior to the elective surgery.

10.4 HYPERPARATHYROIDISM SECONDARY TO RENAL FAILURE (RENAL OSTEODYSTROPHY)

The pathogenesis of the secondary hyperparathyroidism complicating renal failure has been more clearly defined as not only phosphate retention, but also defective production of 1,25 dihydroxyvitamin D (calcitriol). In addition to monitoring phosphate intake and modulating dialysis to maintain normal serum phosphate, it has become common practice to provide intravenous calcitriol to all patients undergoing regular dialysis. This has substantially reduced the severity of the secondary hyperparathyroidism of renal osteodystrophy. There remain, however, a number of patients who present with end-stage renal disease of long-standing duration, with previously unrecognized and untreated secondary hyperparathyroidism. Many of these patients will have classic radiographic features of hyperparathyroidism. An occasional patient will present with a fragility fracture, often of the proximal femur, complicating both the hyperparathyroidism and the vitamin D deficiency. These patients clearly require operative intervention as quickly as practicable, but the likelihood of a successful outcome from surgery is diminished by severe secondary hyperparathyroidism. When possible, this should be corrected by administration of calcitriol, but this may take weeks to months to fully correct the hyperparathyroidism. In that circumstance, elective subtotal parathyroidectomy should be performed as early as possible following the orthopedic procedure.

10.5 PAGET'S DISEASE OF BONE

Case Report — *A 73-year-old man was referred to a neurologist for evaluation of lower extremity weakness. Spine radiographs detected a lesion of the 12th thoracic vertebra, i.e., an ivory-like vertebra characteristic of Paget's disease. The patient was referred to an orthopedic surgeon, but while waiting for his appointment, developed acute paraplegia. An endocrinologist was consulted to determine when medical therapy for Paget's disease should be instituted in relation to the decompression surgery. The endocrinologist persuaded the orthopedic surgeon to delay surgery for 24 hours while the patient was treated with a 90 mg dose of Pamidronate administered intravenously over a 4-hour period. The next day, the orthopedic surgeon and endocrinologist saw the patient on rounds together and the patient stated that he felt he was getting some feeling back in his legs. Objective evidence of improvement was equivocal, but the endocrinologist again persuaded the orthopedist to delay surgery a further 24 hours. Now objective evidence of neurologic recovery was noted and surgery was again postponed. The patient had a complete remission of lower extremity symptoms over the next 7 to 10 days. Symptoms did not recur and elective laminectomy was performed 3 months later.*

While paraplegia complicating the vertebral involvement with Paget's disease is uncommon, there are increasing reports of "cure" of this paraplegia with medical therapy for the Paget's. Therefore, it seems very reasonable to delay seemingly urgent surgery until the patient has received at least one course of therapy. Many orthopedic surgeons have also noted that medical therapy prior to surgery for Paget's reduces the vascularity of the skeletal lesion and minimizes intraoperative blood loss. Therefore, whenever possible, patients with Paget's disease should have surgery delayed until at least one course of therapy has been given.

The patient described above represents one end of the clinical spectrum of Paget's disease of bone. As is the case with osteoporosis and primary hyperparathyroidism, most patients with Paget's disease now present without symptoms. The disease is detected either as a result of an increase in total serum alkaline phosphatase, or the finding of skeletal changes characteristic of Paget's disease on a radiograph taken for reasons other than any concern about Paget's disease. There are now four bisphosphonates available in the United States for oral treatment of Paget's disease. These are etidronate, alendronate, tiludronate, and risedronate. In addition, pamidronate is approved as intravenous therapy for Paget's disease. These therapies for Paget's disease are expensive, but are otherwise safe and well tolerated in the vast majority of patients. Many patients experience a sustained remission of Paget's disease, defined as a sustained reduction in serum alkaline phosphatase in asymptomatic patients, after just one course of therapy. Therefore, once Paget's disease has been diagnosed, even asymptomatic patients should receive therapy with one of the above-mentioned bisphosphates. When patients are on therapy, their serum alkaline phosphatase should be monitored three times at monthly intervals to confirm that the therapy is effective. If there is no significant drop in the alkaline phosphatase after three months of therapy, the bisphosphonate used should be changed. After a course of therapy has been completed, alkaline phosphatase should be monitored every six months and therapy reinstituted if the alkaline phosphatase starts to rise again or if the patient develops symptoms that might be referable to the Paget's disease. Skeletal deformities of Paget's disease are slow to develop, and progress slowly. It is presumed that these deformities will not progress on medical therapy, nor will they regress on therapy.

10.6 OSTEOMALACIA

Case 1 *— A 73-year-old woman was referred for evaluation of osteoporosis. She had complained of back pain. Radiographs demonstrated skeletal demineralization and a low BMD. The patient had complained of bone pain for almost 12 months and had progressive weakness. These complaints are atypical for osteoporosis. Further history indicated that she had 5 bowel motions per day; this she regarded as normal because she had this frequency of bowel motion for as long as she could remember. Physical examination confirmed generalized skeletal tenderness and mild proximal muscle weakness. Laboratory studies indicated that plasma calcium was 9.1 mg/dl, the inorganic phosphate 2.7 (reference interval 2.5 to 4.5), and the alkaline phosphatase 170 (normal less than 115). A 24-hour urine calcium excretion was 30 mg and serum 25 hydroxyvitamin D level was 7 (reference interval 10 to 55 ng/ml). Therapy with 25 hydroxyvitamin D was initiated and within 4 weeks the patient had complete resolution of skeletal pain and muscle weakness. Serial measurement showed substantial increase of BMD.*

Case 2 *— A 34-year-old woman was treated symptomatically for a diagnosis of systemic lupus erythematosus for a period of 2 years. During therapy, she complained of progressive weakness with progressive muscle, bone, and joint pains. A bone scan was performed which showed multiple areas of increased tracer uptake throughout the skeleton and a diagnosis of Paget's disease of bone was entertained. Biochemical profile indicated the total alkaline phosphatase was 1,500, which was consistent with a diagnosis of Paget's disease, and serum calcium was at the upper limit of normal at 10.3 mg/dl. The serum intact PTH at 1,500 pg/ml was severalfold higher than the normal range (10 to 65), and the patient was referred because of the seemingly unusual combination of Paget's disease of bone and primary hyperparathyroidism. Review of the bone scan did not show typical features of Paget's disease, but more generalized increased uptake consistent with a systemic metabolic bone disease. The patient had marked skeletal tenderness and very marked proximal myopathy. On close questioning, she reported that 10 years earlier she'd had gastric surgery for treatment of obesity and she had lost 50% of her total body weight in the last 10 years. The presumptive diagnosis of osteomalacia was confirmed by the 24-hour urine calcium of 10 mg, and an undetectable serum 25-hydroxyvitamin D. Radiographs showed changes of severe secondary hyperparathyroidism. Radiographs of the ribs suggested the presence of Looser zones. This patient was treated with 25-hydroxyvitamin D, with gradual improvement in her symptoms.*

The two patients described here represent the opposite end of the clinical spectrum of vitamin D deficiency with frank clinical osteomalacia manifested by bone pain and tenderness and proximal muscle weakness. Symptoms of osteomalacia respond rapidly and completely to vitamin D replacement. 25-hydroxyvitamin D is the major storage form of this hormone and vitamin D deficiency can be confirmed by low or undetectable levels in the blood. Because 25-hydroxyvitamin D is the major storage form of the hormone, it is the most appropriate form to use for replacement therapy. Responses can be obtained with the parent vitamin D (cholecalciferol), but larger doses are required and it takes longer for the symptoms to dissipate. One could consider therapy with 1,25-dihydroxyvitamin D, which is substantially more potent than 25-hydroxyvitamin D, but since this does not replenish the body stores of vitamin D, therapy must be continued for long periods of time. In contrast, once body stores of vitamin D are replenished with 25-hydroxyvitamin D, therapy can become intermittent. More importantly, one should seek out the cause of the vitamin D malabsorption/malnutrition and correct that, if at all possible. In the first of the two patients described above, the diagnosis of nontropical sprue was confirmed and the appropriate treatment is a gluten-free diet. The appropriate treatment for the second patient is reversal of the surgical procedure used to treat her obesity. The patient refused that therapy.

10.7 SUMMARY AND CONCLUSIONS

Improved understanding of the pathophysiology of metabolic bone disease, improved diagnostic modalities, and improved therapeutic options have all combined to lessen the surgical role for orthopedists in patients with metabolic bone disease. However, since the orthopedist is still most often the first physician consulted by the patient or primary care physicians for possible metabolic bone disease, it is essential that the orthopedists become fully conversant with all new modalities. When metabolic bone disease is complicated to the point that surgical intervention is required, the orthopedist must pay close attention to concomitant medical therapy.

SUGGESTED READINGS

Marcus, R., Feldman, D., and Kelsey, J., Eds. *Osteoporosis*, Academic Press, New York, 1996.

Avioli, L.V. and Krane, S.M., Eds. *Metabolic Bone Disease and Clinically Related Disorders.* Third Edition, Academic Press, New York, 1998.

Eastell, R. Drug Therapy: Treatment of Postmenopausal Osteoporosis, *New England Journal of Medicine,* Vol 338(11), 736, 1998.

Thomas, M.K., Lloyd-Jones, D.M., Thadhani, R.I., Shaw, A.C., Deraska, D.J., Kitch, B.T., Vamvakas, E.C., Dick, I.M., Prince, R.L., and Finkelstein, J.S., Hypovitaminosis D in medical inpatients, *New England Journal of Medicine,* Vol 338(12), 777, 1998.

Delmas, P.D. and Meunier, P.J., The management of Paget's disease of bone. *New England Journal of Medicine*, Vol 336(8), 558, 1997.

Kleerekoper, M. Clinical course of primary hyperparathyroidism, In: *The Parathyroids. Basic and Clinical Concepts*, Bilezikian, J.P., Levine, M.A., and Marcus, R., Eds., Raven Press, New York, 1994.

Section III

Clinical Topics

11 The Normal and the Diseased Joint

Wilmer L. Sibbitt, Jr.

CONTENTS

11.1 THE NORMAL JOINT

In the otherwise rigid framework of the osseous skeleton, the joint allows movement, albeit in a highly controlled and directed fashion. Some joints move very little or not at all, and these joints usually fulfill a structural role in the adult skeleton. All joints are highly organized and contain connective tissue which is uniquely differentiated and structured to the particular function of each joint. The tremendous forces

0-8493-9237-3/99/$0.00+$.50

TABLE 11.1
Classification of Joints

Type	Description	Movement	Structure	Examples
Synarthroses	Fused joints	None	Calcified fibrous or cartilaginous elements	Skull
Amphiarthroses	Fibrocartilage joints	Limited	Fibrocartilage discs Hyaline cartilage Fibrous capsule	Intervertebral joints Pubic symphysis
Diarthroses	Synovial joints	Moveable	Hyaline cartilage Synovial membrane	Joints of the extremities

associated with movement and weight bearing are transmitted across joints, and when subject to these forces, even small structural abnormalities can result in progressive pathology and morbidity. Because of the complex structure and relative avascularity of articular tissue, the joint is highly susceptible to injury from trauma, inflammation, infection, and other pathological processes. In clinical orthopedics, the most important joints in terms of disease processes and trauma are the synovial joints and the intervertebral discs.

11.1.1 Types of Joints

Joints can be classified into three distinct groups: 1) fused joints (synarthroses), 2) fibrocartilage joints (amphiarthroses), and 3) synovial joints (diarthroses) (see Table 11.1). The fused joint is immovable; the fibrocartilage joint has limited motion; and the synovial joint is fully moveable.[1,2] Although this classification is based on degree of movement, it also has direct anatomical implications. *Synarthroses* are bound together by calcified fibrous or cartilaginous elements and are found chiefly in the skull. *Amphiarthroses* are composed of fibrocartilage discs, hyaline cartilage on the osseous end plate, and a tough fibrous capsule. The intervertebral discs are typical examples of these joints. *Diarthroses* are characterized by hyaline cartilage and the presence of a highly vascularized synovial membrane and are of particular importance in the extremities.

11.1.2 Synovial Joints

Diarthrodial (synovial) articulations are the most common joints and are of paramount importance in determining the primary movements and stability of the osseous skeleton.[3] Diarthrodial joints have a distinct anatomy consisting of bone, cartilage, synovial membrane, joint capsule, ligaments, and neurovascular elements (Figures 11.1 and 11.2).

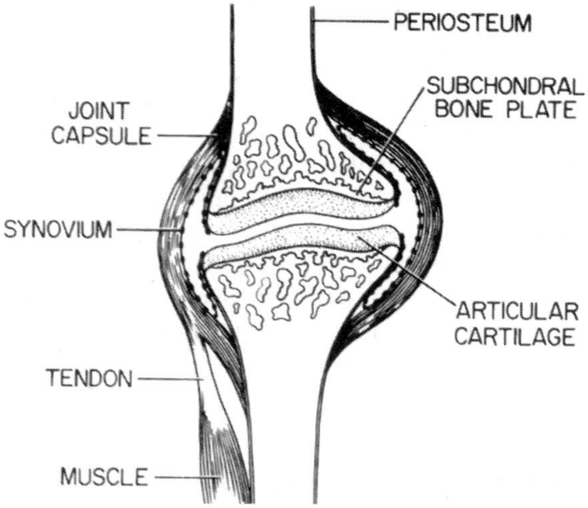

FIGURE 11.1 The Diarthrodial Joint. The articulating surfaces of the typical diarthrodial joint are covered with hyaline cartilage and the entire structure is enveloped in the joint capsule, a fibrous structure which merges with periosteum, tendons, ligaments, and fascia. The synovial membrane lines the joint cavity, but does not cover the articular cartilage. (Reproduced with permission of the American College of Rheumatology.)

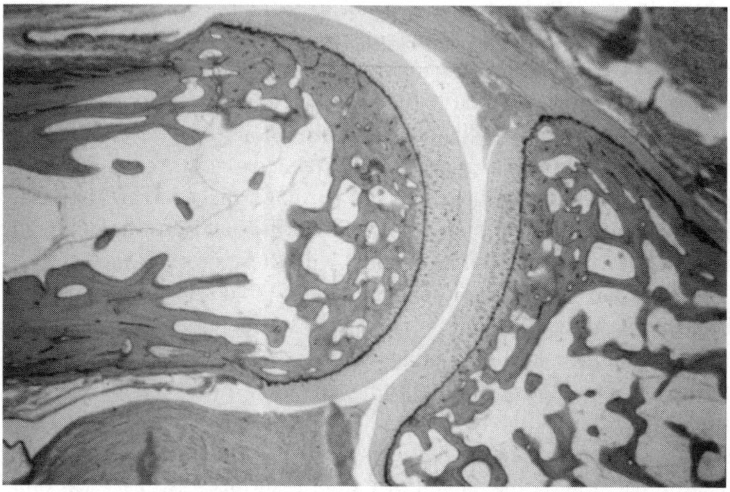

FIGURE 11.2 The Normal Diarthrodial Joint. This midsagittal section of the distal interphalangeal joint reveals the cancellous medullary bone of the metaphysis, the compact cortical bone of the end plate (subchondral bone), the apposing surfaces of hyaline cartilage, the thin, tenuous layer of synovial membrane, and the dense connective tissue of the fibrous capsule. (Reproduced with permission of the American College of Rheumatology.)

11.1.3 Bone

An end-plate of dense cortical bone supports the overlying cartilaginous structures and is often called *subchondral bone* or *subchondral end plate*.[4] The subchondral end plate is thinner than the cortical bone of the metaphysis and contains mature Haversian systems which run parallel with the joint surface, rather than along the long axis of the bone. The end plate and the thin sheets of underlying cancellous bone are arranged at right angles to force of compression, allowing ten times greater deformability than corresponding areas of the cortical shaft. This property allows the subchondral bone to absorb considerable impact without collapsing. Directly below the subchondral bone is an extensive structure of cancellous bone which is less dense than the end plate, but contains typical vascular and hemopoietic elements.

11.1.4 Cartilage

The cartilages within the synovial joint include the hyaline cartilage which covers the joint surface and fibrocartilage which composes menisci and related structures within the joint.[5] The articular cartilage appears white on gross inspection, but assumes a more yellowish cast with age. Hyaline cartilage is usually less than 5 mm thick and is completely avascular and contains no neural elements. Thus, the sensation within the joint must derive from neural structures in adjacent tissues such as the subchondral bone, the synovium, and joint capsule. The metabolic requirements of the cartilage are completely met by the synovial fluid.

Hyaline cartilage has distinct histological zones consisting of: 1) tangential or gliding zone (cells with long axes parallel to surface), 2) transitional zone (cells rounded and random), 3) radial zone (cells lined up in irregular columns), and 4) a calcified zone (separated from radial zone by the "tidemark") (Figure 11.2). The cartilage matrix is composed of 80% water and various protein constituents including type II collagen, other minor collagens, anchorin, chondronectin, and proteoglycans.[6] The chondrocytes are surprisingly metabolically active and continually produce and degrade proteoglycan and collagen in the cartilage matrix. The chondrocytes are exquisitely sensitive to factors such as interleukin-1 and prostaglandins, and may alter the structure of cartilage if stimulated with these or other factors.[7]

The hyaline cartilage is firmly integrated into the cortical end plate and extends from the osseous surface into the joint space. Hyaline cartilage is characterized by a smooth, resilient, and self-lubricating surface which glides almost without friction over the hyaline cartilage of the apposing articular surface. With significant load, the cartilage "sweats," that is, it spontaneously dehydrates, forming a layer of lubricating water on the cartilage surface which, along with the synovial fluid, facilitates the frictionless movement of the joint surfaces against each other.[8,9] The expression of a lubricating layer of water under load is called *hydrostatic lubrication*. At lesser loads, the synovial fluid contributes a *lubricating glycoprotein* which binds to the cartilage surface and acts as a potent anti-friction agent. This type of lubrication is a form of coating lubrication termed *boundary lubrication*.[10]

Menisci are fibrocartilage discs which are present in the knee, temporomandibular, sternoclavicular, distal radioulnar, and acromioclavicular joints.[11] The menisci are usually firmly attached to the joint capsule and adjacent bone. The fibrocartilage in the joint is mostly avascular, but does possess a small vascular arcade at the site of bony attachment. Presumably, the fibrocartilage derives its nutrition from the synovial fluid as well as from this small extension of the osseous vascular arcade. The menisci have collagen fibers arranged circumferentially to distribute the forces of weight bearing. The water content of the fibrocartilage in the joint is similar to that of hyaline cartilage, but the predominant collagen is type I, rather than type II. The menisci are important structures that stabilize the joint (especially hinge joints), absorb external stresses, and bear load.

The joint is also stabilized by the extent and contour of the articular surfaces, surrounding muscles and tendons, and the tough bands of dense connective tissue comprising the ligaments and joint capsule. The articular contour is determined by the type of diarthrodial joint which includes ball and socket (hip), condylar-four-bar linkage (knee), mortised hinge (ankle), ball on disc (shoulder), and convex-concave (wrist) among many other forms. The articular contour determines not only the stability of the joint, but also the type and extent of motion. Some joints, such as the hip, can move in almost any direction, but are limited by the structure of the bony components comprising the ball and socket. Any movement beyond the normal contours of the joint will result in disarticulation, constrained only by the strength of the surrounding muscles, tendons, intrinsic ligaments, and joint capsule.

11.1.5 The Joint Capsule and Ligaments

The *joint capsule* is a tough, fibrous structure composed of dense connective tissue which envelops the entire joint.[1] The joint capsule inserts onto the cortical surface the bone shaft, usually adjacent to the marginal aspects of the hyaline cartilage. In this transition from capsule to bone, parallel bundles of collagen fibers from the joint capsule approach the bone surface and are integrated into a fibrocartilage matrix which is calcified near the cortical surface. The parallel collagen fibers then continue into the cortical osseous tissue and gradually are indistinguishable from the surrounding structures of cortical bone. This anatomical insertion allows a complete distribution of forces and prevents pull-out failure.

Ligaments are thickened bands of connective tissue within the joint capsule and often form discrete structures which are anatomically described as separate entities, although in most cases they remain integral components of the joint capsule.[12] Ligaments are composed of extremely dense connective tissue, containing few fibroblasts but massive collections of parallel collagen fibers which provide increased tensile strength along the axis of the fiber. The ligaments also insert onto the osseous surfaces and stabilize the joint by: 1) limiting range of motion, 2) preventing passive or active disarticulation, and 3) providing stability in the absence of muscular contraction or in the presence of unbalanced muscular contraction.

11.1.6 The Synovial Membrane

The synovial membrane lines the entire joint capsule, but does not normally extend over the hyaline cartilage.[13] The membrane also does not cover fibrocartilaginous structures such as the menisci. The synovial membrane is sufficiently redundant to permit joint motion, yet is limited enough that it is not entrapped between the articular surfaces during motion or weight bearing. The membrane is composed of a synovial cell layer and an adipose layer. The adipose layer, consisting of adipocytes and loose connective tissue, adheres closely to the inner surface of the joint capsule and is extensively vascularized. This rich blood supply directly supports the synoviocytes and indirectly nourishes the avascular joint contents, including cartilage. The synoviocytes produce synovial fluid which passively circulates within the joint and is spontaneously absorbed and utilized by all tissues within the joint.

The normal synovial lining layer is one to three cells thick, and is composed of synoviocytes (synovial cells). Synovial cells are classified into types A and B based on differences in anatomy, cytochemical staining, and function.[14,15] The type A synoviocyte resembles a tissue macrophage and is characterized by a heterochromatin-rich nucleus, abundant cytoplasmic vacuoles, and a poorly developed rough endoplasmic reticulum. Type B synovial cells are the most common synoviocyte (approximately 70% of the total synovial cells) and resemble connective tissue fibroblasts. They are characterized by a pale nucleus, few vacuoles, a well-developed Golgi apparatus, and a prominent rough endoplasmic reticulum. A type C cell, intermediate between fibroblasts and macrophages, has also been identified and may have functions intermediate between A and B cells. The type A cells appear to function in a macrophage-like fashion, while the type B cells produce many of the important proteins found in synovial fluid.

The adipose layer contains blood vessels, adipose cells, loose connective tissue, nerve endings, and immune cells. The blood vessels form a rich vascular supply and are responsible for nourishing the intra-articular tissues and providing a conduit for the movement of fluid and inflammatory cells into the joint. The loose connective tissue allows for accommodation of the synovial membrane to joint movement. The synovial membrane is innervated by mechanoreceptors, nerve plexus, and free endings of unmyelinated nerves which are sensitive to the presence of inflammatory mediators. Immune cells which inhabit the normal synovial membrane include macrophages, dendritic cells, and lymphocytes, although the number and type of immune cells may vary in the presence of various inflammatory diseases.

11.1.7 Synovial Fluid

Synovial fluid performs a number of important functions, including: 1) nourishment of joint components, 2) providing lubrication factors for the joint cartilage, 3) allowing easy movement of the synovial membrane with weight bearing and joint motion, and 4) permitting the movement of inflammatory cells into the joint after trauma or infection.[16] Synovial fluid consists mainly of transudated fluid originating from the small capillaries of the synovial membrane. The small molecules present in synovial fluid closely resemble those in serum and include electrolytes, urate, urea, albumin, and small globulins. Certain molecules are increased within the joint fluid, such as hyaluronate and specialized proteins associated with lubrication.[10] Larger proteins such as fibrinogen, large globulins, and certain complementary components are excluded except in the presence of synovial membrane inflammation.[17] Antibiotics and anti-inflammatory drugs move into the synovial space from the blood by free diffusion and this rate is accelerated in the presence of inflammation. Increased pressure within the joint space from large synovial effusions may decrease the movement of small molecules into the joint space.

11.1.8 Intervertebral Discs

Intervertebral discs are a form of amphiarthrosis and link the vertebral bodies to one another.[1] Although the intervertebral facet joints, which are synovial joints, determine the range of motion in the spine and provide the largest measure of stability, the intervertebral discs are load-bearing structures which absorb both impact and load-force transmitted to the axial skeleton. The discs, the fibrous attachments, and the surrounding ligaments also provide a measure of stability independent of that provided by the facet joints. In fact, the disc must be normal for the facet joints to articulate properly. In disease states, the intervertebral discs can contribute significantly to morbidity and disability.

The intervertebral disc has a distinct anatomy consisting of three major components: 1) an outer fibrous restraining band (annulus fibrosis), 2) the central semi-fluid mass (nucleus pulposis), and 3) the superior and inferior surfaces (the vertebral cartilaginous plates).[2] The annulus fibrosis, composed of largely type I collagen, consists of concentric fibrous lamellae composed of alternating sheets of collagen and is enveloped and contiguous with the anterior and posterior longitudinal ligaments.

The nucleus pulposis consists of a largely acellular, viscid gel, composed of loose fibrous strands of collagen in a gelatinous proteoglycan matrix.[2,18,19] The cartilaginous end plates are composed of hyaline cartilage, but are remarkable in the fact that there is no discrete articular surface, that is, the *tangential or gliding zone* and its overlying *lamina splendens*, usually composed of fine fibers parallel to the surface, are completely absent. Instead of directly bearing load on an opposing cartilaginous structure, the vertebral cartilaginous end plate serves as an anchor for the fine filaments of the nucleus pulposis and the more extensive fibers of the annulus fibrosis.

The entire structure bears load by compressing the nucleus pulposis axially, which expands the width of the disc. The annulus fibrosis prevents the nucleus pulposis from escaping laterally and the load is thus distributed evenly without appreciable shock on the vertebral subchondral bone. When the load is removed, there is a loss of axial compression and the annulus fibrosis resumes its unloaded shape, forcing the nuclear gel back toward the center. The disc then regains its height. Failure of the vertebral discs or the vertebral facet joints can result in severe nerve root or cord compression, or may result in an abnormal distribution of load resulting in rapid degenerative changes or compression fracture.

11.2 THE DISEASED JOINT

The joint is a complex structure subject to the enormous forces of weight bearing and motion, and is extremely susceptible to injury. Congenital abnormalities, trauma, infection, neoplasms, metabolic disease, degenerative diseases, neurological disease, and inflammatory disease can all induce severe pathology within the joint. The broadest classification of diseases of joints are into three categories: 1) noninflammatory, 2) inflammatory, and 3) psychogenic (see Table 11.3). The following discussion will center on those conditions which are acquired and will exclude congenital abnormalities, acute trauma, mechanical abnormalities, neoplastic diseases, and infections which are examined in more detail in other chapters.

11.2.1 Evaluation of the Diseased Joint

The examination of the joint should include the following: 1) *careful history* (stiffness, pain, weakness, fatigue, trauma, joint swelling), 2) *inspection* (swelling, deformity, contracture, erythema), 3) *palpation* (tenderness, swelling, heat, spurs, crepitus), 3) *active and passive range of motion*, 4) *examination for ligamentous instability*, 5) *careful examination of all other joints*, 6) *observation of the patient during activities* (walking, bending, lifting), 7) *careful neurological examination including muscular strength*, 8) *radiographs of the affected area*, and 9) *synovial fluid analysis*. [20,21] Synovial fluid analysis is especially valuable and should always be undertaken during an initial evaluation if a palpable effusion is present.

11.2.2 Synovial Fluid Analysis

Physical examination, radiographs, appropriate blood tests, and synovial fluid examination together will usually result in the correct diagnosis of joint diseases.[22-25] Synovial fluid analysis is especially valuable because it can provide direct access to the joint in a benign manner and often will demonstrate abnormalities not obvious on physical or radiographic examination. Because of this, all joint effusions of unknown etiology should be aspirated and the synovial fluid analyzed. Immediately after arthrocentesis, the fluid should be transferred to a heparinized tube. Oxalated or citrated tubes should not be used because they may interfere with the crystal examination. Synovial fluid left in a syringe or non-heparinized tube may clot, resulting in false-negative microscopic examination.

Routine examination of synovial fluid should include 1) gross appearance, and 2) microscopic, 3) chemical, and 4) microbiological analyses (Table 11.2). The appearance of normal synovial fluid is usually off-white, but clear with impressive

TABLE 11.2
Routine Analysis of Synovial Fluid

Appearance	Microscopic	Microbiologic	Chemical
Volume	Total cell count	Gram stain	Glucose
Color	Differential cell count	Routine culture	
Clarity	Crystal examination	Special cultures	
Viscosity	(polarized and phase-contrast microscopy)	(fungi, viruses, mycobacteria)	
"Mucin clot"			

TABLE 11.3
Analysis of Synovial Fluids

Criteria	Normal	Non-Inflammatory (Group I)	Inflammator (Group II)	Purulent (Group III)	Hemorrhagic (Group IV)
1. Volume (ml)	<4	Often >4	Often >4	Often >4	Often >4
2. Color	Yellow	Xanthochromic	Xanthochromic white	White	Hemorrhagic
3. Clarity	Transparent	Translucent	Translucent or opaque	Opaque	Opaque
4. Mucin clot	Good	Fair to poor	Poor	Poor	Good
5. Spontaneous clot	None	Often	Often	Often	Often
6. Leukocytes (mm^{-3})	<150	<3,000	3,000-50,000	50,000-300,000	Variable
7. Red cells	Low	Low	Low	Low	Extremely high
8. Glucose	Normal	Normal	Normal or low	Low	Normal

viscosity. Microscopic examination should include total and differential cell counts and a crystal examination under polarized and phase-contrast microscopy.[23] Microbiological analysis is particularly valuable when the white cell count in the fluid is elevated and should include gram stain and routine bacteriological culture, although fungal, viral, and tuberculosis cultures are necessary in certain instances.[24] Of the chemical tests, usually joint glucose content is the only one with some interpretative value, although somewhat nonspecific. Occasionally, specialized studies are required such as countercurrent immunoelectrophoresis, complement, protein, or specialized enzymes, but these should not be done routinely.

Synovial fluids can be classified into five groups: 1) normal, 2) noninflammatory (Group I), 3) inflammatory (Group II), 4) purulent (Group III), and 5) hemorrhagic (Group IV) (Table 11.3). The diagnosis can rarely be made from synovial analysis alone, but results help classify the joint disease into a number of broad categories (Table 11.4). Occasionally, synovial biopsy may be necessary to confirm the diagnosis.

11.2.3 Diseases of Joints

The broad categories of joint disease include noninflammatory, inflammatory, and psychogenic. Noninflammatory joint diseases include osteoarthritis, metabolic arthritis, osteonecrosis, neuroarthropathy, and sympathetic dystrophies. Inflammatory diseases include the so-called autoimmune diseases such as rheumatoid arthritis, systemic lupus erythematosus, scleroderma, reactive arthritis, and other non-autoimmune diseases including septic arthritis and immune complex arthritis. Psychogenic diseases include primary fibrositis, restless leg syndrome, and hysteria. Although many of the major forms of arthritis will be discussed to some degree, particular emphasis will be placed on osteoarthritis. This disease is in many ways exemplary of the respective main categories of noninflammatory joint disease.

TABLE 11.4
Joint Disease and Synovial Fluid Analysis

Noninflammatory (Group I)	Inflammatory (Group II)	Purulent (Group III)	Hemorrhagic (Group IV)
Osteoarthritis	Rheumatoid arthritis	Bacteria	Trauma
Trauma	Reactive arthritis	Fungi	Neuroarthropathy
Osteochondritis dissecans	Viral arthritis	Tuberculosis	Blood dyscrasias
Sickle cell	Rheumatic fever	Joint prosthesis	Tumor
Osteonecrosis	Behcet's syndrome	Crystal synovitis	Anticoagulants
Osteochondromatosis	Fat droplet synovitis		Myeloproliferative diseases
Amyloidosis	Crystal synovitis		Thrombocytosis
	Systemic lupus erythematosus		
	Polyarteritis nodosa		
	Scleroderma		
	Polymyalgia rheumatica		
	Corticosteroid therapy		

11.3 NONINFLAMMATORY DISEASES OF JOINTS

11.3.1 Osteoarthritis

Osteoarthritis is not a single disease entity, but a collection of diseases which result in similar biochemical and structural changes in the joint cartilage, subchondral bone, and synovial membrane. Osteoarthritis is also known as degenerative joint disease, arthrosis, and osteoarthrosis. Osteoarthritis is classified as a noninflammatory disease, yet certain inflammatory changes are noted in the synovial membrane and surrounding articular tissues. Thus, the term *osteoarthritis* is more correct than the term *degenerative joint disease*, which implies a passive disease with little contribution of cellular activity.[26] As will be seen later, osteoarthritis is not a passive degenerative disease, but is an active process involving the direct participation by cartilage, synovial, and bone cells in the alteration of joint structure.[27] The term *osteoarthritis* also implies that anti-inflammatory drugs might be helpful to relieve the symptoms of this disease, as indeed they are.[28] Osteoarthritis is not, however, characterized by the intense cellular inflammation of the more classic inflammatory arthritides.

11.3.2 Clinical Symptoms and Signs

The diagnosis of osteoarthritis is usually made on the basis of the physical examination and radiographs, both of which are usually highly specific.[29-31] However, only 30% of patients with radiographically characteristic osteoarthritis complain of symptoms referable to the affected joints. Importantly, the presence of osteophytes alone occurs more often in those patients who may remain asymptomatic, while joint space narrowing, subchondral bone cysts, and eburnation with or without osteophytes most occur in those patients with symptoms characteristic of osteoarthritis.[32]

Osteoarthritis generally causes *pain* isolated to the affected joint, occurring with joint use and improved by rest. The pain is usually not sharp or localized, but most often is vague and aching in nature. As the disease progresses, the pain may become constant, especially at night. In some instances the symptoms of pain are disabling. *Stiffness* is a prominent feature of this disease and is especially evident upon rising in the morning and after periods of inactivity during the day. The stiffness of osteoarthritis is of short duration, usually lasting 15 to 20 minutes, compared to that of rheumatoid arthritis which persists for greater than 1 hour. The stiffness of osteoarthritis is often described as *articular gelling*.

Giving way of a joint may occur with seizing of the denuded articular surfaces, muscle spasm, muscle or capsular contracture, or obstruction of joint motion from impinging osteophytes or loose cartilage fragments. The patient often complains of a *cracking* or *popping* sensation (crepitus) within the affected joint which may or may not improve with continued use.

Physical examination may reveal no obvious changes or may demonstrate *acute or subacute inflammation* which sometimes resembles gout or rheumatoid arthritis. Subacute inflammation usually occurs in the hands and is associated with erosive (inflammatory) osteoarthritis.[30] Acute or subacute inflammation, sometimes associated with massive *effusions*, can also occur in the peripheral joints other than the hands and is associated with the presence of calcium pyrophosphate deposition disease or other related crystal arthropathies.[33,34] *Synovial thickening* may also occur in erosive (inflammatory) osteoarthritis, but is more characteristic of rheumatoid arthritis and other chronic inflammatory arthritides than of osteoarthritis.[35] *Crepitus* is usually palpated as the joint is put through its range motion and is related to the changed architecture of the osteoarthritic joint. The joint contour is often altered due to the presence of *marginal osteophytes* and remodeling of the adjacent bone (squaring). In the case of erosive osteoarthritis, the axial orientation of the joint may be changed, causing a deformity.[32]

The *pattern of joint involvement* in osteoarthritis is characteristic, involving the distal interphalangeal joints (Heberden's nodes), the proximal interphalangeal joints (Bouchard's nodes), the first carpometacarpal joint (shelf sign), the trapezioscaphoid joint, first metatarsophalangeal joint (bunion), the acromioclavicular joint, and temporomandibular joints.[36] The medial and patellofemoral compartments are most frequently affected in the knee, although the lateral compartment can also be involved, especially in the presence of crystal deposition disease.[32,37,38] Involvement of the hip, *malum coxae senilis* or *morbus coxae senilis*, induces decreased range of motion and an *antalgic gait* and is common, especially in the elderly.[39] *Isolated involvement* of one joint with osteoarthritis implies severe injury to that specific joint and may occur subsequent to trauma, infection, osteonecrosis, congenital deformity, joint instability, or some other localized process.[40-42]

11.3.3 Osteoarthritis of the Spine

The spine is also commonly affected in the various forms of osteoarthritis.[43] Osteoarthritis of the spine results from degenerative changes in the intervertebral fibrocartilaginous discs, damage to the vertebral bodies, and degeneration of the posterior apophyseal joints.[18,19] Subluxation of the apophyseal joints may occur from the instability induced by disc space narrowing. Osteophytosis of the anterior surface of the vertebral bodies is common and in the cervical spine may induce dysphagia. Occasionally, osteoarthritic changes in the intervertebral discs are termed *degenerative disc disease* or *spondylosis* to distinguish these changes from those in diarthrodial joints. Although this distinction recognizes the slightly different radiologic changes of osteoarthritis in diarthrodial verses amphiarthrodial joints, it is on the whole merely a semantic distinction.

Osteoarthritis of the spine causes pain and stiffness, as it does in other affected joints, but more frequently is associated with radiculation and muscle spasm. *Nerve root compression* or *spinal stenosis* may occur from encroachment of the neural space by osteophytosis, prolapse of the nucleus pulposis of a degenerated intervertebral disc, or subluxation from apophyseal joint instability.[43] These changes most frequently occur in the cervical spine, but can also occur in the other areas as well, especially the lumbar spine. Upper or lower motor neurons may be affected depending whether peripheral nerve, nerve root, or spinal cord are being compressed, resulting in radiculation, weakness, pain, and disability. Occasionally, compression of the spinal or vertebral arteries may occur, resulting in central cord syndrome or direct cerebral abnormalities.

A specialized form of osteoarthritis is *ankylosing hyperostosis*, which is also known as *Forestier's disease* and *diffuse idiopathic skeletal hyperostosis* (DISH).[44,45] DISH is characterized by a florid hyperostosis of the spine resulting in anterior osseous ridges with fusion and calcification of the anterior longitudinal ligament and peripheral disc margins, especially in the anterior and right lateral aspects of the spine (Figure 11.3). Pain is usually minimal and the findings on radiographs are often incidental. To differentiate DISH from ordinary osteoarthritis and ankylosing spondylitis, the following criteria must be present: 1) flowing ossification along the anterolateral aspect of at least four contiguous vertebra, 2) preservation of disc height, 3) absence of vacuum phenomena or vertebral body marginal sclerosis, and 4) absence of apophyseal and sacroiliac joint erosions, sclerosis, or fusion. DISH can also have peripheral manifestations characterized by hyperostoses or "whiskering" in the heel, elbows, ilium, shoulders, hips, knees, and ankles.

11.3.4 Laboratory and Radiologic Examination

The laboratory evaluation of osteoarthritis is usually unremarkable. Erythrocyte sedimentation rate, blood counts, urinalysis, and autoimmune serologies are negative. *Synovial fluid* is usually noninflammatory (Group I) with only a slight increase in white blood cells, sloughed collagen fibers, and, in patients with recurrent effusions, cholesterol crystals. Synovial fluid analysis is important to exclude crystal synovitis, especially calcium pyrophosphate deposition disease, basic calcium phosphate, and gout.

The radiographic changes of osteoarthritis are variable, but tend to increase with the degree of joint pathology (Figure 11.4). In the early stages of osteoarthritis the radiographs are usually normal. Typical changes include irregular narrowing of the joint space, subchondral bony sclerosis (eburnation), marginal osteophyte formation,

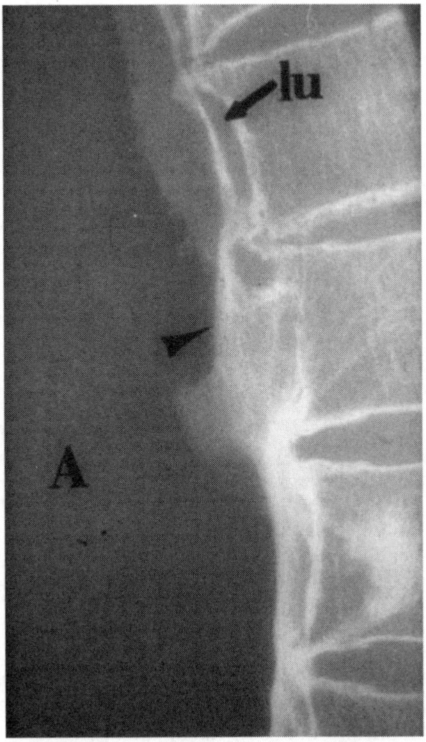

FIGURE 11.3 Diffuse Idiopathic Skeletal Hyperostosis (DISH). This radiograph demonstrates DISH with flowing longitudinal ossification (arrowhead) with a gap of radiolucency (arrow) beneath this new bone. The resulting appearance (dripping candle wax) is typical of this disease. (Reproduced with permission of the American College of Rheumatology.)

bone cysts (pseudocysts), bony collapse, and, finally, gross deformity with subluxation and loose bodies.[27,29-36] Osteophyte formation is the most nonspecific of these signs and may occur in the absence of other more typical changes.[32] In these cases osteophytes are probably not an indicator of osteoarthritis, but rather an osteoblastic process related to ligamentous insertions. Standard radiographs are usually sufficient to detect the abnormalities associated with osteoarthritis, but computed tomography (CT) and magnetic resonance imaging (MRI) are often useful when evaluating the spine.

11.3.5 Pathology of Osteoarthritis

The pathological changes of osteoarthritis closely parallel those abnormalities evident on roentgenographic studies. The earliest change noted in the articular cartilage is focal loss of metachromasia (decreased proteoglycans) which is associated with a softening of the cartilage, described as focal chondromucoid softening (Figure 11.5).[26,27,42,46] With the loss of proteoglycans, the cartilage loses elasticity and the sheer forces disrupt the normal collagen fibers, resulting in microfissures, which in turn are associated with a proliferation of chondrocytes on the borders of these lesions (Figure 11.6).

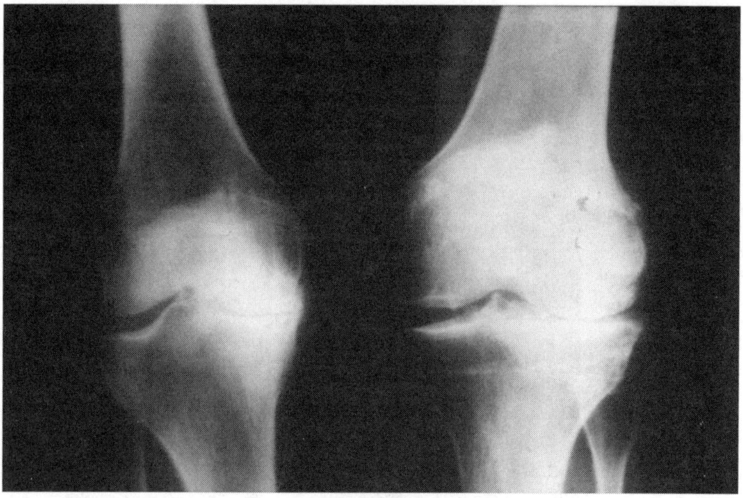

FIGURE 11.4 Radiograph of Osteoarthritis. This posteroanterior projection demonstrates severe narrowing of the medial compartment on the left and similar changes of the lateral compartment on the right. Sclerosis of the adjacent bone is evident, as well as remodeling of the joint surfaces with flattening on the femoral condyles and elongation of the margins of the tibia. On the right lateral aspect of the tibia, subchondral cysts are present (pseudocysts). The irregular joint space narrowing, pseudocysts, and reactive new bone formation all suggest osteoarthritis (degenerative joint disease) rather than an inflammatory arthritis. (Reproduced with permission of the American College of Rheumatology.)

The role of the chondrocytes may not be passive, but may actually result in further absorption of matrix and more rapid progression of the disease.[7] In some cases the chondrocytes form clusters, producing proteoglycan, but little or no collagen. As the disease progresses, the surface of the cartilage is disrupted further, resulting in fibrillation of the collagen fibers and then frank erosion. New mixed hyaline and fibrocartilage is created by nests of proliferating chondrocytes, especially over the surface of osteophytes. Eventually the cartilage may be completely denuded, exposing the underlying bony end plate.

New bone formation occurs at two sites: 1) the osteophytic excrescences, and 2) subchondral and subcortical bone.[47] Marginal osteophytes may develop into isolated protuberances in the joint space or may follow the capsular and ligamentous attachments at the joint margins. The osteophyte is composed of cortical and cancellous bone which extends from and is contiguous with the normal subchondral and cancellous bone of the joint.[42] The osteophyte is covered by a layer of composite hyaline and fibrocartilage which is subsumed by the synovial space. *Eburnation*, a smooth, ivory-like appearance to the bone, occurs especially in areas of denuded subcortical bone and is histologically characterized by bony proliferation, empty lacuna, and increased bone density.

Cystic areas of bone commonly occur beneath the eburnated cortical surface and contain fragments of dead bone, cartilage, amorphous debris, and, occasionally, pockets of mucoid fluid. These *pseudocysts* are characterized by microfractures in

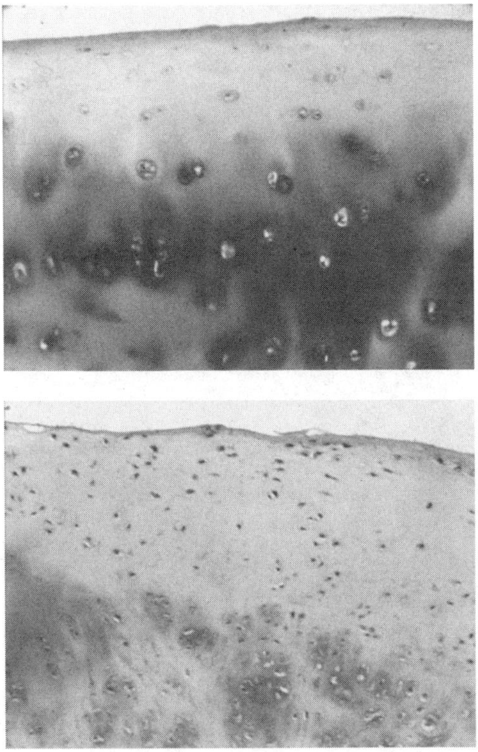

FIGURE 11.5 Normal and Osteoarthritic Hyaline Cartilage. The upper figure demonstrates normal hyaline cartilage stained with Safranin-O which binds to acid mucopolysaccharide. As can be seen, acid mucopolysaccharide is diffusely present except for the area closest to the articular surface (lamina splendans). In contrast, osteoarthritic cartilage demonstrates diffuse hypercellularity, extensive loss of mucopolysaccharide, and early disruption of the articular surface. (Reproduced with permission of the American College of Rheumatology.)

the overlying cortical bone and cartilage, and allow intra-articular pressure to be transmitted directly to the underlying bone, which presumably results in further bone degeneration.[48] Focal ossific metaplasia occurs at the base of the articular cartilage and results in remodeling of the joint contour in which new bone is added to a portion of the articular cortex, while adjacent areas are reabsorbed in a focal fashion. Much of the deformity of osteoarthritis is related to new bone formation and the collapse of adjacent bone, processes which may be associated with both hypovascularity and hypervascularity. Other forms of osteoarthritis, despite their diverse etiologies, have similar pathology.[49-59]

11.3.6 Osteonecrosis

Osteonecrosis is a condition characterized by the ischemic death of the cellular constituents of bone and bone marrow. This condition is also known as avascular necrosis, aseptic necrosis, and osseous ischemia.[61-65] Etiologies include trauma (especially of

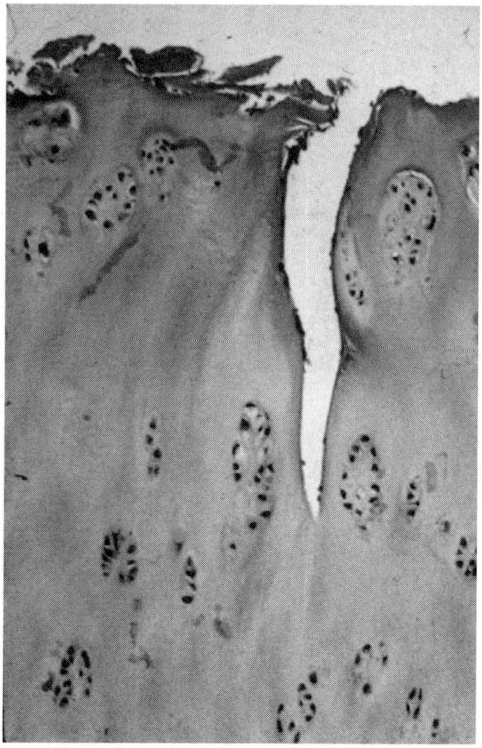

FIGURE 11.6 Osteoarthritic Cartilage. This microscopic section demonstrates the early changes of osteoarthritis with clumping of chondrocytes, small tangential clefts on the surface of the already altered hyaline cartilage, and a deeper vertical fissure. (Reproduced with permission of the American College of Rheumatology.)

the hip), chemotherapy, corticosteroids, decompression injuries, and others. Pathologically, the disease has a number of different stages.[66,67] Early in the course the patient is asymptomatic and severe symptoms usually do not appear until late in the disease when subchondral collapse is imminent or has occurred. In Stage 0, I, or II core decompression with cortical grafting may be successful in preventing further collapse, but these patients usually are asymptomatic until irreversible damage has occurred.[68] Osteonecrosis is first invisible to standard roentgenograms, but can be detected by MRI or radionuclide bone scan. Later on, radiographic changes include demineralization, sclerosis, mottled densities, and, eventually, structural collapse (subchondral fracture) (Figure 11.7). Stages III and IV are characterized by severe, disabling symptoms which often necessitate total joint arthroplasty.

11.3.7 Reflex Sympathetic Dystrophy

Reflex sympathetic dystrophy (RSD) is characterized by 1) pain and tenderness in an extremity, 2) signs and symptoms of vasomotor instability, 3) swelling in the affected extremity, and 4) dystrophic skin changes.[69] RSD is also known as causalgia,

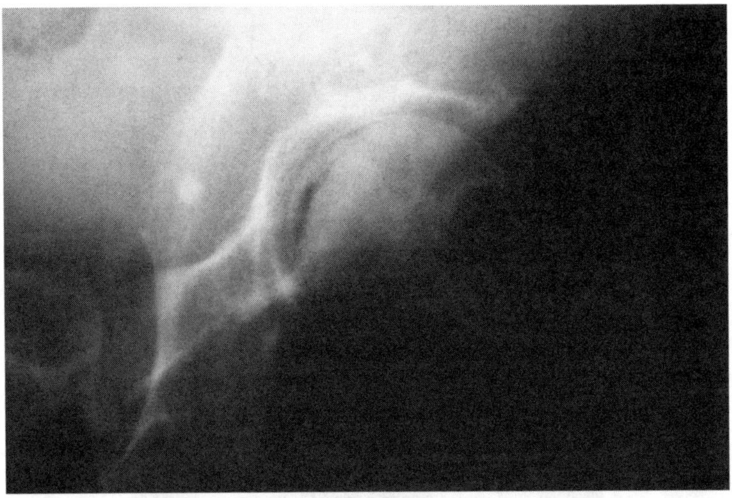

FIGURE 11.7 Osteonecrosis. This radiograph demonstrates the evolving changes of osteonecrosis (avascular necrosis, aseptic necrosis) in the hip. The joint space is maintained, the subchondral bone has lost its sharp margins, and the underlying trabeculae are hazy. A radiolucent line is present under the subchondral bone and represents cleavage or fracture through an area of partially reabsorbed and weakened bone. As this lesion progresses, the articular surface will fracture, sclerosis will develop, and the femoral head will flatten or collapse, resulting in severe pain and disability. (Reproduced with permission of the American College of Rheumatology.)

Sudeck's atrophy, should-hand syndrome, algodystrophy, traumatic angiospasm, and post-traumatic osteoporosis.[70] RSD can be disabling and induces swelling and contracture of an affected extremity. The etiologies of RSD are quite diverse. In orthopedic practice, RSD most often occurs after surgery or injury to an extremity, and is often manifested in a patient who has persistent pain and swelling despite adequate orthopedic therapy for the original disorder.[71]

Radiographs may demonstrate patchy or mottled osteopenia and erosive changes suggesting rheumatoid arthritis or neoplasm may be present.[72] 99m-Technetium bone scans demonstrate increased uptake and increased or decreased blood flow in the affected extremity.[73] This syndrome is thought to involve overstimulation of both the peripheral autonomic and central nervous systems, although local inflammation may also play a role.[69,74] Prevention of the syndrome is of the greatest importance and can usually be accomplished by early mobilization. RSD can be treated with physical therapy, sympathetic blockade, corticosteroids, vasodilator drugs, and analgesics.[75] Therapy should be instituted early, as the more advanced cases of hard contracture are difficult to reverse.

11.3.8 Neuropathic Joint

The neuropathic joint is a rapidly progressive destructive arthropathy of peripheral joints associated with an underlying neuropathy.[76] Synonyms include neurarthropathy, neuropathic arthropathy, neurotrophic arthropathy, Charcot joint, and neurogenic

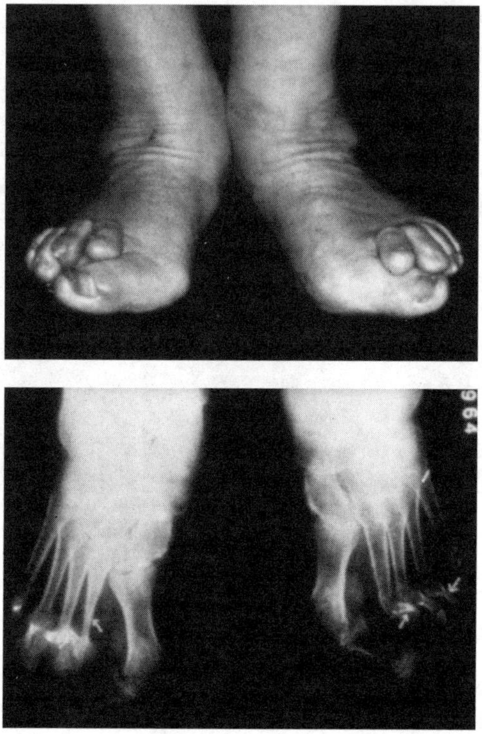

FIGURE 11.8 Neuropathic Joint. The most common neuropathic joints encountered by the orthopedic surgeon occurs in the setting of diabetic neuroarthropathy. The upper photograph demonstrates the typical changes of neuroarthropathy in the foot with spread of the forefoot, hallux valgus, and overlapping of adjacent toes. The radiograph shows complete disorganization of the metatarsophalangeal joints and tapering of the metatarsal shafts (osteolysis). Involvement of the midfoot and forefoot is most common, but occasionally the ankle or knee can also be affected. (Reproduced with permission of the American College of Rheumatology.)

arthropathy.[77] Neuropathic joints can occur as a complication to a host of different conditions but in modern industrialized societies occur most commonly in patients with diabetes mellitus.[78-82] In these patients, the joint destruction is largely confined to the foot and ankle[83] (Figure 11.8).

Most patients have minimal or vague pain and eventually seek help after they develop a limp and swelling in the midfoot, forefoot, or ankle. In some patients painless deformity, especially collapse of the midfoot (rocker bottom feet), is already present. Synovial fluid is usually noninflammatory, but may be xanthochromic and hemorrhagic, or may contain CPPD crystals.[84] Physical examination reveals swelling, typical deformities and the presence of a sensory neuropathy.

Radiographs demonstrate swelling, osteoporosis, para-articular debris, bony fragmentation, fractures, absorption of subchondral bone, and sclerosis. Malalignment with angular deformity and subluxation contribute to deformity. In diabetes, resorption of the distal metatarsals or phalanxes may occur (osteolysis). Although repetitive trauma to any denervated unprotected extremity is important, invasion of

TABLE 11.5
Disease Associations of Hypertrophic Osteoarthropathy (HPO)

Primary HPO	
Pachydermoperiostosis; Touraine-Solente-Gole syndrome	
Secondary HPO	
Pulmonary neoplasms	Lung abscess
Bronchiectasis	Chronic bronchitis
Empyema	Chronic pneumonitis
Pneumoconiosis	Pulmonary tuberculosis
Mediastinal Hodgkin's disease	Sarcoidosis
Congenital malformations of heart	Cystic Fibrosis
Ulcerative colitis	Regional enteritis
Amebic colitis	Subphrenic abscess
Cirrhosis	Idiopathic steatorrhea
Neoplasms of small intestine	Sprue
Multiple colonic polyposis	Carcinoma of GI track
Cholangiolitic cirrhosis	Hepatic amyloidosis
Thyroid disease	Pregnancy
Connective tissue diseases	Purgative abuse
Hyperparathyroidism	Thyroid acropachy

the surrounding bone by hypervascular tissue associated with neuropathy may be the cause of the resorptive changes. CPPD crystals may also contribute to the destructive arthropathy. Treatment includes appropriate stable footwear, splinting, arthrodesis, and treatment of the underlying neuropathy. Total joint replacements, although sometimes successful, are generally contraindicated for neuropathic disease.

11.3.9 Hypertrophic Osteoarthropathy

Hypertrophic osteoarthropathy (HPO) is characterized by clubbing of the fingers and toes, periostitis of the long bones, and arthritis.[85] Primary HPO is hereditary and occurs most often in children.[86] Secondary HPO can be insidious as the hypertrophic pulmonary osteoarthropathy, or can manifest as a rapidly progressive syndrome with joint pain and stiffness associated with malignant disease.[87-89] Diseases associated with HPO are shown in Table 11.5. Periostitis may be asymptomatic or may induce a deep, aching pain, burning, and tenderness along the shafts of the long bones. The arthritis may be oligo- or polyarticular and may be associated with effusions. Synovial fluid is noninflammatory (Group I). Radiographs demonstrate subperiosteal new bone layering in the distal diaphyseal regions and 99m-Tc diphosphonate bone scans demonstrate a pericortical linear accumulation along the long bone and phalanges. Pathology is characterized by mild inflammation and hypervascularization. Treatment includes anti-inflammatory agents, chemical vagotomy, corticosteroids, and treatment of the underlying disorder.

REFERENCES

1. Gray, H.: *Anatomy of the Human Body,* 29th ed. Edited by C.M. Gross. Philadelphia, Lea & Febiger, 1973.
2. Mankin, H.J. and Radin, E.: Structure and function of joints. In: *Arthritis and allied conditions. A Textbook of Rheumatology.* Edited by William J. Koopman. Philadelphia, Williams & Wilkins, 1997, pp.175-192.
3. Hammerman, D., Rosenberg, L.D., and Schubert, M.: Diarthrodial joints revisited. *J. Bone Joint Surg.* 52A:725-774, 1970.
4. Davies, D. and Palfray, A.: Studies on the anatomy and function of bones and joints. In: *Pathology of Rheumatoid Arthritis.* Edited by F. Evans. Berlin, Springer-Verlag, 1966, pp.130-143.
5. Mankin, H.J.: The articular cartilage, cartilage healing, and osteoarthrosis. In: *Adult Orthopedics.* Edited by R.L. Cruess and W.R.J. Renme. New York, Churchill-Livingstone, 1984, pp. 163-270.
6. Lane, J.M. and Weiss, C.: Current comment: review of articular cartilage collagen research. *Arthritis Rheum.* 18:553-562, 1975.
7. Dingle, J.T.: The effect of synovial catabolism on cartilage synthetic activity. *Connect. Tissue Res.* 12:277-286, 1984.
8. Gardner, E.: The physiology of joints. *J. Bone Joint Surg.* 45A:1061-1066, 1963.
9. Mow, V.C. and Mansour, J.M.: The nonlinear interaction between cartilage deformation and interstitial fluid flow. *J. Biomech.* 10:31-39, 1977.
10. Swann, D.A. and Radin, E.L.: The molecular basis of articular lubrication. I. Purification and properties of a lubricating fraction from bovine synovial fluid. *J. Biol. Chem.* 274:8069-8073, 1972.
11. Brantigan, O.C. and Voshell, A.F.: Mechanics of ligaments and menisci of the knee joint. *J. Bone Joint Surg.* 23A:44-66, 1941.
12. Amiel, D. et al.: Tendons and ligaments: a morphological and biochemical comparison. *J. Orthop. Res.* 1:257-265, 1984.
13. Gradially, F.N.: Fine structure of the joints. In: *The Joints and Synovial Fluid.* Edited by L. Sokoloff. New York, Academic Press, 1978, pp.110-120.
14. Mueller-Ladner, U., Gay, R.E., and Gay, S.: Structure and function of synoviocytes. In: *Arthritis and Allied Conditions. A Textbook of Rheumatology.* Edited by William J. Koopman. Philadelphia, Williams & Wilkins, 1997, pp. 243-254.
15. Krane, S.M.: Aspects of the cell biology of the rheumatoid synovial lesions. *Ann. Rheum. Dis.* 40:433-448, 1981.
16. McCarty, D.J.: Synovial Fluid. In: *Arthritis and Allied Conditions. A Textbook of Rheumatology.* Edited by William J. Koopman. Philadelphia, Williams & Wilkins, 1997, pp. 81-102.
17. Cho, N.H. and Neuhaus, O.W.: Absence of blood clotting substances from synovial fluid. *Thrombosis et Diathesis Haemorrhagica* 5:108-111, 1960.
18. Coventry, M.B.: Anatomy of the intervertebral disc. *Clin. Orthop.* 67:9-15, 1969.
19. Park, W.W. and Schiff, D.C.M.: The applied anatomy of the intervertebral disc. *Orthop. Clin. North. Am.* 2:309-324, 1971.
20. Polley, H.F. and Hunder, G.G.: *Rheumatological Interviewing and Physical Examination of the Joints,* 2nd ed. Philadelphia, W.B. Saunders, 1978.
21. McCarty, D.J.: Differential diagnosis of arthritis: analysis of signs and symptoms. In: *Arthritis and Allied Conditions. A Textbook of Rheumatology.* Edited by William J. Koopman. Philadelphia, Williams & Wilkins, 1997, pp.35-46.

22. Schumacher, H.R. et al.: Reproductivity of synovial fluid analyses. *Arthritis Rheum.* 29:770-774, 1986.
23. Gatter, R.A.: The compensated polarized light microscope in clinical rheumatology. *Arthritis Rheum.* 17:253-255, 1974.
24. Krey, R.P. and Bailen, D.A.: Synovial fluid leukocytosis: a study of extremes. *Am. J. Med.* 67:436-442, 1979.
25. Gatter, R.A.: *A practical handbook of joint fluid analysis*. Philadelphia, Lea & Febiger, 1984.
26. Ilardi, C.F. and Sokoloff, L.: The pathology of osteoarthritis: ten strategic questions of pharmacologic management. *Semin. Arthritis Rheum.* 11(Suppl. 1):3-7, 1981.
27. Fabry, G. and Mulier, J.C.: Biochemical analyses in osteoarthritis of the hip: A correlative study between glycosaminoglycan loss, enzyme activity, and radiologic signs. *Clin. Orthop.* 153:253-264, 1980.
28. Tokunaga, M. et al.: Change of prostaglandin E level in joint fluids after treatment with flurbiprofen in patients with rheumatoid arthritis and osteoarthritis. *Ann. Rheum. Dis.* 40:462-465, 1981.
29. Havdrup, T., Hulth, A., and Telhag, H.: The subchondral bone in osteoarthritis ad rheumatoid arthritis of the knee. A histological and microradiographical study. *Acta Orthop. Scand.* 47:345-350, 1976.
30. Utsinger, P.D. et al.: Roentgenologic, immunologic, and therapeutic study of erosive (inflammatory) osteoarthritis. *Arch. Intern. Med.* 138:693-697, 1978.
31. Yazici, H. et al.: Primary osteoarthrosis of the knee or hip. *JAMA* 231:1256-1260, 1975.
32. Hernborg, J.S. and Nilsson, B.E.: The relationship between osteophytes in the knee joint, osteoarthritis, and aging. *Acta Orthop. Scand.* 44:69-74, 1973.
33. Halvorsen, P.B. and McCarty, D.J.: Patterns of radiographic abnormalities associated with basic calcium phosphate and calcium pyrophosphate dihydrate deposition in the knee. *Ann. Rheum. Dis.* 45:603-605, 1986.
34. McCarty, D.J. et al.: Diseases associated with calcium pyrophosphate dihydrate crystal deposition — a controlled study. *Am. J. Med.* 56:704-714, 1974.
35. Goldenberg, D.L., Egan, M.S., and Cohen, A.S.: Inflammatory synovitis in degenerative joint disease. *J. Rheumatol.* 9:204-209, 1982.
36. Moskowitz, R.W.: Clinical and laboratory findings in osteoarthritis. In: *Arthritis and Allied Conditions. A Textbook of Rheumatology.* Edited by William J. Koopman. Philadelphia, Williams & Wilkins, 1997, pp. 1985-2012.
37. Goodfellow, J., Hungerford, D.S., and Wood, C.: Patello-femoral joint mechanics and pathology. 2. Chondromalacia patellae. *J. Bone Joint Surg.* 58B:291-299, 1976.
38. Meachim, G.: Age-related degeneration of patellar articular cartilage. *J. Anat.* 134:365-371, 1982.
39. Macys, J.R., Bullough, P.G., and Wilson, P.D., Jr.: Coxarthrosis: a study of the natural history based on a correlation of clinical, radiographic, and pathologic findings. Semin. Arthritis Rheum. 10:66-80, 1980.
40. Peyron, J.G.: Epidemiologic and etiologic approach of osteoarthritis. *Semin. Arthritis Rheum.* 8:288-306, 1979.
41. Bird, H.A., Tribe, C.R., and Bacon, P.A.: Joint hypermobility leading to osteoarthrosis and chondrocalcinosis. *Ann. Rheum. Dis.* 37:203-211, 1978.
42. Thompson, R.C., Jr. and Bassett, C.A.L.: Histological observations on experimentally induced degeneration of articular cartilage. *J. Bone Joint Surg.* 52:435-443, 1970.
43. Arnoldi, C.C., Brodsky, A.E., and Cauchoix, J.: Lumbar spinal stenosis and nerve root entrapment syndromes-Definition and classification. *Clin. Orthop.* 115:4-5, 1976.

44. Utsinger, P.D., Resnick, D., and Shapiro, R.: Diffuse skeletal abnormalities in Forestier disease. *Arch. Intern. Med.* 136:763-768, 1976.
45. Resnick, D. et al.: Diffuse idiopathic hyperostosis (DISH) (ankylosing hyperostosis of Forestier and Rotes-Querol). *Semin. Arthritis Rheum.* 7:153-187, 1978.
46. Christensen, S.B. and Reimann, I.: Differential histochemical staining of glycosaminoglycans in the matrix of osteoarthritic cartilage. *Acta Pathol. Microbiol. Scand.* 88:61-68, 1980.
47. Milgram, J.W.: Morphologic alterations in the subchondral bone in advanced degenerative arthritis. *Clin. Orthop.* 173:293-312, 1983.
48. Radin, E.L., et al.: Response of joints to impact loading. III. Relationship between trabecular microfractures and cartilage degeneration. *J. Biomech.* 6:51-57, 1973.
49. Sokoloff, L.: Endemic forms of osteoarthritis. *Clin. Rheum. Dis.* 11:187-202, 1985.
50. Mainardi, C.L. et al.: Proliferative synovitis in hemophilia: biochemical and morphological observations. *Arthritis Rheum.* 21:137-144, 1978.
51. O'Brien, W.M., La Du, B.N., and Bunim, J.J.: Biochemical, pathological and clinical aspects of alcaptonuria, ochronosis, and ochronotic arthropathy: Review of world literature (1584-1962). *Am. J. Med.* 34:813-838, 1963.
52. Golding, D.N. and Walshe, J.M.: Arthropathy of Wilson's disease. A study of clinical and radiological features in 32 patients. *Ann. Rheum. Dis.* 36:99-111, 1977.
53. Hamilton, E. et al.: Idiopathic hemochromatosis. *Q.J. Med.* 145:171-182, 1968.
54. Schumacher, H.R.: Articular cartilage in the degenerative arthropathy of hemochromatosis. *Arthritis Rheum.* 25:1460-1468, 1982.
55. Nesterov, A.I.: The clinical course of Kashin-Beck disease. *Arthritis Rheum.* 29:660-664, 1986.
56. Bluestone, R. et al.: Acromegalic arthropathy. *Ann. Rheum. Dis.* 30:243-258, 1971.
57. Moskowitz, R.W. et al.: Experimentally induced corticosteroid arthropathy. *Arthritis Rheum.* 13:236-243, 1970.
58. Glick, R. and Parhami, N.: Frostbite arthritis. *J. Rheumatol.* 6:456-460, 1979.
59. Jones, J.P., Jr.: Osteonecrosis. In: *Arthritis and Allied Conditions. A Textbook of Rheumatology.* Edited by William J. Koopman. Philadelphia, Williams & Wilkins, 1997, pp. 1923-1944.
60. Roeder, L.F., Jr. and DeLee, J.C.: Femoral head fractures associated with posterior hip dislocations. *Clin. Orthop.* 147:121-130, 1980.
61. Jones, J.P., Jr.: Fat embolism and osteonecrosis. *Orthop. Clin. North Am.* 16:595-633, 1985.
62. Jacobs, B.: Epidemiology of traumatic and nontraumatic osteonecrosis. *Clin. Orthop.* 130:51-67, 1978.
63. Ficat, R.P. and Arlet, J.: *Ischemia and bone necrosis*. Baltimore, Williams & Wilkins, 1980.
64. Johnson, L.C.: Histogenesis of avascular necrosis. In: *Proceedings of the Conference of Aseptic Necrosis of the Femoral Head.* U.S. Public Health Service. St. Louis, Missouri, 1964, pp. 55-79.
65. Glimcher, M.J. and Kenzora, J.E.: The biology of osteonecrosis of the human femoral head and its clinical implications. I. Tissue biology. *Clin. Orthop.* 138:284-309, 1979.
66. Alavi, A., McCloskey, J.R., and Steinberg, M.E.: Early detection of avascular necrosis of the femoral head by 99-technetium diphosphonate bone scan: a preliminary report. *Clin. Orthop.* 127:137-141, 1977.
67. Bassett, L.W. et al.: Magnetic resonance imaging in the early diagnosis of ischemic necrosis of the femoral head: preliminary results. *Clin. Orthop.* 214:237-248, 1987.

68. Camp, J.F. and Colwell, C.W., Jr.: Core decompression of the femoral head for osteonecrosis. *J. Bone Joint Surg.* 68(A):1313-1319, 1986.
69. Kozin, F. et al.: The reflex sympathetic dystrophy syndrome (RSDS) III. Scintigraphic studies, further evidence for the therapeutic efficacy of systemic corticosteroids, and proposed diagnostic criteria. *Am. J. Med.* 70:23-30, 1981.
70. Kozin, F.: The reflex sympathetic dystrophy syndrome. *Bull. Rheum. Dis.* 36:1-8, 1986.
71. Cooney, W.P., Dobyns, J.H., and Linscheid, R.L.: Complications of Colle's fracture. *J. Bone Joint Surg.* 62A:613-619, 1980.
72. Jones, G.: Radiological appearances of disuse osteoporosis. *Clin. Radiol.* 20:345-353, 1969.
73. Gaucher, A. et al.: The diagnostic value of 99m-Tc-diphosphonate bone imaging in transient osteoporosis of the hip. *J. Rheumatol.* 6:774, 1979.
74. Drucker, W.R. et al.: Pathogenesis of post-traumatic sympathetic dystrophy. *Am. J. Surg.* 97:454-465, 1979.
75. Kozin, F. et al.: The reflex sympathetic dystrophy syndrome. 1. Clinical and histologic studies: Evidence for bilaterality, response to corticosteroids, and articular involvement. *Am. J. Med.* 60:321-331, 1976.
76. Ellman, M.H.: Neuropathic joint disease (Charcot Joints) In: *Arthritis and allied conditions. A Textbook of Rheumatology.* Edited by William J. Koopman. Philadelphia, Williams & Wilkins, 1997, pp. 1641-1660.
77. Bruckner, F.E. and Howell, A.: Neuropathic joints. *Semin. Arthritis Rheum.* 2:47-69, 1972.
78. Frykberg, R.G.: Neuropathic arthropathy: The diabetic Charcot foot. *Diabetes Educator* 9:17-20, 1984.
79. O'Conner, B.L., Palmoski, M.J., and Brandt, K.D.: Neurogenic acceleration of degenerative joint lesions. *J. Bone Joint Surg.* 67A:562-572, 1985.
80. Steinberg, C.L., Duthie, R.B., and Piva, A.E.: Charcot-like arthropathy following intra-articular hydrocortisone. *JAMA* 181:851-854, 1962.
81. Chillag, K.J. and Stevens, D.B.: Idiopathic neurogenic arthropathy. *J. Pediatar. Orthop.* 5:597-600, 1985.
82. Soudry, M. et al.: Total knee arthroplasty in Charcot and Charcot-like joints. *Clin. Orthop.* 208:199-204, 1986.
83. Kraft, E., Spyropoulos, E., and Finby, N.: Neurogenic disorders of the foot in diabetes mellitus. *AJR* 124:17-24, 1975.
84. Helms, C.A., Chapman, G.S., and Wild, J.H.: Charcot-like joints in calcium pyrophosphate dihydrate deposition disease. *Skeletal Radiol.* 7:55-58, 1981.
85. Altman, R. D.: Hypertrophic osteoarthropathy. In: *Arthritis and Allied Conditions. A Textbook of Rheumatology.* Edited by William J. Koopman. Philadelphia, Williams & Wilkins, 1997, pp. 1751-1761.
86. Hedayanti, H., Barmada, R., and Skosey, J.L.: Acrolysis in pachydermoperiostosis. *Arch. Intern. Med.* 140:1087-1088, 1980.
87. Marinez-Lavin, M.: Digital clubbing and hypertrophic osteoarthropathy: a unifying hypothesis. *J. Rheumatol.* 14:6-8, 1987.
88. Jajic, I. et al.: primary hypertrophic osteoarthropathy (HPO) and changes in the joints. *Scand. J. Rheumatol.* 9:89-96, 1980.
89. Ali, A. et al.: Distribution of hypertrophic pulmonary osteoarthropathy. *Am. J. Roentgenol.* 134:771-780, 1980.

12 Neuromuscular Function and the Skeleton

George E. Omer, Jr.

CONTENTS

12.1 NORMAL PERIPHERAL NERVE AND SKELETAL MUSCLE FUNCTION

Nerve cells, termed neurons, have the unique ability to communicate precisely, rapidly, and over long distances with one another and with other tissues, such as muscles. A typical neuron has four morphologicalty distinct regions: dendrites, cell body, axon, and presynaptic terminal.[1] Dendrites are processes that branch off the cell body and serve as the main apparatus for receiving input from other neurons. The cell body, or perikaryon, contains the nucleus and is the metabolic center of the neuron; in the cell body proteins are synthesized, assembled into macromolecules and transported down the axon via axoplasmic transport. The cell bodies are situated in the spinal cord (motor), the dorsal root ganglion (sensory), and sympathetic ganglia (sympathetic). A cell body is related to only one axon. The axon usually contains more than 90% of the total cytoplasmic surface of the neuron.[2] The axon, or nerve fiber, is the primary conducting unit of the neuron and arises from a specialized region of the cell body, the axon hillock, and from which the all-or-none action potential is initiated. The presynaptic terminals are fine specialized endings of the axon nearest its target organ or termination site; they are responsible for transmitting information from the neuron to the dendrites of another neuron or to a postsynaptic receptor such as the neuromuscular junction.

The proteins required to maintain the structural integrity of the axon, to support action potential propagation, and to enable neurotransmitter release at the presynaptic

0-8493-9237-3/99/$0.00+$.50

terminals are produced only in the cell body.[1,2] Special intracellular transport systems, or neurotubules, bring molecules synthesized in the cell body to the axon and nerve terminals, and return degradation products from the axon and terminals to the cell body for molecular reprocessing.[3] Materials move on the intracellular transportation system in three ways: fast and slow anterograde transport, and fast retrograde transport. Transport from the cell body down the axon is known as anterograde transport. There is a steady loss of constituents as they are carried peripherally, with the result that only 70% of the synthesized materials reach the axon terminal.[2] Fast anterograde axonal transport (20 to 410 mm/day) is dependent upon an adequate supply of energy, and is blocked by anoxia, metabolic inhibitors, or toxic substances.[1,3] Anterograde transport includes components of the cytoskeleton, including microfilaments and microtubules. The microtubules have a close relationship with the fast axonal transport system.[3] Slow anterograde axonal transport (0.1 to 30 mm/day) transports a more limited and specific group of proteins than fast axoplasmic transport. In contrast, transport from the periphery to the cell body is termed retrograde transport. The retrograde transport velocity (1 to 300 mm/day) is fast, but somewhat slower than the fast anterograde transport. At least 50% of materials originally transported by anterograde transport to the axon terminal are recycled and transported back to the cell body.[2,3] Retrograde transport transmission mechanism is similar to that of anterograde transport and requires energy. An important function of retrograde transport is the transfer of information regarding the status of the axon, its terminals, its target cells, and its environment.[2,3] That information is transferred by special neurotrophic factors, which are proteins supplied by the target territory, incorporated by the axon terminals, and transported by retrograde transport to the cell body. Intracellular transport systems depend upon adenosine triphosphate (ATP) derived primarily from oxidative metabolism. Segmental extraneural pressure may interfere with anterograde as well as retrograde axonal transport.[4] Further, axon transport is blocked within 10 to 30 minutes after a nerve is made anoxic as by switching to a nitrogen atmosphere.[1]

The axon has a core of axoplasm surrounded by a continuous plasma membrane called the axolemma.[5,6] The axoplasm contains a variety of elements, including microtubules and neurofilaments. Axons are surrounded by glial cells identified as microglia and macroglia.[1] Microglia arise from macrophages and are phagocytes that are mobilized after injury, infection, or disease. In the peripheral nervous system, the primary macroglia are Schwann cells. Each Schwann cell myelinates a region of one axon. Therefore, axons are either myelinated or nonmyelinated, depending upon their relationship with Schwann cells.[5] Schwann cells insulate the axons by forming a myelin sheath composed of 70% lipid and 30% protein. The myelin and cytoplasm within a Schwann cell are arranged in a series of concentric subcellular compartments surrounding the axon. This myelin sheath insulates the Schwann cell from the endoneurium.[1,2,6] The Schwann cell basal lamina, together with adjacent parts of the endoneurial connective tissue, form an endoneurial tube.[6] The myelinated nerve fiber consists of only one axon, which is associated with only one Schwann cell at any level along its course. A single peripheral axon can be myelinated by as many as 500 Schwann cells.[1] Schwann cells line up longitudinally at intervals of 0.1 to 1.0 mm, and the intervals are termed the nodes of Ranvier, where finger-like cellular processes interdigitate. Only at the node of Ranvier is there an exchange of ions between the axon and the surrounding extracellular fluid, resulting in a higher impulse velocity.[2,6] In nonmyelinated nerve fibers, Schwann cells accumulate multiple axons that are arranged in internal troughs. In nonmyelinated nerve fibers, ion exchange is continuous across the axolemma, resulting in a slower impulse velocity.

Information flows within and between neurons by chemical and electrical signals. The neuronal cell membrane is a lipid bilayer into which various membrane proteins are incorporated. The integral proteins within the membrane are incapable of mixing with water while the proteins in the extracellular and intracellular space attract water. Ions pass through the membrane by way of ion channels or pores composed of proteins that are present in the membrane. Ion channels can have selective permeabilities based on the size, charge, or hydration of the specific ion. In all neurons there is an electrical potential difference between the two sides of the cell membrane. In the resting state, there is a negative potential within the cell compared to the external environment. This resting potential is usually between –50 and –80 mV. The resting potential results from an unequal distribution of monovalent ions on either side of the cell membrane. Resting nerve cells are permeable to Na+, K+, and Cl–.[1] The sodium (Na+) potassium (K+) pump is an integral membrane protein that uses energy, in the form of adenosine triphosphate (ATP), to pump three Na+ out of the neuron for every two K+ it brings into the neuron. In the resting neuron the active fluxes, driven by the sodium-potassium pump, and the passive fluxes, driven by diffusion, are balanced so that the net flux of Na+ and K+ is zero. The resting membrane potential is actually a steady-state potential, because energy is needed to maintain the ion gradients across the membrane.[1]

Electrons process and transmit information using electrical signals produced by temporary changes in the current flow into and out of the neuron.[2,4] Electrical signals are either graded potentials or action potentials. A graded potential is a local change in a neuron's membrane potential. The amplitude of the voltage change is variable and directly related to the intensity of the external signal. Graded potentials are three types: (1) receptor (or generator) potentials are found in specialized sensory cells such as pain receptors or mechanoreceptors; (2) synaptic potentials are changes evoked at a synapse by ionic currents through the membrane of the postsynaptic cell; and (3) pacemaker potentials found in the heart and smooth muscle. These are spontaneous changes caused by the intrinsic properties of the cell rather than external stimuli. As a graded potential travels down the axon it decreases in amplitude. The distance where the voltage has decreased to 37% of its maximum is defined as the length constant. Graded potentials are utilized only for communication over short distances within a neuron. In contrast, the action potential transmits coded messages rapidly and over long distances to other neurons or effector organs such as muscle. An action potential is an explosive change in the membrane potential from its normal resting potential to a very positive value. In the neuron membrane, gated ion channels open or close as a result of structural changes that occur in response to various stimuli. The three major signals that can gate ion channels are voltage, chemical transmitters, and mechanical signals (pressure or stretch). Nongated channels are always open and are responsible for the resting membrane potential. The sodium Na+ channels responsible for the action potential are voltage-gated. Membrane depolarization causes a conformational change that opens the channels, allowing Na+ to diffuse into the cell according to its electrochemical gradient. Action potentials are propagated down the axon by a combination of passive current flow and active membrane changes. Once the membrane along any point of the axon has been depolarized beyond threshold, an action potential is generated in that region in response to the opening of voltage-gated Na+ channels. This local depolarization then spreads passively along the axon, causing the adjacent region of the membrane to reach the necessary threshold for generating an action potential. The depolarization is spread by passive current flow that results from the potential difference between the active and the inactive regions of the axon membrane. Once the depolarization of the inactive region of the membrane approaches threshold, the voltage-gated Na+ channels in this region open, Na+ rushes into the axoplasm, and an action potential is initiated. The actively generated depolarization then spreads by passive local circuit flow to the next region of the membrane, and the cycle is repeated. Vertebrate axons are wrapped in myelin, which effectively acts as an insulator, increasing the membrane resistance and decreasing the membrane capacitance; this results in an increased rate of passive current flow. Although myelin interferes with action potential initiation, there are specialized regions of the axon that are not wrapped in myelin termed the nodes of Ranvier, at which there is a high concentration of voltage-gated Na+ channels. Action potentials are evoked at the nodes, and local currents flow quickly, largely unattenuated, down the myelinated region of the axon (the internode) from one node to the next, where a new action potential is evoked. Thus, action potential production jumps via saltatory propagation from node to node. This is a very effective means of increasing the conduction velocity.[1] Larger diameter axons have a lower current threshold and their axoplasm is less resistant to current flow; therefore, a graded increase in stimulus strength will excite the larger axons first. The primary difference between myelinated and unmyelinated nerve fibers is the conduction velocity.

Each nerve fiber, or axon, is ensheathed in loose connective tissue termed the endoneurium. Bundles of nerve fibers are termed fascicles. The terms funiculus, fasciculus, and fascicle are synonymous. Fascicles are protected by an external multilamellated sheath termed the perineurium. The perineurium has a diffusion barrier to a number of extrinsic macromolecules and maintains an optimal intrafascicular environment with a well-developed microvascular system. Bundles of fascicles are embedded in a well-vascularized areolar connective tissue membrane termed the epineurium. The epineurium protects nerve fibers from friction, compression and stretch, and is much thicker near joints. The nerve trunk is surrounded by loose connective tissue called mesoneurium that allows considerable gliding. An example would be the 14.5 mm of movement of the median nerve when the wrist is ranged through full extension and flexion.[7]

During normal development, nerves reach the muscle at the myotubal stage, where the acetylcholine sensitivity is distributed over the entire membrane. In the vicinity of the neuromuscular junction, nerves ramify repeatedly into terminal branches that abruptly taper by losing their myelin sheaths to give rise to nerve endings. Skeletal muscle is under the control of a nerve that enters the muscle at its motor point.[8] Each nerve cell axon then branches many times, and every muscle fiber is contacted by one nerve terminal. This point of contact is called the motor end plate. In the muscle fiber, the postsynaptic membranes/subneural apparatuses are composed of synaptic troughs with junctional folds. This subneural apparatus appears much earlier than the accumulation of nuclei and elaboration of membranes found later at the endplate region of the muscle.[9,10] There is rapid maturation of the muscle, myotubes become muscle fibers and the increase in the specific activity of pre- and post-synaptic enzymes is directly related to the increasing complexity of the endplates. Chemosensitivity is restricted to the endplate region. The density of acetylcholine receptors at the endplate becomes 1,000 to 10,000 times higher than in the extra-junctional area.[11]

A single nerve axon and all muscle fibers it contacts constitute a motor unit. Both the number of muscle fibers within a motor unit and the number of motor units within a given muscle are quite variable. A motor unit is stimulated to contract by an electrical impulse, or action potential, which originates from the cell body of the nerve. This potential is propagated down the entire length of the axon from the spinal cord to the peripheral skeletal muscle motor point. The nerve forms a synapse with the muscle at a specialized region known as the motor end place. An electrical impulse passing along the cell membrane of the axon is transformed to a similar electrical signal in the membrane of the muscle fiber. This transmission is not achieved by direct electrical transmission; the process involves chemical transmission across a gap of extracellular space separating the two membrane systems. As the axon approaches the synapse, the nerve terminal spreads out over an area of the muscle membrane called the sole plate. An axon terminal and muscle membrane/sole plate interdigitate across a series of membrane foldings called primary synaptic folds, which greatly amplify the area of membrane juxtaposed between nerve and muscle. At all times, the muscle membrane is separated from the nerve membrane by a space of approximately 50 nm, called the synaptic cleft.[8]

Signals are passed from nerve to muscle by chemical transmitters. The chemical acetylcholine is stored in the presynaptic axon in small membrane-bound sacs called vesicles. When the electrical impulse arrives in the terminal axon, the membrane allows the flow of calcium ions into the cell. An increase in the intracellular calcium concentration causes the vesicles to fuse with the terminal axon membrane and to release acetylcholine into the synaptic cleft. The acetycholine must then diffuse across the synaptic cleft and bind to a specific receptor on the surface of the muscle membrane. The binding of the acetylcholine to its receptor allows currents to flow into the muscle membrane and depolarize the cell. Depolarization triggers an action potential that passes the length of the muscle membrane. The action potential in the muscle membrane is similar to the action potential in a nerve. The acetylcholine is deactivated by the enzyme acetylcholinesterase or other less specific cholinesterases located in the extracellular space and associated with the basement membrane. The breakdown products may be reabsorbed by the terminal axon to be used in the resynthesis of additional transmitter substances.[8]

Skeletal muscle cells develop from a mesodermal cell population arising from the somite. The somite is formed from the mesoderm between the digestive canal and the surface of the body in the embryo. The most primitive muscle cells are termed myoblasts. These fusiform cells respond to molecular messengers to undergo mitosis. Skeletal myoblasts eventually withdraw from the cell cycle and never enter another cell division.[9] After final mitosis, the myoblasts synthesize many proteins specific for striated muscle. The myoblasts become elongated and fusiform in shape. Skeletal myoblasts align themselves into rows, and fuse to form multi-nucleated, cross-striated cells termed myotubes. The underlying mechanism of cell fusion/recognition is unknown.[9] Differentiation continues as the centrally placed nuclei of the myotube migrate to the periphery, and the myotubes differentiate into muscle fibers. By the seventh week of gestation, distinct muscle and tendinous structures can be identified.[8] Even before contact between the motor nerve and the skeletal muscle is established, both systems can be recognized as cholinergic: the nerve terminal can synthesize and release acetylcholine, and the muscle fiber is able to respond to acetylcholine. If the myotubes do not become innervated, their differentiation is arrested and the myotubes atrophy and become replaced by fat.[9]

The basic structural element of skeletal muscle is the muscle fiber. Each striated muscle fiber contains numerous nuclei, which usually are located at the periphery of the fiber. In addition, separate cells called satellite cells lie along the surface of the muscle at the periphery of each fiber. The satellite cells are considered to be stem cells capable of proliferation and regeneration when there is damage to the muscle fiber.[12] Each muscle fiber contains a sarcoplasm which is similar to the cytoplasm of other cells. The sarcoplasm contains a cellular matrix and organelles. The organelles include the Golgi apparatus, found near many of the nuclei, and the mitochondria, which are abundant near the nuclei. The other important organelle is the sarcoplasmic reticulum, a continuous membrane system that corresponds to the endoplasmic reticulum of other cell types. Other components of the sarcoplasm include lipid droplets, glycogen, and myoglobin. Individual muscle fibers are surrounded by a plasma membrane known as the sarcolemma. External to the sarcolemma, or plasmalemma, is a separate basement membrane, or basal lamina, that is 100 to 200 mm thick.[8,10] This membrane consists of an inner layer, the lamina rara or lucida, and an outer, more dense layer, the lamina densa. The basement membrane contains a number of protein and carbohydrate components contributed by both the muscle fiber and fibroblasts. Among its components are collagen, laminin, fibronectin, and other specific glycoproteins. The basement membrane then merges with a reticular layer and the extracellular matrix. The basement membrane, the reticular layer, and the close layer of matrix and collagen fibers together constitute the endomysium, which is well supplied with capillaries.

If the plasma membrane/sarcolemma and basement membranes of a muscle fiber are separated, the internal structures of the cell are seen to consist of many long, slender, parallel elements called myofibrils. The long myofibrils are about 1 μm in diameter and have a distinct banding pattern.[8] Vertebrate striated muscle is named for the transverse striations or bands seen when the muscle fibers are viewed by a light microscope. Band patterns are composed of dark A-bands alternating with lighter I-bands. The sarcomere is the repeating muscle unit and is defined from the dark Z line in the middle of each I-band. The A-bands are the middle portion of each sarcomere, and in the center of each A-band there is a lighter region called the H zone. Thick myosin-containing filaments, 1.65 μm long and about 12 nm in diameter, extend the length of the A-band and align transversely in a hexagonal lattice. Thinner actin-containing filaments (8 nm diameter) extend 1.05 μm on each side of the Z line as far as the H zone, and within the A-band they occupy the trigonal positions of the myosin-filament lattice. Electron micrographs show projections from the myosin filaments that are able to bridge the gap to the actin filaments and thus are called cross bridges. The cross bridges project from the thick filaments toward the thin filaments at regular intervals of approximately 14.3 nm.[10] The polarity of the molecular packing at the ends of the myosin filaments and in the actin filaments is such that the interaction produces a force in only one direction, that which increases filament overlap.[10]

Cross bridges use the energy made available from the hydrolysis of adenosine triphosphate to undergo a conformational change and cause the thick filaments to slide past the thin filaments. The cross bridges cycle many times as they become released from the actin on the thin filament, spring back to their initial conformation, and are ready to repeat the process in rapid succession. Both actin and myosin molecules have a recognizable polarity, which is essential to muscular contraction. To allow shortening of the sarcomere, the polarity must be different in the thick filaments on either side of the M line so that the thick filament arrays of the I-bands on either side of the A-band are pulled toward each other and toward the center of the A-band. Similarly, the thin filaments must have opposite polarity on either side of the Z line so that they are pulled in between the thick filaments by the cross bridges to allow shortening. These activities form the basis for the sliding filament with swinging cross bridge, which specifies a theory of muscle contraction.[8]

Electrical impulses pass down the muscle membrane to reach the interior of the muscle by an extensive and intricate membrane system. Transverse tubules penetrate from the surface into the muscle fibers near the level of the A-band and I-band junctions in mammalian muscle. These tubules are perpendicular to the axis of the cells and are termed transverse. The transverse tubules interact with another large system of membrane-bound sacs called the sarcoplasmic reticulum, which stores calcium inside its membrane system and, therefore, keeps calcium out of the muscle cytoplasm. The membranes of the sarcoplasmic reticulum actively accumulate calcium from the muscle cytoplasm. Control of the intracellular calcium concentration is the mechanism for regulating the on-off contractile function of the contractile proteins. An electrical impulse originating within the muscle membrane and tubular systems causes the momentary release of calcium from the sarcoplasmic reticulum into the muscle cytoplasm. Calcium release, in turn, is the trigger that causes the contractile proteins to interact and to generate force. The membrane system, including the surface membrane, transverse tubules, and sarcoplasmic reticulum, provides a mechanism for rapid conduction of an electric signal from the cell surface throughout the entire muscle fiber.[8] Those metabolic characteristics of skeletal muscle fibers that are associated with contractile activity are not rigidly fixed, but can be altered by changing the pattern of activity of a skeletal muscle. The characteristic properties of the muscle membrane, i.e., its electrical constants, become rigidly fixed during early development of the muscle and cannot be readily changed. While the chemical sensitivity of the muscle fiber outside the endplate is influenced by a number of procedures, the properties of the synaptic region are not subject to modulation.[9]

Slow and fast mammalian muscles are innervated at a single site on the membrane. The nerve terminals in fast muscles are long and spread over longer distances than those to slow fibers, which are short and less smooth. Slow and fast muscle fibers can be distinguished by differences in fiber diameter, width of the Z-line, mitochondrial content, appearance of myofibrils, and elaboration of the internal membrane system.[9] Fast muscles (Type II) have high enzyme activity for anaerobic glycolysis while slow muscles (Type I) have a high capacity for oxidative metabolism. It is not known if these fiber distributions are genetically based or are a response to sustained training. All skeletal muscles have three kinds of messenger RNA and are therefore able to synthesize all different types of myosin, and it is only later in development that the muscle cell continues to synthesize one type and no longer synthesizes the others. Differentiation occurs after innervation. The different properties of the muscle fibers develop under the influence of their innervation and the motor nerve is able even in the adult animal to determine the properties of the undifferentiated muscle fibers.[9]

Muscle fibers have a variety of architectural arrangements for specific functions, such as parallel, unipennate, bipennate, or fusiform. Fiber arrangement within the muscle is an important determinant of its functional and contractile properties. Fiber arrangement can be parallel or oblique to the long axis of the muscle. In general, maximal force production is proportional to the physiologic cross-sectional area of a muscle, but the total amount and speed of shortening are proportional to indiviual muscle fiber length.[8] Muscle fibers are organized by the surrounding connective tissue. The endomysin is the fine-textured connective tissue layer that surrounds individual muscle fibers. Muscle fibers, or myofibrils, are arranged together into bundles, usually 10 to 20, called muscle fascicles.[10] The endomysium separates individual myofibrils within a fascicle. The thicker connective tissue surrounding fascicles is termed the perimysium. The connective tissue surrounding the whole muscle is called the epimysium. The epimysium covers the muscle loosely in order to permit the changes in length during the contraction-extension cycle of muscle function.[8,12]

12.2 THE INJURED NERVE AND DENERVATED SKELETAL MUSCLE

In the severed axon, both the proximal and distal stumps immediately develop marked edema. The distal stump of the nerve fiber, separated from its source of nourishment, undergoes a series of events termed Wallerian degeneration. The axon and myelin sheath degenerate, and Schwann cells and microglia remove the debris. Morphologic changes occur within 24 hours after injury, and all unmyelinated axons degenerate within one week.[13] By 3 weeks after injury, most of the axon and myelin have been digested by the Schwann cells, and by 8 weeks, the debridement is largely complete.[14] There is progressive decrease in the fascicular cross-sectional area, with subsequent collapse of the individual endoneurial tubes. This shrinkage of the distal stump is maximal at about 3 months after injury. Endoneurial tubes within the distal segment of a disrupted nerve may wither to 10% of their original diameter, and to what extent the endoneurial tube can expand in response to ingrowing axons is unknown.[15] In denervated skeletal muscle the nuclei become rounded and swollen and their chromatin is dispersed. Some of the nuclei take up positions in the center of the muscle fiber. Fibrosis surrounding shrinking muscle fibers occurs, and at the ultrastructural level there are alterations in the sarcoplasmic reticulum and myofilaments. The sarcoplasmic reticulum initially increases in volume, but this is followed by a decrease in volume. There is an alteration in the conduction rate of the action potential.[9] Individual muscle fibers show spontaneous asynchronous contractions arising from spontaneous fluctuations in membrane potential. Denervation leads to a spread of acetylcholine sensitivity along the entire surface of the nerve fiber, secondary to the appearance of acetylcholine receptors outside the endplate region.[9] The lack of activity of denervated muscles probably contributes to denervation hypersensitivity. In inactive muscles, the diameter of the muscle fibers decreases just as in denervated muscles,[9] so that the injured and denervated muscle is in double jeopardy for fibrotic immobilization.

During World War II, Sir Herbert Seddon introduced a simple classification of traumatic nerve injuries.[16] Minimal injury is termed neurapraxia and may be secondary to localized ischemic demyelination. Moderate injury is termed axonotmesis. It is characterized by interruption of the axons and their myelin sheath; the endoneurial tubes remain intact and guide the regenerating axons to their appropriate peripheral connections. Severe injury, termed neurotmesis, involves a nerve that either has been completely severed or is so seriously disorganized that spontaneous regeneration is impossible. Most traumatic injuries, including compression, friction, stretch, lacerations, fractures, dislocations, or gunshot wounds, can result in any one or combinations of these three types of injury patterns.

Sir Sydney Sunderland[17] provided the following classifications in relation to the internal structure of the nerve trunk: (1) First-degree trauma — loss of axon conduction; this corresponds to neurapraxia; there are no fibrillation or denervation changes in the affected muscles.[1] (2) Second-degree trauma — transection of the axon with an intact endoneurial sheath inside an intact perineurium; this corresponds to axonotmesis. Fibrillation and other electromyographic signs of denervation are found in the muscles, and the denervated muscles atrophy.[1] (3) Third-degree trauma — transection of axon and endoneurial sheath inside an intact perineurium. There is complete loss of motor and sensory functions in the region served by the nerve. In addition, the involved muscles remain in a denervated state for a longer period of time and additional time may be required for functional recovery when the muscles are reinnervated. In general, the more proximal the injury the worse the prognosis for functional recovery.[1,4] (4) Fourth-degree trauma — transection of many axons with their endoneurial sheath and the perineurium; the nerve trunk continuity is maintained by epineurial tissue. Axon regeneration is complicated by extensive intraneural scarring and complete disruption of the fascicular structure. Wallerian degeneration occurs in the usual pattern. (5) Fifth-degree trauma-transection of the entire nerve trunk; usually a neuroma forms on the proximal stump.

Peripheral nerves are only as functional as the pertinent sensory receptors and muscle-tendon motors. Multiple nerve involvement jeopardizes functional recovery of the entire extremity more than an isolated nerve injury. Severe vascular deficiency, chronic osteomyelitis, osseous nonunion, and articular incongruity all contribute to fibrotic infiltration, adhesions, and limited joint motion. Clinical studies of peripheral nerve recovery in humans show considerable variation because return of useful function depends as much on the total response of the extremity to the injury as on the regeneration of the injured nerve.[18] In addition, skeletal muscle biopsy does not differentiate between secondary disuse or partial denervation.[19] Seddon's classification is more related to traumatic injury, while Sunderland's classification is more related to disrupted histopathology. Neither classification provides clear prognostic information related to the traumatic injury, and most peripheral nerve histopathology is classified following clinical observation and electrodiagnostic studies. It is important to know the percentage of peripheral nerves that should recover from various types of traumatic injuries and the time required for return of clinical function.

In both closed and open injuries, approximately 70% of nerve injuries that retain anatomic continuity result in spontaneous recovery.[15,18] Approximately 85% of closed nerve injuries associated with fractures of long bones will have spontaneous clinical recovery.[15] Approximately 69% of nerve palsies resulting from either low velocity or high velocity gunshot wounds will have spontaneous recovery.[15,18,20] The time frame for spontaneous recovery of nerve lesions resulting from fractures and dislocations or crush injuries is 1 to 4 months; the comparable period for gunshot wounds is 3 to 9 months.[15,18] These results suggest that neurapraxia lesions resolve in 1 to 4 months and axonotmesis lesions resolve in 3 to 9 months. Significant spontaneous recovery is gained in approximately 90% of nerve injuries when a normal nerve action potential is recorded across a neuroma in continuity at 3 months after injury. External neurolysis is usually not indicated, because only 30% of successful cases recover function outside the projected time frame for spontaneous recovery.[15,18] The effectiveness of internal neurolysis is questionable because as little as 6 to 8 cm of nerve divested of mesoneurium may constitute a loss of segmental blood supply sufficient to produce necrosis of that segment of the nerve.[15]

12.3 PERIPHERAL NERVE REPAIR

There are only two principles in the manual techniques for suture repair: (1) align the fascicles, and (2) avoid tension in all suture lines.[21] The manual techniques used for nerve suture are the only factors affecting the return of function that is fully under the control of the attending surgeon.

The surgeon must control instruments, suture material, and operating field magnification. Magnification (20×) is most pertinent when the nerve stumps are debrided in a chronic lesion. The nerve stumps must be debrided to tissue that demonstrates normal funicular patterns free of scar (Figure 12.1) Suture material should be nonreactive to body tissues and small in diameter with durable swaged-on microneedles. Suturing of epineurium with 8-0 or 9-0 nylon and perineurium with 9-0 or 10-0 nylon is appropriate. Non-magnetic stainless steel microscopic instruments are available to handle the small needles and fine-caliber suture.

Open wounds with associated nerve palsy require debridement. Incisions should be placed so as to be able to directly observe the neurovascular structures. Although

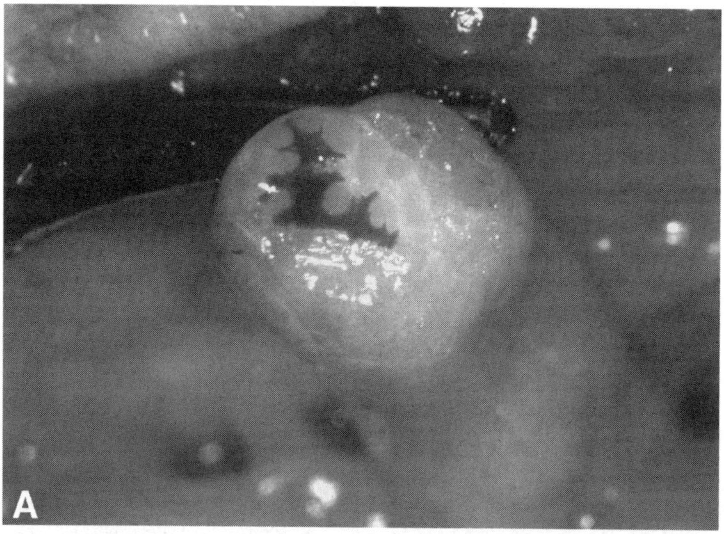

FIGURE 12.1 (A) The scarred end of a peripheral nerve following severe injury with a time delay before suture. From Omer, G.E., Jr.: Peripheral Nerve Injuries and Gunshot Wounds, Chap 41:398-405; (in) Omer, G.E., Jr., Spinner, M., and Van Beek, A.L. (Eds): *Management of Peripheral Nerve Problems,* W.B. Saunders, Philadelphia, 2nd ed., 1998 (Figure 41-4, page 401). With permission.

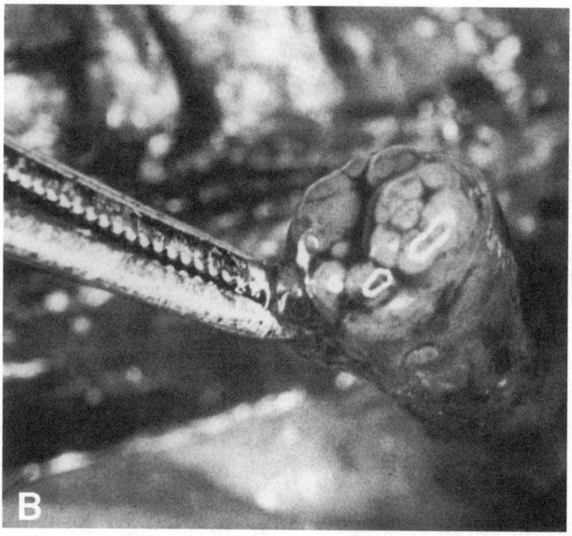

FIGURE 12.1 (B) Fascicular groups are exposed following debridement. From Omer, G.E., Jr. and Pirela-Cruz, M.A.: Complications of Peripheral Nerve Injuries, Chap 30:811-856 (in) Epps, C.H., Jr. (Ed): *Complications in Orthopaedic Surgery,* J.B. Lippincott, Philadelphia, 3rd ed., 1994 (Figure 30-3, page 818). With permission.

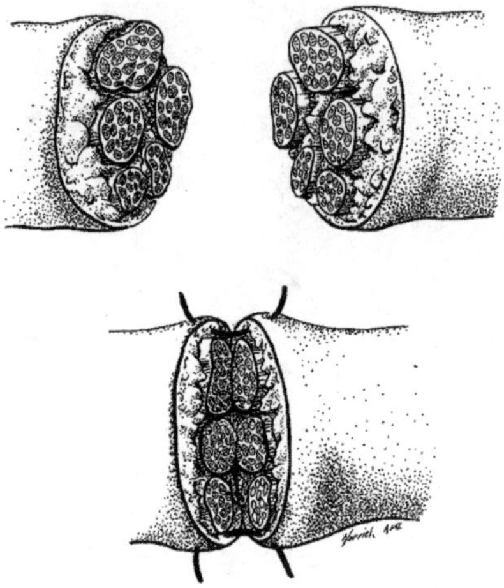

FIGURE 12.2 (A and B) Epineurial circumferential closure technique for nerve suture. From Omer, G.E., Jr. and Pirela-Cruz, M.A.: Complications of Peripheral Nerve Injuries, Chap 30: 811-856 (in) Epps, C.H., Jr. (Ed): *Complications in Orthopaedic Surgery,* J.B. Lippincott, Philadelphia, 3rd ed., 1994 (Figure 30-4, page 819). With permission.

appropriate treatment for a severed nerve is neurorrhaphy, many factors such as a nerve gap prevent ideal treatment.[18] In the open injury with fractures and soft tissue loss, the nerve is often disrupted with partial loss. Two fine wire sutures are aligned in the epineurium of the proximal and distal nerve stumps. Each wire suture is then sutured to adjacent soft tissue to prevent retraction. Later, the disrupted nerve can be identified radiologically.

12.3.1 Epineurial Suture

Flourens (1828) and Baudens (1836) are credited with first using the epineurial suture technique (Figure 12.2) for nerve repair.[22] If an acute injury, the wound must be debrided. If a significant amount of scarring is found within the nerve stump, transection is repeated until fascicular groups are easily identified (Figure 12.1). Magnification is most important during debridement of the nerve stumps. The branching and intermingling of the fascicular groups in a nerve trunk make it difficult to match the proximal and distal fascicular pattern if a segment of nerve 2.5 cm or greater has been removed.[23] The most difficult technical step is transection of the nerve to achieve a flat stump for both nerve ends, thereby obtaining a flush joint for the anastomosis. Surface markings, such as longitudinal blood vessels, are used to align the proximal and distal nerve stumps and prevent malrotation of the fascicular pattern. The epineurial suture technique is performed with fine nylon suture. Initial sutures are placed 180° around the circumference (at the 9 o'clock and 3 o'clock positions), and the aligned anterior arc of epineurium is repaired with interrupted sutures. The nerve then is rotated 180° by passing one of the initial coaptation sutures posteriorly and turning the unrepaired posterior epineurium into view for interrupted sutures. The tourniquet should be released before the final sutures are placed to

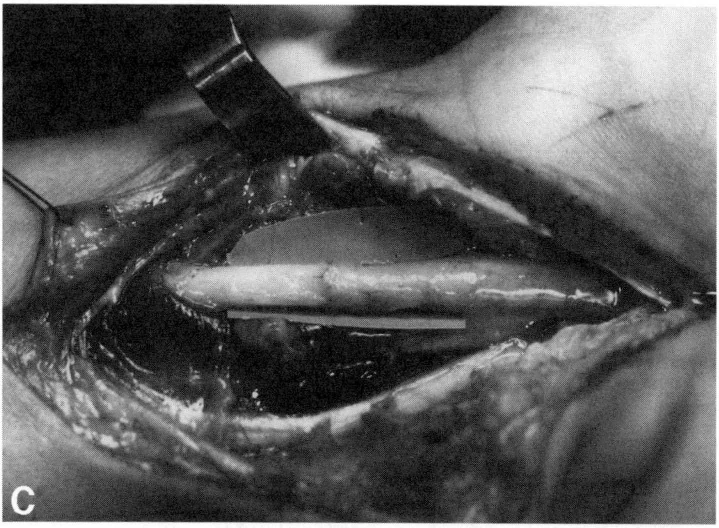

FIGURE 12.2 (C) Lacerated medial nerve, with surface match for epineurial closure. From Moneim, M.S.A. and Omer, G.E., Jr.: Clinical Outcome Following Acute Nerve Repair, Chap 43: 414-419 (in) Omer, G.E., Jr., Spinner, M., and Van Beek, A.L. (Eds.): *Management of Peripheral Nerve Problems,* W.B. Saunders, Philadelphia, 2nd ed., 1998 (Figure 43-lA, page 415). With permission.

evacuate any potential hematoma between the nerve stumps. Histological examination of nerve repairs done without magnification or fine suture material has demonstrated fascicular malalignment, while the amount of tension used in the anastomosis is directly related to the resulting connective tissue/scar proliferation.[24]

12.3.2 Fascicular (Funicular, Bundle, Group Fascicular) Suture

In 1917, Langley recommended fascicular sutures (Figure 12.3) to obtain a better clinical result for sensory and motor function.[15] Smith is credited for popularizing the use of the operating microscope in 1964 for nerve repairs.[25] Technically, the funicular repair is similar to the epineurial repair but requires greater magnification. Accurate alignment and approximation of fascicular patterns are critical for maximal neuronal regeneration. Group fascicular repair is used for larger nerves where the nerve has definable groups of fascicles. Usually, the size and grouping of proximal fascicules are used to match the distal fascicules; there is no practical method to identify motor or sensory groups except their pattern in the stumps.[15] Suture of the intraneurial epineurium (the condensed connective tissue around groups of fascicles) is performed with 9-0 or 10-0 suture, and magnification is essential for accurate placement of the sutures. The needle should never be placed in the fascicular content and should only be placed through external or internal perineurium.[26] The epineurium need not be repaired and can be excised for 1 cm proximal and distal from the suture lines to ensure that this outer layer does not interpose between the approximated

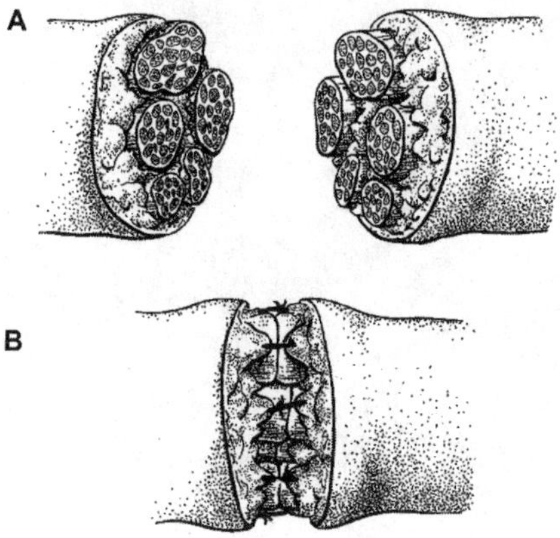

FIGURE 12.3 (A) and (B) Intraepineurial repair (Fascicular bundle) technique. (C) Nerve laceration with identification of fascicular bundles for matching. (D) Fascicular bundle repair technique with sutures through the intraneural epineurium. Figure 12.3A,B,C,D from Omer, G.E., Jr. and Pirela-Cruz, M.A.: Complications of Peripheral Nerve Injuries, Chap 30: 811-856 (in) Epps, C.H., Jr. (Ed): *Complications in Orthopaedic Surgery,* J.B. Lippincott, Philadelphia, 3rd ed., 1994 (Figure 30-5, page 821). With permission.

fascicules. Critical comparison of clinical results in patients, including objective measurements and analysis, has not demonstrated significant differences between epineurial and fascicular neurorhaphies when appropriate suture material, instruments, and magnification are used.[27,28]

12.3.3 Interfascicular Graft Suture

The first documented nerve graft was performed by J.J. Philipeaux and A. Vulpian in 1870.[15] In 1972, Millesi introduced interfascicular nerve grafts (Figure 12.4).[29] This current technique does not attempt to cover totally the surface of the proximal and distal stumps; instead, it is an "extended" fascicular suture. The injured nerve is prepared for anastomosis by trimming the nerve stumps to acceptable fascicular patterns. Autogenous material is preferred for nerve grafts; the sural nerve and the medial or lateral antebrachial cutaneous nerves are the preferred sources. A sketch of the fascicular pattern of the nerve stumps is made to plan the connecting graft. The donor nerve is reversed to preserve all nerve fibers that will enter the graft. The donor nerve will fill gaps between groups of fasciculi that have the approximate cross-sectional area of the donor nerve. The donor nerve is sectioned to fit the gap in the disrupted nerve without tension or redundancy. One suture connects the intraneurial epineurium of the selected fasciculus to the circumferential epineurium of the donor graft nerve at both the proximal and distal ends. Occasionally, as determined under magnification, an additional 10-0 suture is necessary to establish optimal alignment and transverse contact.

In a long nerve graft, the distal suture line may scar and block before the axons reach that level. Clinically, this becomes apparent as the advancing Tinel's sign stops and does not proceed distally. If there is more than a 30-day delay at that point, the

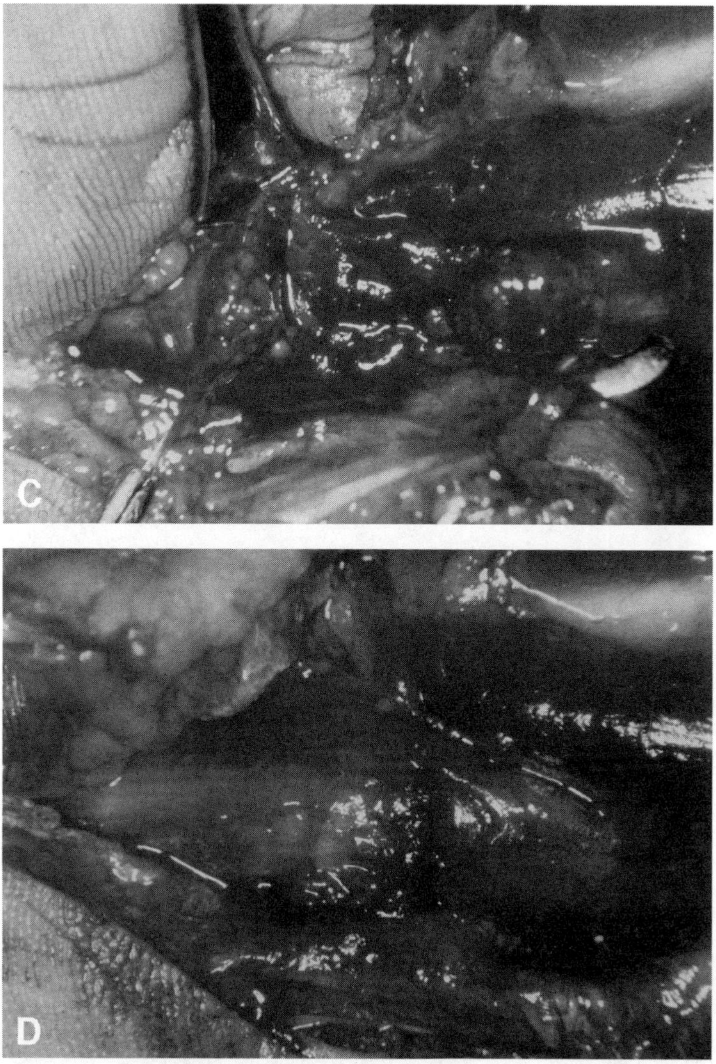

FIGURE 12.3 (continued)

distal suture site should be exposed and electrodiagnostic techniques used (nerve action potentials) to evaluate the neuroma-in-continuity. If there is no distal electrical conduction, the distal suture site should be resected and a second neurorhaphy performed.[15]

12.3.4 Prognostic Factors

Age is the most significant single factor in recovery after nerve suture.[30] Young patients have a greater intrinsic capacity for sensory reeducation and motor adaptability. The more extensive and severe the injury is to the involved extremity, the longer is the time required for tissue homeostasis. Multiple nerve involvement is a

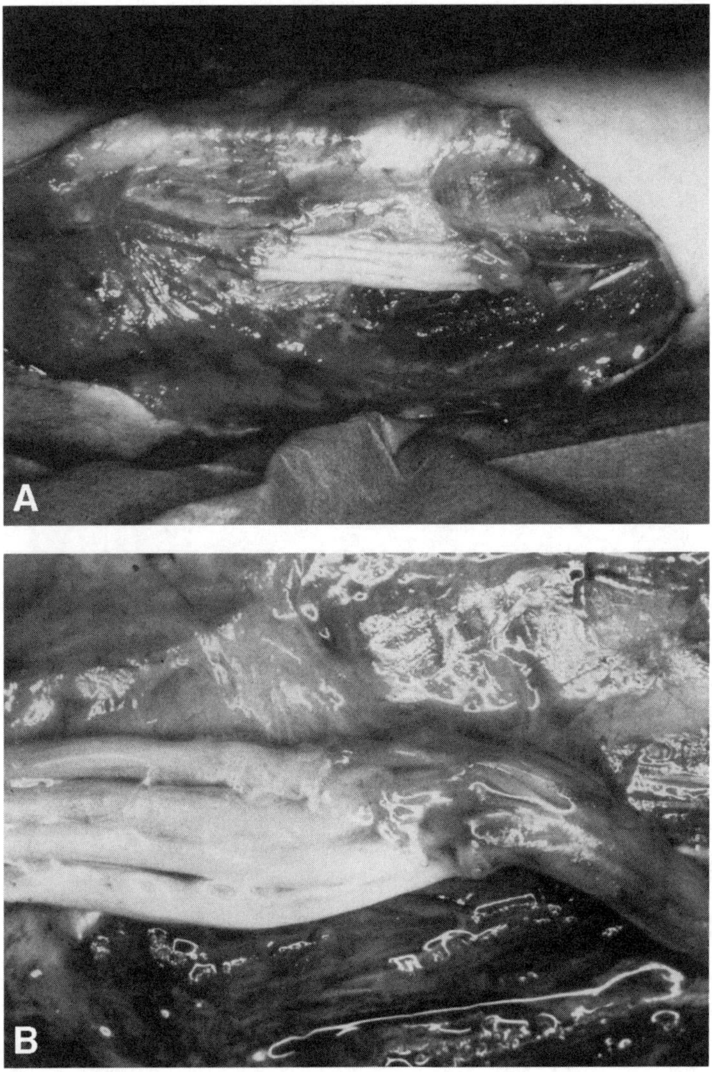

FIGURE 12.4 (A) Sural Nerve cables placed between fascicular groups as the technique for autogenous nerve graft. (B) Sutures are placed in the intraepineurium to stabilize the fascicular groups. From Omer, G.E., Jr.. and Pirela-Cruz, M.A.: Complications of Peripheral Nerve Injuries, Chap 30: 811-856 (in) Epps, C. H., Jr. (Ed): *Complications in Orthopaedic Surgery,* J.B. Lippincott, Philadelphia, 3rd ed., 1994 (Figure 30-6, page 822). With permission.

more serious problem for functional recovery than an isolated nerve injury. The more proximal the injury involving the nerve, the longer the distal tissues will be denervated and the slower will be recovery of function. The time interval between injury and nerve suture is important in all injuries.

The British Research Council introduced a grading system in 1954 that attempted to assess the recovery of an entire peripheral nerve in relation to total extremity

TABLE 12.1
The British Medical Research Council Rating Scale

Motor Recovery	Sensory Recovery	Description
M5	S4	Complete recovery
M4	S3+	All synergetic and independent movements are possible
		Some recovery of two-point discrimination within autonomous area
M3	S3	All important muscles act against resistance
		Return of superficial cutaneous pain and tactile sensibility throughout the autonomous area with disappearance of any previous overreaction
M2	S2	Return of perceptible contraction in both proximal and distal muscles
		Return of some degree of superficial cutaneous pain and tactile sensibility within the autonomous area of the nerve
M1	S1	Return of perceptible contractions in proximal muscles
		Recovery of deep cutaneous pain sensibility within the autonomous area of the nerve
M0	S0	No contraction
		Absence of sensibility within the autonomous area

From Seddon, H.J. (Ed): *Peripheral Nerve Injuries,* Medical Research Council Special Report Series, No.282, London, Her Majesty's Stationery Office, 1954.

function[15,31] (Table 12.1). Our experience has been that primary end-to-end repair gives 60 to 65% good motor (M4 or better), and 80 to 85% good sensory (S3+ or better) results. Repair with grafts gives 25 to 30% good motor (M4 or better) and 60 to 65% good sensory (S3+ or better) results.[31]

12.4 NERVE REGENERATION AFTER REPAIR

When an axon is severed, the cell body of that neuron goes through structural and functional changes reflecting an alteration in metabolic activity emphasizing the production of proteins needed for axonal repair and growth. The closer the injury is to the cell body, or the greater the loss of axoplasm, the more severe the reaction. Axonal degeneration occurs over one or several internodal segments in the proximal stump, leaving the endoneurial tubes of the distal centimeter of the proximal stump occupied only by Schwann cells. The fate of the axons proximal to the injury depends upon the survival of the cell body. If the cell body degenerates, the entire proximal length of the axon undergoes Wallerian degeneration. If the cell body survives, the proximal nerve fibers undergo a reduction in axon diameter and myelin thickness. This permanent reduction in axon diameter and myelin thickness is accompanied with a slowing of the conduction velocity.[1]

After transection, proximal myelinated axons produce a great number of collateral and terminal sprouts that advance distally. Collateral sprouts arise from the nodes of Ranvier at the level where the axons are still intact, while terminal sprouts arise from the tips of the remaining axons. The growing sprouts from a single axon form an anatomic unit called the regenerating unit.[1,2,4] The regenerating units consist of clusters of nonmyelinated axons originating from the same myelinated axon and surrounded by a single Schwann cell and its basal lamina. After a period of time, the average number of sprouts per regenerating unit diminishes because some axons fail to make functional contact with a peripheral target.[1,2,4] Following transection and repair of the nerve trunk, there is considerable misdirection, so that one endoneurial tube can contain sprouts from several different parent axons.[4] The rate of axonal outgrowth varies with species, type of injury, and level of occurrence. On average, the outgrowth rate is about 1 to 2 mm per day. The initial direction of axon growth seems to be determined by the neuron, but the direction of further growth appears to be determined by factors in the tissue through which the axon grows. Neurotrophism, from the Greek *trophikos*, or nursing, was originally coined to describe an interaction between developing neurons and their targets, in which a substance produced by the target is taken up by innervating axons and transported back to the neuron, preventing its death.[5,32] The neurotrophic concept was introduced by examination of the actions of nerve growth factor, the first neurotrophic factor to be isolated. Neurotropism, from the Greek *trope*, or a turning, is used to describe regeneration of an axon up a concentration gradient of a diffusible substance to reinnervate a specific target.[32] It has been studied since the time of Ramon y S. Cajal (1890) to draw regenerating axons en masse to a distal nerve stump, generating specificity at the tissue level. Present studies indicate that it might be impossible to make a clear distinction between the two factors because substances that are secreted by the non-neuronal cells after an injury can act like a tropic factor, although they normally have a trophic influence.[3]

If adult muscle is injured, new muscle fibers will develop. The derivation of the myoblasts is unknown. However, the initial process of muscle regeneration can start and proceed in the absence of innervation.[12] In addition, myotubes cannot develop differentiated muscle fibers, i.e., slow or fast, without innervation. Once the muscle fibers become innervated, the nerve fibers that fail to make connections are redundant and die back.

Functional recovery still is unsatisfactory in adults. There is an obvious need for an alternative approach to peripheral nerve injuries to improve clinical results. Increased knowledge of molecular mechanisms regulating axonal outgrowth may prove to be the key factor in the future. The current development of central nervous system research with special reference to brain plasticity may prove to be another key factor in the future. There are indications that factors like visuospatial cognitive capacity are important for recovery of functional sensibility following nerve injury in adults. It is difficult to place a time frame on functional retraining and recovery, because it depends on nerve regeneration plus other factors such as age, intelligence, patience, perseverance, and motivation. The patient's ability to use new and altered patterns of motor and sensory innervation is a slow process that continues for at least 5 years following initial return of function. Clinical studies of neural recovery in the human show considerable variation, because return of useful function depends as much on the total response of the involved extremity to the injury as the regeneration of the injured nerve.

REFERENCES

1. Bodine, S.C. and Lieber, R.L., Peripheral nerve physiology, anatomy, and pathology, in *Orthopaedic Basic Science*, Simon, S.R., Ed., American Academy of Orthopaedic Surgeons, Chicago, 1994, Chap. 8:325-396.
2. Lundborg, G. and Dahlm, L.B., Structure and function of peripheral nerve, in *Operative Nerve Repair and Reconstruction*, Gelberman, R.H., Ed., J.B. Lippincott Co., Philadelphia, 1991, Chap. 1: 3-.
3. Hurst, L.C. and Badalamente, M.A., Biochemical properties of peripheral nerve, in *Operative Nerve Repair and Reconstruction*, Gelberman, R.H., Ed., J.B. Lippincott Co., Philadelphia, 1991, Chap. 4: 55-72.
4. Lundborg, G. and Dahlin, L.B., Pathophysiology of peripheral nerve trauma, in *Management of Peripheral Nerve Problems*, 2nd ed., Omer, G.E. Jr., Spinner, M., and Van Beek, A.L., Eds., W.B. Saunders, Philadelphia, 1998, Chap. 37:353-364.
5. Sunderland, S., *Nerves and Nerve Injuries*, 2nd ed., Churchill Livingstone, Edinburgh, 1978, Chap. 1-2:3-60.
6. Thomas, P.K. and Ochoa, J., Microscopic anatomy of peripheral nerve fibres, in *Peripheral Neuropathy*, Dyck, P.J., Thomas, P.K., Lambert, E.H., and Bunge, M.B., Eds., W.B. Saunders, Philadelphia, 1984:39-96.
7. Wilgis, E.F.S. and Murphy, R., The significance of longitudinal excursion in peripheral nerves, *Hand Clinics*, 2 (4): 761-766, 1986.
8. Garrett, W.E., Jr. and Best, T.M., Anatomy, physiology, and mechanics of skeletal muscle, in *Orthopaedic Basic Science*, Simon, S.R., Ed., American Academy of Orthopaedic Surgeons, Chicago, 1994, Chap. 3: 89-125.
9. Vrbova, G., Gordon, T., and Jones, R., Eds., *Nerve-Muscle Interaction*, Chapman and Hall, London, 1978 (Halstead Press, John Wiley & Sons, New York), 1978.
10. Peachey, L.D., Adrian, R.H., and Geiger, S.R., *Skeletal Muscle*, American Physiological Society, Bethesda, Maryland, 1983, 685 pages.
11. Fertuck, H.C. and Salpeter, M.M., Localisation of acetylcholine receptors by 1251 labelled bungarotoxin binding at mouse end plates, *Proc. Nat. Acad. Sci.*, 71, 1974: 1376-1378.
12. Carlson, B.M., The regeneration of skeletal muscle — a review, *American Journal of Anatomy*, 137,1973: 119-150.
13. Orgel, M.C., Experimental studies with clinical application to peripheral nerve injury: A review of the past decade, *Clinical Orthopaedics*, 163, 1984: 98-106.
14. Ducker, T.S., Metabolic factors in surgery of peripheral nerves, *Surg. Clin. North Am.*, 52, 1972:1109-1122.
15. Omer, G.E., Jr. and Pirela-Cruz, M.A., Complications of peripheral nerve injuries, in *Complications in Orthopaedic Surgery*, 3rd ed., Epps, C.H., Jr., Ed., J.B. Lippincott, Philadelphia, Vol. 2, 1994, Chap. 30:811-856.
16. Seddon, H.J., Three types of nerve injury, *Brain,* 66: 237-288, 1943.
17. Sunderiand, S., A classification of peripheral nerve injuries producing loss of function, *Brain,* 74: 491-516, 1951.
18. Omer, G.E., Jr., The prognosis for untreated traumatic injuries, in *Management of Peripheral Nerve Problems*, 2nd ed., Omer, G.E., Jr., Spinner, M., and Van Beek, A.L., Eds., W.B. Saunders, Philadelphia, 1998, Chap. 38: 365-370.
19. Guelinckx, P.J., Sinsel, N.K., and Dom, R., Contemporary muscle morphology as related to nerve pathology, in *Management of Peripheral Nerve Problems*, 2nd ed., Omer, G.E., Jr., Spinner, M., and Van Beek, A.L., Eds., W.B. Saunders, Philadelphia, 1998, Chap. 65: 663-668.

20. Omer, G.E., Jr., War injuries of the hand, in *The Hand*, Tubiana, R., Ed. W.B. Saunders, Philadelphia, 1988, Vol. 3, Chap. 82: 903-924.
21. Omer, G.E., Jr., Acute management of peripheral nerve injuries, *Hand Clinics*, 2 (1):193-206, 1986.
22. Omer, G.E., Jr. and Spinner, M., Peripheral nerve testing and suture techniques, *Amer. Acad. Orthop. Surg.*, lnstru. Course Lect, 24:122-143, 1975.
23. Watchmaker, G.P., Gumucio, C.A., Crandall, R.E., Vannier, M.A., and Weeks, P.M., Fascicular topography of the median nerve: A computer based study to identify branching patterns, *J. Hand. Surg.*, 16-A:53-59, 1991.
24. Edshage, S., Peripheral nerve suture, a technique for improved intraneural topography, evaluation of some suture materials, *Acta Chir. Scand.* (Suppl 331), 1964.
25. Smith, J.W., Microsurgery of peripheral nerves, *Plast. Reconstr. Surg.*, 33: 317-329, 1964.
26. Van Beek, A.L. and Pirela-Cruz, M.A., Microsurgical nerve repairs, in *Management of Peripheral Nerve Problems*, 2nd ed., Omer, G.E., Jr., Spinner, M., and Van Beek, A.L., Eds., W.B. Saunders, Philadelphia, 1998, Chap. 26:260-269.
27. Omer, G.E., Jr., O'Brien, W.J., Murray, H.M., Torkelson, E.O., and Orgel, M.G., The technical factors influencing the results of the epineurial technique for peripheral nerve repair, *Peripheral Nerve Repair and Regeneration*, 3: 67-80, 1986.
28. Urbaniak, J.R., Fascicular nerve repair, *Clin. Orthop.*, 163: 57-64, 1982.
29. Millesi, H., Messl, G., and Berger, A., The interfascicular nerve grafting of the medial and ulnar nerves, *J. Bone and Joint Surg.*, 54A: 727-750, 1972.
30. Ducker, T.B., Pathophysiology of peripheral nerve trauma, in *Management of Peripheral Nerve Problems*, Omer, G.E., Jr. and Spinner, M., Eds., W.B. Saunders, Philadelphia, 1980, Chap. 29:475-486.
31. Moneim, M.S. and Omer, G.E., Jr., Clinical outcome following acute nerve repair, in *Management of Peripheral Nerve Problems*, 2nd ed., Omer, G.E., Jr., Spinner, M., and Van Beek, A.L., Eds., W.B. Saunders, Philadelphia, 1998, Chap. 43: 414-419.
32. Brushart, T.M., Trophic and tropic influences on peripheral nerve regeneration, in *Management of Peripheral Nerve Problems*, 2nd ed., Omer, G.E., Jr., Spinner, M., and Van Reek, A.L., Eds., W.B. Saunders, Philadelphia, 1998, Chap. 43: 414-419.

13 Biomechanical Principles Applied to Skeletal Function

Thomas A. DeCoster and Brian Robinson

CONTENTS

13.1 PRINCIPLES AND DEFINITIONS OF MECHANICS

The musculoskeletal system provides both support and motion. The science of biomechanics involves the effects of forces and energy on biologic systems. By applying Newtonian mechanics to these biologic models, we gain an understanding of their function and behavior. The treatment of problems of the musculoskeletal system is facilitated by a knowledge of biomechanical principles. This chapter reviews fundamental principles related to orthopaedic aspects of the musculoskeletal system. Definitions of biomechanical terminology have been included as applied to the biologic model. Examples provided relate these principles to cartilage, bone, muscle, and ligament tissue, and are intended to serve as tools in the understanding and effective management of patients.

0-8493-9237-3/99/$0.00+$.50

13.1.1 Definitions

Anisotropic — Material whose mechanical properties vary with orientation of loading (bone).

Brittle — Materials that remain elastic to failure and therefore have little or no plastic deformation (ceramics, PMMA).

Creep — Progressive deformation under constant load over time (polyethylene).

Ductile — Material that undergoes major plastic deformation prior to failure (adolescent bone).

Dynamics — The mechanics of moving objects.

Elasticity — Capacity of material to resume original shape after application of a load (medial collateral ligament).

Endurance limit — Load that produces failure of an object subjected to 10 million cycles (5th metatarsal fatigue fracture).

Equilibrium — A state of balance for a body at rest. The sum of all forces acting on the body equals zero, and sum of all moments about any point is zero.

Fatigue — The process by which a material fails due to cyclical loading at levels below ultimate stress (5th metatarsal fatigue fracture).

Force — Any action that tends to cause a change in motion of an object (biceps contraction).

Friction — The force between two bodies in contact that resists motion between the bodies.

Inertia — The tendency of a body to oppose any force tending to move it from a position of rest or to change its uniform motion.

Isotropic — Material that possesses the same mechanical properties in all directions (metals, ceramics).

Kinematics — The study of motion of bodies.

Kinetics — The study of motion of bodies and forces involved.

Mass — The quantity of matter of an object.

Mechanics — The science of motion and structure of material objects.

Modulus of elasticity — Uniaxial stress divided by uniaxial strain in the elastic phase of a material (Young's modulus).

Moment — The measure of a tendency to move a body about a point or axis; $F \times d$, where F is a force and d the perpendicular distance from line of action of the force to the point or axis of rotation.

Moment of inertia — A fixed constant of an object that is a measure of the resistance of the body to change in its state of rotation.

Momentum — The property of an object equal to mass times velocity.

Plasticity — The permanent deformation of a material to applied stress without total failure or breakage (greenstick fracture).

Rotation — Motion about one axis.

Statics — The mechanics of a body at rest or equilibrium.

Stiffness — The tendency to resist deformation.

Strain — Change in dimension of a material caused by an applied force, measured as change in length divided by original length.

Strain rate — The rate of deformation (strain) to an applied load (stress) per second.

Strength — Resistance to failure.

Stress — Force being applied to a material measured as pressure or force per unit area perpendicular (normal stress) or parallel (shear stress).

Stress fracture — A misnomer; erroneously used as a synonym for fatigue fracture. All fractures are the result of an applied stress.

Toughness — The capacity to store energy prior to failure.

Translation — A motion where two points of a body move in a parallel manner (fracture displacement).

Ultimate stress — The stress at which material fails (fracture).

Viscoelastic — A substance in which material properties vary over time. The relationship between stress and strain is time dependent (anterior cruciate ligament).

Wolff's postulate — Bone has the capacity to change its structure in response to applied loads over time.

Yield stress — The amount of force per unit area required for material to begin plastic deformation.

13.1.2 Principles

To understand how fractures occur or how articular cartilage becomes damaged, it is useful to develop a framework to analyze the stresses and strains produced when forces and moments are applied to the body. A typical stress-strain curve is depicted in Figure 13.1. For most materials there is a direct stress-strain relationship. Initially there is a linear relationship (line 0-Y), followed by a nonlinear relationship that ultimately leads to material failure when significant stress is applied. The slope of the initial linear phase is the modulus of elasticity (E) measured as the change in stress divided by change in strain anywhere along the linear portion of the graph. The response of a material to an applied stress within the linearly elastic region is completely reversible. The point beyond which stress is no longer proportional to the strain is defined by the yield point (Y). If a material is stretched beyond this, further deformation is no longer purely elastic and when the load is removed this results in a small but permanent deformation (plasticity) of the specimen (D). The ultimate stress (U_{stress}) is the point at which the material fails (F). Strength of a material is defined by the maximum stress that a material achieves. The toughness of a material is defined by the amount of energy a material can absorb prior to failure. This corresponds to the entire shaded area under the curve. By knowing these relationships and understanding their significance, stress-strain relationships and other biomechanical parameters can be determined for biologic specimens such as bone. It is important to note that a material (bone) is analyzed by a stress-strain curve, whereas a structure (an individual femur) is analyzed by a load-deformation curve.

The ultimate tensile stress (U_{stress}) is the stress at failure that occurs with only one cycle. However, with repeated cycles, failure will occur at lower stress. Figure 13.2 demonstrates the relationship between load and number of cycles to

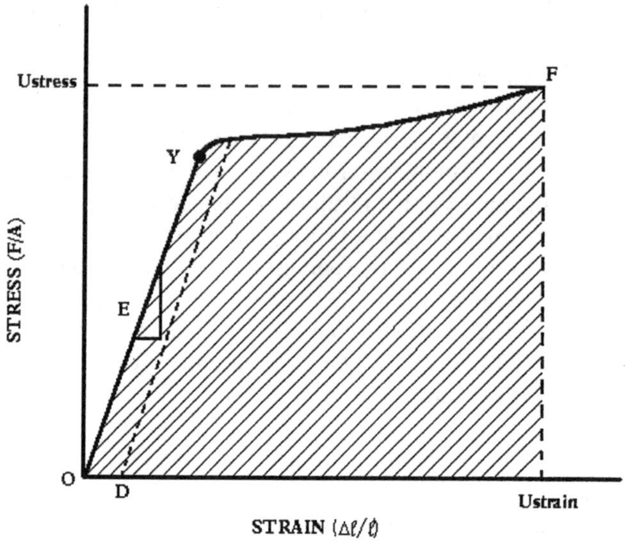

FIGURE 13.1 Typical stress-strain relationship for a material with an initial linear elastic phase to the yield point (Y) followed by plastic deformation to failure (F). The slope of the elastic phase (E) is the modulus of elasticity. Toughness of a material is the area under the curve (shaded).

failure. The fatigue limit (FL) is the point at which failure will not occur no matter how often the cycle is repeated. Practically, the endurance limit is estimated as the load that produces failure in 10 million cycles.

Linear elasticity is useful for evaluation of static elements such as buildings, bridges, and orthopedic implants. However, biologic tissues do not behave similarly. Biologic tissues such as bone, cartilage, and ligaments have viscoelastic properties which are time dependent. When a material exhibits deformation with time under an applied load it is termed creep. Figure 13.3 shows the measured deformation of two different structures subjected to a constant load over time. The deformation of material A does not change with time, whereas deformation has occurred in material B. Material B has undergone creep and demonstrates viscoelastic behavior. The lower graph (curve D) demonstrates the concept of stress relaxation. Stress relaxation occurs when the force required to maintain deformation of a viscoelastic material decreases with time.

When the yield point is very close to the ultimate failure point, the plastic phase is short and the material is considered brittle. A rubber band is elastic (long elastic phase), brittle (short plastic phase), and ductile (high strain to failure). The ends of a snapped rubber band fit back together nearly perfectly, a phenomenon observed in brittle materials. A brittle material such as polymethylmethacrylate (PMMA) has a short elastic phase and virtually no plastic phase. A material with a very long plastic phase, such as taffy, would be considered relatively ductile but not very brittle.

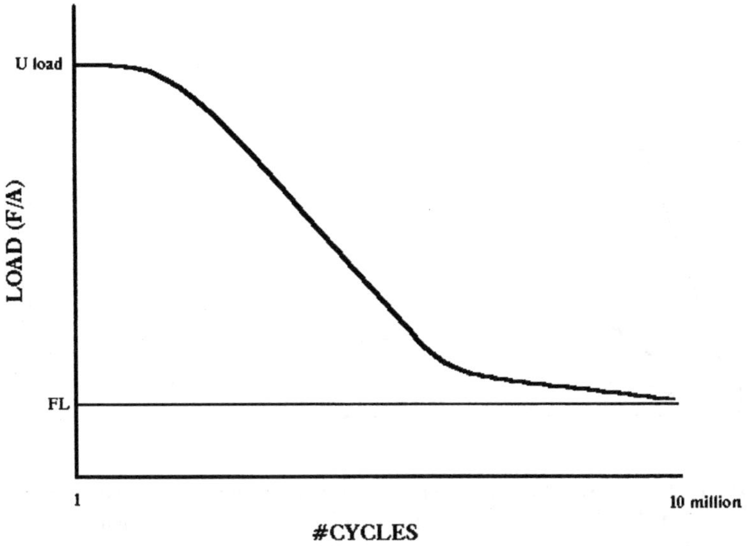

FIGURE 13.2 Fatigue limit (FL) is demonstrated by decreased load to failure with increasing number of load cycles.

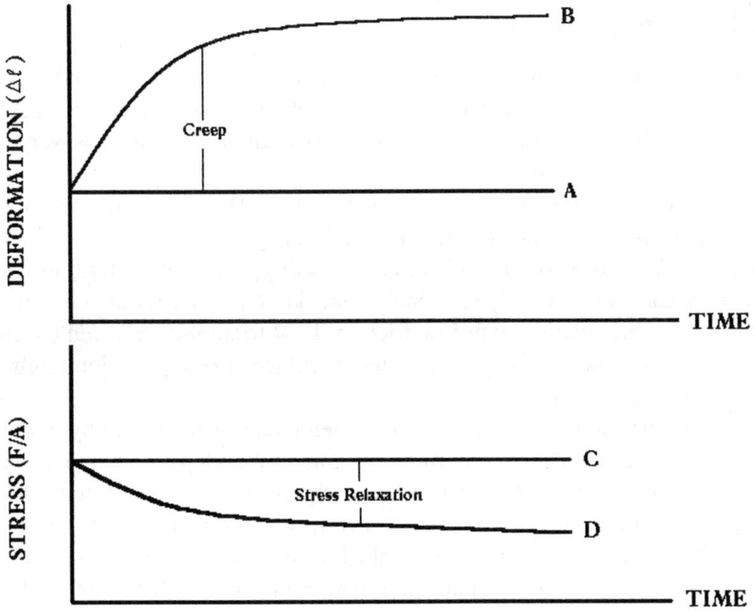

FIGURE 13.3 Viscoelastic properties of both creep (increasing deformation under constant load over time, curve B) and stress relaxation (decreasing stress under constant load over time, curve D). The response of materials and structures which are not viscoelastic are represented by lines C and A.

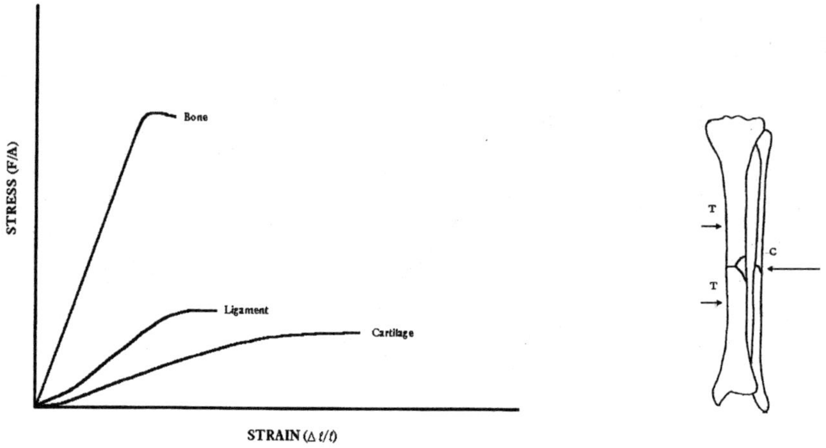

FIGURE 13.4 Relative stress-strain curves for bone, ligament and tendon. Tibia fracture pattern associated with three-point bending (C is compression and T is tension). See text for further details.

13.2 BIOMECHANISMS OF MUSCULOSKELETAL TISSUE

13.2.1 Articular Cartilage

Some of the basic mechanical properties of articular cartilage tissue can be identified from analysis of measurement of strain to applied stress (Figure 13.4). Articular cartilage is resistant to compressive loads and is quite ductile. It is very fatigue resistant and is a viscoelastic tissue.

The function of synovial joints is to allow motion. These joints must also transmit load and be resistant to breakdown, particularly in cyclical compressive loading. An average person who walks 10 miles per day will apply over 10 million cycles of load across each knee in a year. One of the keys to successful joint motion is maintenance of articulation with low friction. Low friction is achieved by virtue of the structure and metabolism of articular cartilage, as well as joint lubrication facilitated by synovial fluid.

Synovial fluid flow across cartilage cell membranes is facilitated by joint motion and loading which do not compromise flow, as in a collapsible blood vessel. The elastic modulus of articular cartilage in compression is a direct function of its proteoglycan contact. The fluid expressed from loading facilitates boundary lubrication of the articulating surfaces. When the load is removed, the globular proteoglycan elastically recoils to its original shape and fluid is reabsorbed. The elastic recoil is a result of electrostatic and osmotic properties as well as mechanical properties of the proteoglycan. Hyaluronate injection therapy, a new treatment of osteoarthritis, works by providing superior lubrication for the affected joint.

When load is applied across a joint over time, fluid will flow away from the area of loading and indentation will occur. Deformation over time in response to a constant load, or creep, identifies articular cartilage as a viscoelastic substance. Articular cartilage is extremely resistant to fatigue but structural degeneration will occur when acute loads exceed the ultimate strength or when cyclical loads exceed the fatigue strength.

Articular cartilage has very limited capacity for cellular hyperplasia. This increases its susceptibility to fatigue failure. Osteoarthritis may represent fatigue failure of articular cartilage. Although physiologic loading may benefit cartilage cells, normal activities in the presence of deformity, such as joint incongruity, can result in localized loads above the fatigue limit of cartilage, leading to degeneration of the cells and loss of function.

Rheumatoid arthritis may have the same ultimate loss of joint function as osteoarthritis but the loads generated tend not to be excessive in an absolute sense. The loads are made relatively excessive by a decrease in cartilage endurance, resulting perhaps from a metabolically induced change in the synovial fluid and/or synovium. Thus, rheumatoid arthritis and osteoarthritis both represent states of fatigue failure due to mechanical causes.

One of the primary functions of joints is to transmit loads. When a functional load is applied to a joint there is a muscle or ligamentous force produced which restrains the applied force. The resultant force vector produced by these two forces is known as the joint reaction force. The joint reaction force of the hip is approximately five times greater than body weight and is primarily due to the force of contraction of the abductors across the joint. This relationship can be demonstrated by a free-body diagram of the hip (Figure 13.5). Decreased joint reactive force across the hip is accomplished by increasing the ratio of a/b. Increasing the offset during total hip arthroplasty, by lateralizing the greater trochanter or using a long neck prosthesis, is a clinical example of effectively increasing length a and thereby decreasing the joint reactive force across the total hip arthroplasty.

C - center of hip rotation
W - total weight
F_M - abductor force
F_{JR} - joint reactive force
a - distance from F_M to C
b - distance from C to W

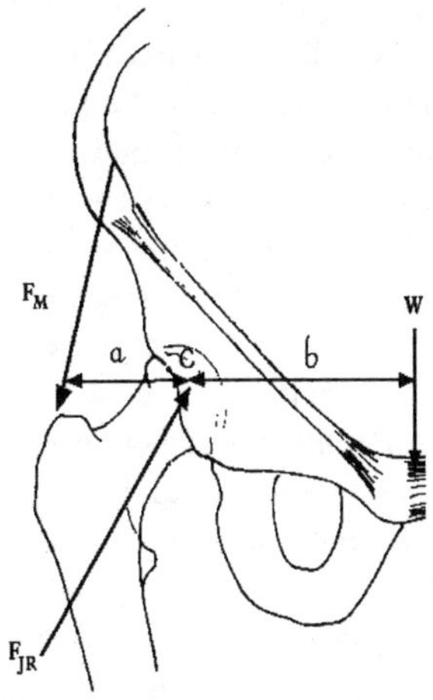

FIGURE 13.5 Hip joint free body diagram.

13.2.2 Bone

The function of bone is to provide structural support, protection of viscera, and stable attachments for muscles. The basic mechanical properties of bone tissue can be identified from an analysis of the ratio of strain to applied stress (Figure 13.4). Bone is quite strong with respect to compression. The ratio of the yield point, and stress to failure in compression is relatively high in bone. Bone, however, fails at a relatively low ratio of strain-to-failure (low ductility). It is susceptible to a low fatigue limit and is mildly viscoelastic. Proof of bone's viscoelastic nature is the fact that bone fails at three times the stress when the load is applied quickly.

A variety of pathological conditions may affect bone. Osteoporosis is a condition where the quantity of bone is diminished per unit volume of bone. In osteoporosis, the stress-strain relationship is unchanged, but load deformation is shifted down. Osteomalacia, a condition of diminished bone quality, would result in a downward shift of the stress-strain curve, as well as of the load deformation curve.

Fractures occur when bone is loaded beyond its ultimate strength and may occur as a result of compression, tension, or torsional loading. Three-point bending, as demonstrated in Figure 13.4, will cause tension to develop in the side labeled T and compression on side C. The resistance to fracture is a function of the magnitude of the bending force, the cross-sectional area of bone, and geometric distribution of the bone. If the load exceeds ultimate strength, fracture will occur and a crack will be initiated. Bone is anisotropic, being weaker in tension than compression. For equal loads, failure will initially occur on the tension side. In cases of a load that is applied extremely slowly or to a pathologically weak bone, the resulting fracture will assume a transverse pattern. A more typical fracture pattern is shown in Figure 13.4 with the butterfly comminution on the side of compression. The secondary fracture lines are at 45° to the long axis of the bone and comprise about two thirds of the diameter of the bone. The addition of axial load to three-point bending will tend to enlarge the percentage of circumferences involved in comminution, as will the magnitude of the forces and rate of loading.

Time-related changes have an important impact on fatigue resistance and help distinguish biological from inert substances. Crack initiation, propagation, and fracture are phases of fatigue fracture. Crack initiation typically occurs after the first 90% of cycles necessary for fatigue failure. Bone as biological tissue tends to lay down new bone over time, and *in vivo* endurance limits are much higher than *in vitro* endurance limits. There is evidence that strain is the physical property most directly related to osteogenesis. This effect is mediated by piezoelectric phenomena. Compression creates a small positive charge, which under certain conditions is osteoinductive.

Iatrogenic trauma to bone occurs with holes or slot defects used for screw placement, bone graft harvest, and surgical exposure. A small hole in a tubular bone, such as that following removal of a 4.5-mm screw from a femur, dramatically increases risk of fracture. Ultimate strength to a torsional load is reduced by half. When a large cortical graft greater than one third the tibial circumference is harvested, an open section tube is created. Ultimate strength to torsional load is reduced by two thirds and energy needed to induce failure is reduced by 90%.

13.2.3 Muscle

Muscle provides the force needed for motion. The mechanical characteristic of muscle that facilitates this function is contractibility.

The strain to applied torsion stress is commonly referred to as distensibility, and muscle is very ductile in tension. It has a long elastic and plastic phase and the strain needed to bring about failure is quite high. Muscle has a high fatigue level and is quite viscoelastic. Muscles undergo progressive elongation in response to a constant load over time (stress relaxation) and demonstrate other viscoelastic properties. Tension applied to a muscle held at constant length deteriorates to zero over time.

In a process fueled by adenosine triphosphate, mediated by calcium influx, and triggered by excitation of electrical signals from the neuromuscular junction, muscle filaments slide together, causing contraction of the muscle and generation of force. Muscle fibers are incapable of active lengthening; their response to an external tension depends on their state of excitation or tone. Although each myofibril contracts completely or not at all, the same is not true of the muscle as a whole. Therefore, the mechanical characteristics of a visibly contracting muscle depend on the magnitude of the active contraction. That in turn depends on the characteristics of the excitation signal, the length of muscle during contraction, and the speed of contraction. Muscle is surrounded by an extensive network of connective tissue (collagen) which aids in the mechanical transmission of forces and provides additional resistance to stretch.

Muscles are attached to bone by tendons, which are composed of parallel bundles of collagen specialized to transmit tension. Tendons are smaller in cross-sectional area than their corresponding muscle, but yield point and ultimate failure occur at higher stress per unit area. The yield and strain-to-failure are less, making the tendon less ductile. This may account for an increased susceptibility of tendons to rupture as compared to muscle.

Tendinitis may be a biological response to plastic deformation. Tension injuries to muscle-tendon units are clinically referred to as strains, in contrast to sprains for ligament tension injuries. This is potentially confusing because "strain" is a universal mechanical response of tissue, as opposed to an injury of a specific structure.

Mechanical characteristics are important in tendon transfers, which are usually designed to replace lost function. Balances must be achieved between agonists and antagonists both in terms of excursion and strength. An extensor must have sufficient strength to stretch a flexor with resting tone even if function requires greater strength in flexion than extension. Muscle force-generating capacity is a function of cross-sectional area. Muscle tone can provide a limit to antagonistic range of motion. In muscles that cross more than one joint, the range of motion of one joint depends on the position of another. For example, if gastrocnemius tightness limits ankle dorsiflexion, then greater dorsiflexion will occur with the knee flexed than extended, because this muscle crosses both the knee and ankle joints. This is one way muscle can act as a dynamic stabilizing link between joints.

13.2.4 Ligaments

Ligaments are fibrous connective tissue bands, with abundant skewed bundles of collagen, that connect bones. The function of ligaments is to enhance joint stability and direct normal tracking with motion. The extremes of range of motion are generally controlled by tension in ligaments or joint surface contours. Ligaments also resist externally applied forces, out of the plane of motion, throughout the normal joint range of motion.

Ligaments play a very important role in limiting secondary range of motion as primary position changes. Similar to relaxed muscle and in contrast to bone and cartilage, ligaments typically exist *in vitro* in a resting state of slack that must be overcome before strains begin. The mechanical parameters of ligament tissue are illustrated in Figure 13.4. Ligaments are commonly exposed to tensile loading and are strongest in resisting tension. Ligaments do not resist compression particularly well and would be easily crushed if exposed to compressive loads.

Ligaments have a long and fairly high plastic phase (ductile) with considerable capacity to absorb energy. Ligament tissue is fatigue resistant and exhibits creep. Bone and ligament tissue strength (stress to ultimate failure) both vary as a function of rate of load application. Although both have increased strength at faster load rates, the ligament will fail first at slow rates, whereas the bone will fail first at rapid rates (Figure 13.4). A ligament avulsion fracture does not require plastic deformation of the ligament, but plastic deformation is possible in the presence of an avulsion fracture. Plastic deformation always occurs in the presence of ligament rupture and is possible as an isolated injury. Some have classified ligament response to tension on the basis of mechanics, with grade I being the elastic phase, grade II the plastic phase, and grade III beyond ultimate strength (Figure 13.6). Clinical correlation of this mechanical grading system can be made by the assessment of the amount of excursion and subjective quality of the end-point as the ligament becomes taut. Physical examination of an injured ligament includes evaluation of excursion and end-point quality. The end-point quality is mainly determined by the ligament becoming taut. Grade I ligament injury is characterized by normal excursion because elastic recoil has occurred with minimal plastic deformation and end-point quality is normal. Grade II injury demonstrates increased excursion because of plastic deformation and normal end-point quality because the ligament is in continuity. Grade III injury represents complete ligament disruption. When this injury occurs, joint excursion is increased until secondary restraints become taut and end-point quality is poor, reflecting the nature of secondary restraints. To make the clinical assessment of ligament injury more objective, instruments such as the KT-1000 arthrometer have been developed to standardize the applied loads and measurement of excursion.

Ligament bundles are in various stages of tautness in any given position of a joint. As load is applied little strain occurs until these bundles become taut. As strain occurs in the elastic phase, slack is taken out of other bundles and energy is absorbed. A constant load in a different joint position may lead to some bundles becoming slack as their particular bony attachments are brought closer together by joint motion and others becoming taut as their points of bony contact are separated. No bundle

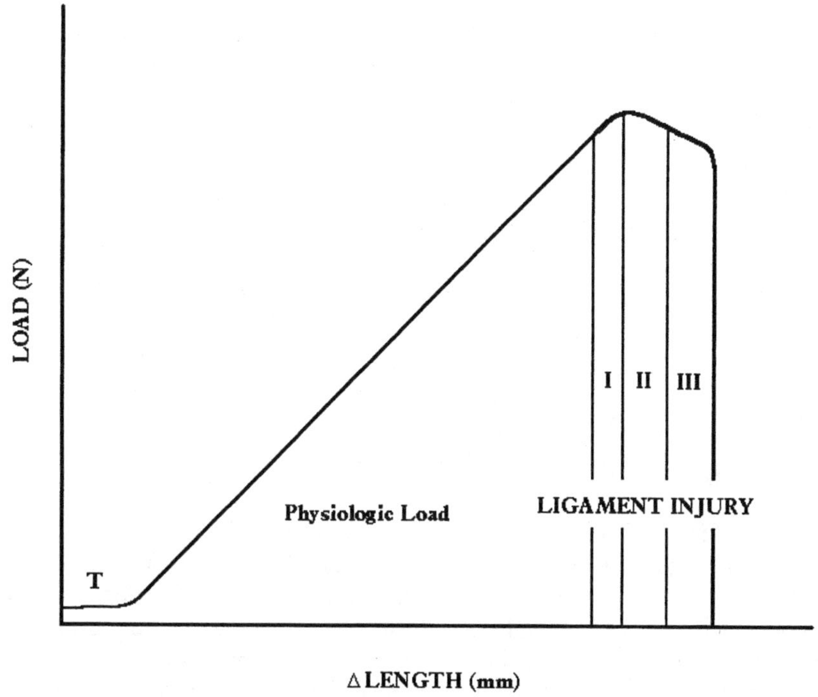

FIGURE 13.6 Typical load deformation curve for a ligament. Note that injury occurs once physiologic load has been exceeded (beyond the yield point).

may be stretched beyond its yield point within a normal range of motion, or plastic deformation would occur leading to progressive joint laxity. This has led to the concept of isometric ligament attachment. Isometry is not strictly accurate. Points of bony attachment do not stay at a constant distance through range of motion in a normal joint. To prevent injury, this normal change in distance must be within the slack and elastic phase of strain allowed by individual ligament fibers. For example, if the points of attachment of an anterior cruciate ligament graft are significantly farther apart in flexion compared to extension, then the graft will either stretch, resulting in laxity, or knee flexion will be restricted, resulting in stiffness.

13.3 SKELETAL FIXATION

Implants are used to provide structural support in the presence of acquired skeletal instability (fracture). The function of fracture fixation devices is to maintain reduction and allow fracture healing. Skeletal implants require sufficient strength to avoid failure from physiological loads but must not prevent normal bone healing to occur.

As with all non-biological materials, fracture fixation devices are susceptible to fatigue failure. Since some transmission of load to the bone is desirable, fracture fixation devices are not exclusively stiff. Thus, motion at the fracture site decreases as union occurs and the bone assumes a greater proportion of applied loads. There is a slow race between fracture union and implant failure. Factors that impede union (excessive motion, large fracture gap, infection, soft-tissue interposition, and hypovascularity) increase the likelihood of fatigue failure of the implant.

Because of the forces applied to implants, strength is an essential requirement to prevent implant failure and loss of reduction. Strain to physiologic load is particularly important in avoiding malunion and nonunion. If the implant is too flexible, then the strain from physiological load is too great, the callus will not ossify and nonunion will result. Alternatively, reduction will be lost, leading to malunion. If the implant is too stiff, then there may be too little bone strain and there may be insufficient stimulus to bone healing and atrophic nonunion with bone resorption will occur.

Mechanical properties of the implant and the bone implant construct vary with type and design of the device. Some basic mechanical principles of screws, plates, intramedullary nails, and external fixation will now be discussed.

13.3.1 Intramedullary Nails

Unlocked intramedullary nails are internal struts and are load sharing because of their frictional attachment to bone. The strength of a circular nail is proportional to the yield strength of the material and the third power of the nail radius. The stiffness is proportional to the elastic modulus and the moment of inertia. An intramedullary nail mechanically represents a cylinder. Thus, the moment of inertia and stiffness are proportional to the fourth power of the radius of the nail. As an example, a 16-mm nail is more than twice as strong and more than three times as stiff as a 12-mm nail.

	12-mm nail	16-mm nail	Increase
Strength α $\mathbf{r}^3$	$(12/2)^3 = 216$	$(16/2)^3 = 512$	2.4
Stiffness α $\mathbf{r}^4$	$(12/2)^4 = 1296$	$(16/2)^4 = 4096$	3.6

The nail-bone construct is very resistant to translation in the coronal and sagittal planes. Prevention of angulatory malunion is mainly dependent on the property of the nail, inasmuch as bone-nail contact is increased by bending loads and the fracture fragments have very little resistance to bending. Closed section nails have ten times greater resistance to torsion than slotted nails. However, prevention of rotational malunion is more dependent on bone-nail contact and fracture stability rather than on the torsional stiffness of the nail.

Nail strength in compression is far in excess of physiological loads. The nail slides in the bone and the bone-nail interface has little resistance to axial load, causing the construct to be dependent upon fracture orientation. A reduced transverse fracture is nearly as resistant to pure compression as an intact bone. In the presence of extensive comminution the construct has very little resistance to compression and is unstable along its length. Small compression forces are primary stimulants to bone healing. Intramedullary nails, load-sharing devices, do not prevent transmission of this mechanical stimulus and thereby stimulate osteogenesis. Addition of proximal and distal locking screws leads to more load bearing by the implant. Delayed union may be treated by removal of locking screws, which makes the construct more load sharing, and in turn stimulates healing at the fracture site.

13.3.2 Plate

Plate fixation of fractures is more likely to result in stress shielding of compression. Therefore, accurate reduction of the fracture is necessary for a successful outcome. The plate must be of sufficient strength to resist axial load. Plate strength in this mode is a function of the material and geometry of the plate. Plate strength in general is not sufficient to withstand the repetitive physiological load of full weight-bearing. The plate is even less resistant to bending and torsion. Plates are quite resistant to tension. Therefore, accurate length and stable reduction of the bone cortex opposite to the plate is very important in resisting bending loads.

Due to rigid fixation of bony fragments, a plate absorbs a compressive load in proportion to the relative stiffness of the plate and bone. The stiffness of a rectangular plate is a function of the elastic modulus of the material and the cross-sectional area of the plate. For example, fixation of a 10-mm bone with a 2-mm thick stainless steel plate will result in load sharing. Stainless steel is about ten times less elastic than bone, but the bone is five times thicker than the plate. Therefore, the plate will absorb two thirds of any applied load and the bone will absorb one third. Increasing the thickness of the plate increases its strength and resistance to fatigue failure but also decreases its elasticity. This is undesirable, because it increases protection against stress and therefore bone resorption. A 4-mm-thick plate would absorb 80% of the load and the bone only 20%. Stress protection continues after fracture healing if the implant has not loosened or been removed.

Refracture after plate removal is a risk for three reasons: 1. There is a section of avascular, and thus dead bone, beneath the plate. 2. Holes left from extracted screws weaken bone structure. 3. Stress protection results in metabolic resorption of bone in proportion to the relative stiffness of the bone-plate construct. Ridges of bone around screw holes and plate edges add strength to the bone in these weakened areas. Removal of a ridge of bone adjacent to extracted plates is cosmetically appealing but weakens the bone in an area of stress concentration and therefore is discouraged. Remodeling after plate removal can completely reverse all three deleterious effects, but this takes several months.

Plate material also influences plate mechanics. Titanium is less stiff than stainless steel and has desirable strength and fatigue characteristics. Stress protection for a given geometry of plate would be less with titanium than with stainless steel. It is unclear whether the increased strain transmission to the fracture site is favorable for fracture healing and clinically relevant.

13.3.3 Screws

Screws gain purchase in bone as a result of the interface between the trailing edge of the thread and bone and the undersurface of the screw head against the cortex. The screw threads work as simple inclined plane machines (Figure 13.7). Interfragmentary compression is achieved by thread purchase only in the far cortex. A screw introduced into a properly prepared hole advances until the undersurface of the head

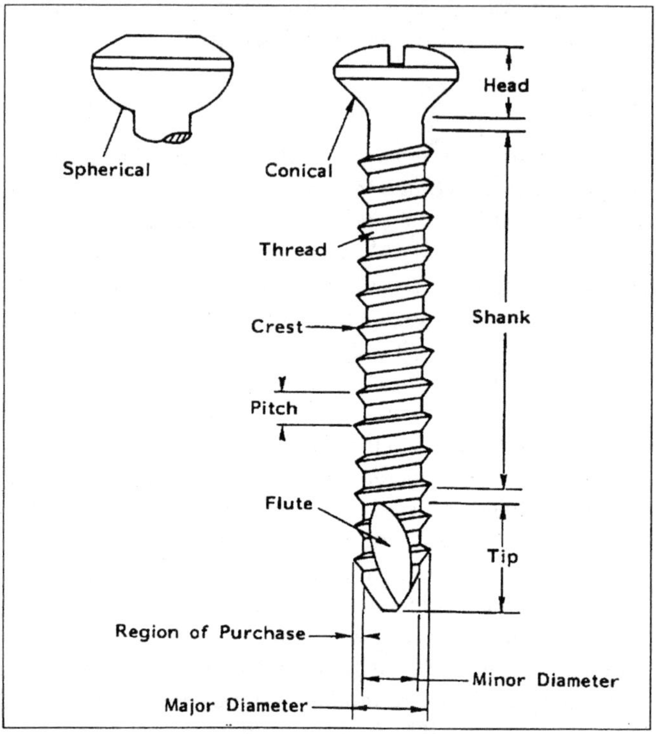

FIGURE 13.7 Bone screw characteristics.

comes into contact with the bone. Further turning of the screw causes it to spin but it remains stationary relative to the near cortex. The far fragment slides up the spiral inclined plane of the screw thread and compression of the fracture is achieved.

The strength of the screw itself is a function of its minor diameter and the material. Failure of a screw can occur at the fracture site, at the thread-bone interface, or at the bone-screw head interface. Failure at the fracture site is a function of surface area contact and hence dependent on fracture pattern, reduction, and bone quality. Similarly, failure at the bone-screw head interface is a function of surface area contact and material strength (i.e., bone and screw). The contact area may be increased by use of a countersink or washer. The most common failure is at the thread-bone interface and is a function of the bone density, contact area, and thread design.

Tremendous compressive forces can be achieved with screw fixation; these are generally well tolerated by the bone ends. The isolated screw is particularly susceptible to loosening, as fixation is so dependent on the small amount of bone at the thread-bone interface that may fail with time. The friction of fracture ends anatomically reduced and held in compression protects the thread-bone interface from the stresses of applied loads. Plates may also be used to neutralize the stresses of applied loads taking advantage of the stress protection phenomena.

13.3.4 External Fixation

External fixation is comprised of pins held by pin-holding clamps connected to rods. Pins are typically subjected to cyclical bending loads. The strength of the pin itself is a function of the least diameter between the near cortex and pin-holding clamp. If threads extend beyond the near cortex, this least diameter is the minor thread diameter. For tapered pins the least diameter is that at the near cortex. Small diameter wires placed under tension have mechanical properties similar to large untensioned half-pins. Complex articulations have been developed to optimize the stabilizing capacity of frames across joints to maintain reduction and allow motion when the frame axis of motion matches the joint.

Frame stability is enhanced by increasing pin diameter and number, increasing connecting rod diameter and number, increasing number of connections between connecting rods, decreasing the distance from fracture to pins, and decreasing distance from bone to connecting rod. External fixators provide non-rigid fixation and exact reduction is not required for successful treatment.

By being external, these frames are accessible to mechanical alteration over the course of fracture healing. As fracture healing progresses, the need for frame rigidity lessens and dynamization of the fixator is desirable in order to prevent nonunion. Slotted sliding connecting rod geometry may allow dynamization by allowing load transmission in compression, while still resisting torsion, angulation, and translation. Longitudinal compression of the fracture ends can be accomplished by increasing the overlap of the connecting rods.

REFERENCES

1. Black, J. *Orthopaedic Biomaterials in Research and Practice.* Churchill Livingstone, New York, 1988.
2. Black, J. and Dumbleton, J.H., Eds. *Clinical Biomechanics—A case history approach.* Churchill Livingstone, New York, 1981.
3. Cochran, G.V. *A Primer of Orthopaedic Biomechanics.* Churchill Livingstone, New York, 1982.
4. Dalton, J.D., Jr., Seaber, A.V., and Garrett, W.E., Jr. Biomechanics of passively stretched muscle: viscoelasticity vs. reflex effects, *Surg. Forum,* 40, 516, 1989.
5. Gozna, E.R. and Harrington, I.J. *Biomechanics of Musculoskeletal Injury.* William and Wilkins, Baltimore, 1982.
6. Mow, V.C. and Hayes, W.C., Eds. *Basic Orthopaedic Biomechanics.* Raven Press, New York, 1991.
7. Nordin, M. and Frankel, V.H., Eds. *Basic Biomechanics of the Musculoskeletal System.* 2nd ed. Lea & Febiger, Philadelphia, 1989.
8. Noyes, F.R., Butler, D.L., Grood, E.S., et al. Biomechanical analysis of human ligament grafts used in knee ligament repairs and reconstructions, *J. Bone Joint Surg.,* 66A, 344, 1984.
9. Pauwels, F. *Biomechanics of the Locomotor Apparatus.* Springer-Verlag, New York, 1980.

14 Healing of Bone and Connective Tissues

Andrew E. Caputo

CONTENTS

14.1 HEALING

Whether bone, tendon, or ligament, the healing of musculoskeletal tissues occurs through similar and specific phases. Despite their biochemical and biomechanical differences, these structures are vascularized collagen frameworks and therefore have

0-8493-9237-3/99/$0.00+$.50

similarities in their healing process. Although the healing process is typically divided into three specific phases, this actually represents a continuum of events.[1] The three phases are inflammation, repair, and remodeling. The first phase, *inflammation*, occurs immediately after injury and lasts for 3 to 4 days. Leukocytes and erythrocytes fill the area and phagocytosis of necrotic tissue occurs. Vasoactive and chemotactic factors are released and cells migrate to the affected area. Vascular invasion facilitates the migration of inflammatory and mesenchymal cells. Fibroblasts produce collagen and rudimentary scar tissue. This phase of healing is associated with the clinical findings of swelling, pain, and warmth. Interestingly, fetal wound healing occurs with minimal inflammation and no scar formation. The second phase is *repair*, which involves the removal of necrotic debris and the replacement with new cell matrix. This phase lasts from the first few days to approximately 4 to 6 weeks. Undifferentiated mesenchymal cells proliferate and produce the matrix. The origin of these undifferentiated mesenchymal cells is often a topic of controversy, as they may arise from local tissue (i.e., periosteum of bone) or arrive by way of invading capillaries. The newly synthesized matrix is often specific to the area and depends on local growth factors and biochemical and biomechanical conditions. The third phase, *remodeling*, involves the reorganization of tissue composition specific to the area and can take up to 12 months. The reorganization at the biochemical level involves the density and specificity of cells and the type and orientation of collagen. Biomechanically, the tissues remodel according to specific characteristics that depend on the local conditions. These tissues must therefore be exposed to stress during the healing process to optimize their functional potential.

The specific differences between the healing of bone, tendon, and ligaments, along with the effect of aging, exercise, and immobilization, will now be discussed.

14.2 LIGAMENT

14.2.1 Structure and Function

Ligaments are a specialized form of dense connective tissue that connects one bone to another. Ligaments represent the static restraint to joints, resisting abnormal stress, yet oriented in position to allow normal motion. Like tendons, ligaments have a dense connective tissue matrix made up primarily of collagen type I (70% of dry weight). Ligaments also contain elastin (less than 1% dry weight) which, as the name indicates, affects the elastic properties of the ligament depending on its amount in various locations. Ligaments have two types of insertions: direct and indirect. Direct insertion is the most common and occurs through four zones of transition: collagen, fibrocartilage, mineralized fibrocartilage, and bone.[2] Failure at direct insertions typically occurs between the mineralized and unmineralized fibrocartilage. Indirect insertion sites involve the attachment of superficial fibers to periosteum. The failure of ligaments is strain rate dependent.[3]

Ligament injuries are often referred to as a specific grade, dependent upon the severity of injury. Grade I includes mild sprains, or an overstretching of the ligament without gross disruption. Grade II injuries are partial tears with some evidence of gross tears; however, the ligament maintains some integrity. Grade III injuries are complete ligament disruptions. The grading of ligament tears assists with the treatment plan for these injuries. Grade I and II tears are generally treated conservatively with physical therapy. Microscopic failure of the collagen fibrils in grossly intact ligaments may be a significant cause of clinical instability. Depending on their location, Grade III tears may require operative intervention. This is the case when a tear would not have healed properly because of the interposition soft tissue, as in an injury to the ulnar collateral ligament of the thumb metacarpal-phalangeal joint, or because of interposition of synovial fluid, as in injury to the anterior cruciate ligament of the knee.

Ligaments are relatively avascular, but their healing response is typical of vascularized musculoskeletal tissues. The correlation of the biomechanical properties of ligaments with healing has been most extensively studied in the knee, which has been reviewed recently.[4] Ligaments receive their blood supply primarily from the adjacent soft tissues and partly from the bone insertion sites. In addition, the cruciate ligaments receive much of their nutrition from synovial fluid. During the reparative phase of healing, the predominant collagen is type III. In the later part of the reparative phase, the amount of collagen type I increases and the collagen fibrils become more parallel. As remodeling proceeds, the healing ligament increasingly acquires biomechanical and biochemical properties found in normal, uninjured tissue. Collagen fibrils acquire a larger diameter, and the total collagen content of the fiber increases. Certain ligaments heal with a final cross-sectional area that is greater than the original ligament. The increased size offsets the diminished material properties, with the final result that structural properties are relatively equivalent.

14.2.2 Response to Exercise and Loading

Ligaments do respond favorably to the stress of exercise. As a result, there is an increase in overall mass, stiffness, and the load at which failure recurs. Material properties are also improved, with increased stress and strain at failure.

14.2.3 Response to Immobilization

Immobilization adversely affects the structure and function of ligaments.[5] After prolonged periods of immobilization, ligaments exhibit a decrease in collagen content and synthesis, in water and proteoglycan content.[6] This leads to a decrease in the overall mass, stiffness and load at failure. Disuse can cause subperiosteal bone resorption at the insertion sites,[7] which in turn can increase the possibility of avulsion injuries.

14.2.4 Response to Aging

Aging also affects the location of injury within the ligament-bone complex. In one study, the major mode of failure was ligament disruption in specimens from young adults and avulsion of bone beneath the ligament insertion site in specimens from older people.[8]

14.2.5 Surgical Repair versus Reconstruction

After a complete disruption, some ligaments can heal without surgical intervention. The effective conservative treatment of complete tears has certain requirements. First, the ligament ends should be approximated without soft tissue or synovial fluid interposition. The joint that the ligament spans must be congruous and not subluxable, as this could lead to an incompetent ligament. Accordingly, improved medial collateral ligament healing was found to occur in animals that had anterior cruciate reconstruction as compared to those that did not have that reconstruction.[9] Lastly, the healing ligament should be exposed to stress in a controlled manner to help contour the remodeling process, yet not impair healing. Whatever the treatment method, a *functional* repair is the best that can be expected, but not "*normal*."

The anterior cruciate ligament (ACL) is most commonly studied because it is frequently injured and hard to heal by conservative or surgical repair. It is currently best treated by reconstruction, that is, replacement with another connective tissue. The most common autograft sources include bone-patellar tendon-bone, hamstring tendons, and quadriceps tendon. After implantation, these grafts undergo ligamentization, i.e., conversion of the tendon graft to resemble a ligament. For this to occur, the tissue must first undergo necrosis and then revascularization. During this process, the graft's structural properties decrease, as seen within the first few months after implantation. Early failure typically occurs at the sites of fixation. Once these sites mature, failure usually occurs in the midsubstance of the new ligament. Allografts have also been used as a source for ligament reconstruction. In animal models, allografts have shown poorer structural properties early and a slower rate of incorporation.[10]

14.3 TENDON

14.3.1 Structure and Function

Tendons are a specialized form of dense connective tissue, which transmit muscle force to bone. Compared to ligaments, tendons have a higher content of collagen type I (95% of dry weight compared to 70%) and do not contain elastin. Like ligaments, tendons contain small amounts of collagen type III, which is associated with healing. Tendons also contain small amounts of proteoglycan, usually in areas where the tendons are exposed to compressive loads (i.e., crossing a joint). These biochemical characteristics help to explain some of the differences in material properties between tendons and ligaments. Tendons are typically stiffer (less strain under given load) and less viscoelastic (less sensitive to changes in strain rate). These properties are important in the direct transmission of muscle force to joint motion.

The insertion sites of tendons have regions of fibrocartilage and calcified cartilage, similar to direct ligament insertions.[2]

Like ligaments, tendons can have a spectrum of injury from mild strains to complete rupture. Injuries to tendons can result from acute avulsion of the insertion site, laceration, or from chronic microtrauma with late rupture. Acute eccentric loading of the muscle tendon often causes tears at the musculotendinous junction, because of the abrupt change in stiffness between the two tissues.

Tendons are either extrasynovial or intrasynovial. Intrasynovial tendons (like the flexor digitorum profundus) are less vascularized and obtain their nutrition from synovial fluid, small feeder vessels (vincula), and the sites of insertion into muscle and bone. Extrasynovial tendons, like the patellar tendon, are more vascularized and gain blood supply from adjacent soft tissues, like the fat pad. Sometimes tendons interdigitate prior to insertion (such as the rotator cuff), and their anatomic boundaries are less defined than is the case with digital flexor tendons.

14.3.2 Injury and Repair

The healing of tendons involves the typical stages of inflammation, repair, and remodeling. Completely lacerated or ruptured tendons can heal without surgery. However, relative apposition must occur along with careful avoidance of abnormal stresses, which could impair proper healing. This approach often requires excessive immobilization. Because immobilization is detrimental and therefore undesirable, the need of operative intervention is frequent. The goals of operative intervention are to reestablish continuity and the proper functional tension, while allowing for early motion to optimize functional capacity. Tendon healing, depending on the location and the circumstances of the injury, involves variable degrees of intrinsic and extrinsic healing. Extrinsic healing means incorporation of structures outside the tendon proper (annular pulleys, subcutaneous tissue); this in turn can cause detrimental adhesions. Early studies have emphasized the healing of tendons by means of recruitment of mesenchymal cells from local tissue.[11] However, intrinsic healing occurs as well, because tendon cells do possess the potential of repair.[12,13] Intrasynovial tendons, like the digital flexor tendons, heal by a combination of extrinsic and intrinsic mechanisms. Extrasynovial tendons heal with predominantly extrinsic mechanisms. Tendons have the ability to undergo intrinsic healing with direct tendon apposition. By the controlled use of passive motion for healing repaired intrasynovial tendons, extrinsic healing and adhesions can be limited, thereby effecting stronger repair.[14] Early controlled active motion allows for more improved remodeling and gains in tensile strength.[15] Early active motion requires repair strong enough to withstand these forces and, what is important, diligent compliance with rehabilitation.

Tendon healing into bone occurs through progressive reestablishment of collagen-fiber continuity eventually resembling Sharpey's fibers.[16] The timing of tendon healing into bone is not only important for tendon repairs, but also for anterior cruciate ligament reconstruction.

14.3.3 Response to Exercise and Loading

In general, tendons respond favorably to exercise, with increases in stiffness, and in the number and density of smaller diameter fibrils. However, this may not be true for all tendons.

14.3.4 Response to Immobilization

Tendons are adversely affected by immobilization. Without stress, tendons demonstrate a loss of biomechanical properties at the insertion sites as well as within the substance of the tendon.

14.4 BONE HEALING

14.4.1 Stages

Like other connective tissues, the healing of bone proceeds through the general stages of inflammation, repair, and remodeling. However, fracture healing has its own well-described phases, or events. These are impact, induction, inflammation, soft callus, endochondral ossification, and remodeling.[1] The initial event is impact, which is the absorption of energy creating the fracture. The second stage is induction, which involves hematoma formation, necrosis of the ends of the fracture fragments, and the influx of inflammatory cells. The fracture site exhibits a low oxygen tension and pH, which together with growth factors facilitate the chemotaxis of inflammatory cells. Stage III, inflammation, is heralded by the appearance of various inflammatory cells such as polymorphonuclear cells, macrophages, and mast cells. Vascular proliferation occurs involving both the periosteal vessels and the nutrient medullary artery. Osteoclasts, originating from a monocyte cell line,[17] appear and remove necrotic bone. This stage ends with the appearance of cartilage and bone, i.e., stage IV, the soft callus stage, when fracture motion decreases (Figure 14.1). The hardness

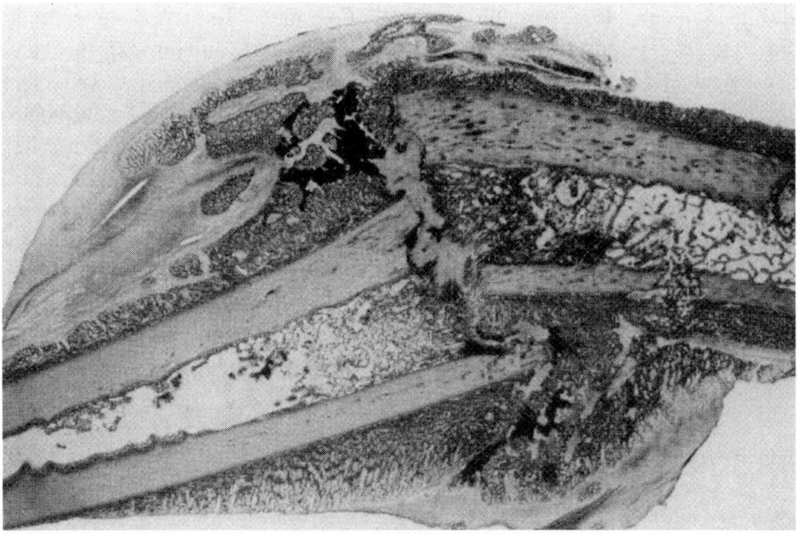

FIGURE 14.1 Light micrograph showing healing of a diaphyseal fracture. The fracture callus consisting primarily of woven bone surrounds and unites the two fracture fragments. As the callus matures, it progressively stabilizes the fracture. Note that the fracture callus contains areas of mineralized and unmineralized cartilage.

of the callus increases as its mineral content increases. Chondroblasts appear in the fracture gap and fibrovascular stroma is converted to chondroid matrix. Endochondral ossification occurs in stage V, where chondroid matrix is converted to woven bone. Radiographic and clinical healing is associated with the end of this stage. The last stage is remodeling, and involves the conversion of woven bone to lamellar bone and the restoration of the medullary cavity and bone diameter.

The periosteum is thicker and more cellular in infants and children, and perhaps for this reason is more active in healing fractures in this age group than adults.

Four biomechanical stages of fracture healing have been described.[18] These include stage I — failure through original fracture site, with low stiffness; stage II — failure through original fracture site, with high stiffness; stage III — failure partially through original fracture site and partially through intact bone, with high stiffness; and stage IV — failure entirely through intact bone, with high stiffness.

14.4.2 Bone Healing in Response to Fixation Methods

The type of surgical intervention determines the type or types of fracture healing. All cases exhibit *primary fracture callus* response, which involves callus formation under the periosteum within the first two weeks. Cast immobilization and nonrigid fixation (i.e., unlocked intramedullary nails) exhibit *external bridging callus* or "endochondral healing," which can bridge fracture gaps. When the bone ends are not in continuity, healing requires bridging callus.

The concept of internal fixation for fracture care is now well recognized, and the principles of anatomical reduction, rigid internal fixation, atraumatic technique, and early range of motion are considered fundamental.[19] Rigid fixation (i.e., with plates) leads to late medullary callus bone formation if the bone ends do not have perfect anatomic apposition.[20] This type of healing can bridge fracture gaps and is the likely outcome of most clinical applications of plate fixation. If perfect apposition is obtained with compression plating, then *primary cortical healing* may occur. This type of healing is slow, cannot bridge gaps, and involves direct osteoclastic resorption and osteon formation.[20] Lamellar bone forms across the fracture line by direct extension of the osteons.[21] Poor apposition will lead to late medullary callus formation and possibly nonunion. One of the concerns with rigid internal fixation is the issue of fatigue fracture secondary to stress shielding of the bone that underlies the plate. Fatigue fracture may be minimized by the use of less rigid internal fixation.

Depending on the construct and stiffness of external fixators and the reduction of the fracture, different types of bone healing may occur. Primary cortical healing can occur with perfect bone apposition and a stiff frame locked in compression. External bridging callus formation may occur with dynamization and intermittent axial load. The use of controlled micromotion has been shown to be advantageous in fracture healing. The application of appropriate axial movement to clinical tibial fractures at a time shortly after injury has been shown to enhance the healing process when external skeletal fixation is used.[22]

Utilization of intramedullary nails has significantly advanced the treatment of long bone fractures. When treated with intramedullary nails, fractures show more periosteal callus than fractures treated with rigid compression plates. Nevertheless, after union occurs, the biomechanical qualities of both are similar.[23] Concern has been expressed about the disruption of the medullary blood supply when intramedullary nails are used. The periosteal arteries supply blood to the outer third of the cortex, and the endosteal vessels supply the inner two thirds of the cortex. Reaming can cause temporary inner cortical necrosis; however, the blood supply is restored in 2 to 3 weeks, with the majority of the regenerative blood supply from endosteum. How much flow is lost depends on the amount and type of reaming.[24] Using intramedullary nails has the advantage that less surgical dissection is needed than for plate fixation. Moreover, intramedullary nails provide a load-sharing construct that allows for early weight bearing.

14.4.3 Collagen Types

Collagen types differ in quality and quantity during fracture healing. Collagen type I is the most prevalent type in bone and is found in high concentrations during the bone forming, or osteogenic, stages of fracture healing. Type II, which is the most prevalent type in cartilage, is found during the chondroid stages. Type III, which is associated with the repair phase of healing for all connective tissues, is prevalent during the mesenchymal stages of fracture healing.

14.4.4 Growth Factors

Various growth factors are involved with the process of fracture healing.[25] These growth factors, their locations and functions are listed in Table 14.1. Growth factor

TABLE 14.1
Growth Factors Involved in Fracture Repair

Growth Factor	Location	Function
Transforming growth factor-β (TGF-β1, TGF-β2)	Platelets, osteoblasts, chondrocytes, bone matrix	1 Increase osteoblast-chondrocyte proliferation 2 Increase proteoglycan synthesis 3 Decrease collagen synthesis
Insulin-like growth factor (IGF) or somatomedin C	Found in bone and cartilage	Stimulates cartilage growth
Platelet-derived growth factor (PDGF)	Platelets, monocytes, endothelial cells	1 Increase osteoblast-chondrocyte proliferation 2 Increase protein synthesis (collagen and noncollagen)
Fibroblast growth factor (FGF)	Inflammatory cells, osteoblasts, chondrocytes	1 Increase cell replication 2 Indirectly increase collagen production
Tumor necrosis factor (TNF)	Macrophages	1 Increase bone resorption 2 Increase cell replication

Reproduced from Kasser (1996), by permission.

production is dependent on the specific stage of fracture healing. For example, TGF-β1 is high during chondrogenesis and endochondral ossification, but low during intramembranous bone formation. TGF-β is known to induce mesenchymal cells to produce type II collagen. Prostaglandins are released in the early phase of bone healing and play a role in early bone resorption, as they stimulate osteoclast activity and cause recruitment of new osteoclasts. Certain cells have been associated with the production of specific growth factors during fracture healing. During the initial stages of fracture healing, macrophages produce growth factors such as TGF-β1, fibroblast growth factor (FGF) and interleukin (IL). PDGF and TGF-β1 are derived from platelet degranulation during hematoma formation. Bone morphogenic protein (BMP) is a growth factor that has recently gained much interest. It is a soluble protein component of bone and when combined with decalcified bone matrix has been shown to induce the formation of bone in extraosseous tissue. In animal models of segmental defects, the use of BMP and decalcified bone matrix has similar effectiveness as autologous iliac crest bone grafting.[26] BMP is currently being tested in large clinical trials for the treatment of nonunions and segmental defects. The receptor cell for BMP is the undifferentiated perivascular mesenchymal cell, which, when stimulated, can produce bone in heterotopic locations.

14.4.5 Nonunion

A delayed union occurs when the fracture healing process slows abnormally. In a nonunion, the process of fracture healing is incomplete. This is often described as the lack of healing at 6 to 8 months, noted radiographically by persistent fracture lines, sclerosis at the fracture ends, a gap, a hypertrophic callus, or a total absence of callus. Most commonly, nonunions are due to either excessive motion or a gap at the fracture site. The incidence of nonunion can also increase with remanipulation of the fracture. Additional factors associated with the development of a nonunion include poor nutrition, smoking, significant comminution and/or soft tissue injury, segmental loss, excessive soft tissue stripping of bone intraoperatively, and rigid fixation with a bone gap. Hypertrophic nonunions are associated with excessive callus formation and are often due to the lack of appropriate immobilization. Atrophic nonunions are recognized by the lack of callus response due to avascularity. Segmental nonunions occur when a segment of bone is missing. A synovial pseudoarthrosis is a false joint or contained sac of fluid that can form in atrophic or hypertrophic nonunions.

How nonunions are treated depends on their cause and the location of the fracture. When a nonunion is due to inadequate immobilization (such as a hypertrophic nonunion), the most important treatment modality is immobilization. This can be accomplished with a cast and electrical stimulation, but open reduction and internal fixation with compression plating is more commonly utilized. After plate stabilization the initial histologic change in hypertrophic nonunions is fibrocartilage mineralization. When a nonunion is atrophic, however, healing requires not only appropriate immobilization, but also removal of the atrophic bone and additional bone graft material.

14.4.6 Electrical Stimulation

The idea of electrical stimulation to enhance healing of fractures and nonunions began with the finding that stress potentials exist in bone. When bone is subjected to a compressive load, the section experiencing compression is electronegative, whereas the section under tension is electropositive. Also, bioelectric or steady-state potentials occur in nonstressed bone in areas of active growth and repair.[27] A dose response of capacitive coupling for the treatment of fractures has been developed.[28] Currently, three basic types of electrical stimulation are used. These are *direct coupling*, which requires implanted electrodes; *inductive coupling*, which is produced by magnetic fields; and *capacitive coupling*, which uses an external capacitor for current generation across the fracture site. Capacitive coupling has been shown to be useful in the treatment of nonunions, except those with synovial pseudarthroses.[29]

14.4.7 Bone Grafting

Bone grafting is utilized to fill in defects secondary to trauma, in congenital abnormalities, or after resection of bone tumors. Of the variety of methods that have been described over the years, the most commonly used are autografts, allografts, and bone substitutes. The selection of the type of bone (cancellous or cortical) depends on the structural needs of the defect. Cortical bone is useful for intercalary defects, such as in diaphyseal defects. Cancellous bone is useful as a space-filler, such as filling in a cyst or packing underneath subchondral bone for depressed intraarticular fractures.

14.4.7.1 Autografts

Autografts, obtained from the patient under treatment, can be cancellous or cortical bone, or a combination of the two. The advantages of autografts over allografts are earlier incorporation and the lack of the risk of disease transmission. The disadvantage is the limited number of available sites and the potential morbidity of the donor site. An important advantage of autografts is that they are osteoconductive and osteoinductive. Osteoconductive means that the graft supplies a structural *framework* for bone formation. Osteoinductive means that the graft supplies factors (cells, growth factors) that *stimulate* bone formation. The osteoinductive potential for autografts depends on the location of the graft and may be altered by the amount of time the graft is out of the host.

Both cortical and cancellous grafts undergo creeping substitution, but in a different sequence.[30] Creeping substitution refers to the replacement of graft bone cells by bone cells that have been newly generated by the host. Cortical graft incorporation involves early osteoclastic resorption with associated increased porosity and decreased mechanical strength. This is followed by creeping substitution of the osteoblasts and associated increased mechanical strength. Cortical bone grafts can produce immediate stability; however, vascular invasion and resorption can decrease the strength of the graft for months to years.[31] In contrast, cancellous bone incorporation begins when early osteoblastic activity deposits osteoid on the necrotic trabeculae (appositional bone formation). This initial bone replacement can take place without the need of cutting cones.[20] Mineralization is followed by later osteoclastic activity. By contrast, cancellous bone incorporation is more complete than cortical grafts. Also, because of increased surface area, cancellous grafts incorporate new cells faster than cortical grafts. The most commonly used cancellous autografts are obtained from the iliac crest (anterior or posterior), distal radius, or proximal tibia. The most common cortical grafts are from the fibula or the anterior iliac crest. Autologous bone marrow preparations have also been tested in the treatment of bone defects.[32]

Autogenous vascularized bone grafts do not undergo necrosis like the nonvascularized bone grafts. Vascularized bone grafts are more efficient than non-vascularized grafts. They can be free (transplanted to a new site and blood flow reestablished by microvascular anastomosis) or pedicled (blood supply never interrupted). Both the fibula and the iliac crest may be utilized as a free or a pedicled graft. Because their blood flow is reestablished as part of the operative procedure, they become part of the recipient bone in a fashion similar to that of a fresh fracture. Vascularized bone grafts are useful clinically in the treatment of segmental bone defects,[33] as they do not undergo necrosis or creeping substitution and the associated loss of mechanical strength. Vascularized grafts are indicated for long segmental defects (usually greater than 5 to 6 cm) or when previous infection or irradiation compromises the recipient bed. They are also indicated for the treatment of osteonecrosis, as in vascularized fibula grafting for avascular necrosis of the femoral head.

Currently, only autografts are vascularized. However, there is ongoing research in the area of vascularized allogenic bone grafts and composite grafts. The most difficult issue with this is the morbidity associated with necessary immunosuppression.

14.4.7.2 Allografts

The most common bone allografts are cortical intercalary grafts and cancellous chips. Cortical allografts have been used for posttraumatic intercalary defects.[34] Osteoarticular allografts include cartilage and have been used successfully for posttraumatic articular defects.[35] The advantage of allografts over autografts is the lack of donor site morbidity; however, possible disease transmission is a concern. Unlike soft tissue allograft transplantation, as with heart or kidney transplants, rejection and the need for immunosuppression are smaller concerns with allograft bone transplantation. Bone allografts require sterile harvesting techniques followed by secondary sterilization to decrease transferable pathogens. Sterilization methods include irradiation or the use of chemical agents. Preservation methods such as freezing or lyophilization also decrease immunogenicity of the graft. Lyophilization makes the graft the least immunogenic, but may cause a decrease in the mechanical integrity of the grafts.

The biomechanical properties of allograft bone can be altered by the methods chosen for its preservation and storage.[36] These effects are minimal with deep-freezing or low-level radiation. However, freeze-drying markedly diminishes the torsional and bending strength of bone allografts but does not deleteriously affect the compressive or tensile strength. Irradiation of bone with more than 3.0 megarad or irradiation combined with freeze-drying appears to cause a significant reduction in breaking strength.

Sterile harvesting with freezing as the secondary method of sterilization is one of the most common methods for allograft recovery and preservation. Osteoarticular allografts require cartilage preservation to maintain cell viability. For this reason, the cartilage surface is exposed to dimethyl sulfoxide or glycerol prior to freezing. This process preserves approximately 40% of chondrocytes.

14.4.7.3 Bone Graft Substitutes

Bone graft substitutes are either proteins derived from organic bone or inorganic materials such as ceramics or polymers. Their function is primarily osteoconductive; i.e., they supply the framework for bone formation and mineralization. The inclusion of growth factors, such as bone morphogenetic protein, or autologous bone marrow, confers some osteoinductive capabilities on the composite bone graft substitute.

The most common types of synthetic or inorganic bone grafts are ceramics that include tricalcium phosphate and hydroxyapatite. They have pore sizes ranging from 100 to 300 μm and are structurally similar to bone. Despite their biocompatibility, the ceramics, especially the calcium phosphates, are extremely brittle. This makes them less attractive for structural applications.

Organic bone grafts can be extracted from either human or bovine sources or produced from recombinant DNA methods.[37] An example is TGF-β, which has been found to enhance fracture healing in rabbits.[38] The most-studied material from these sources is bone morphogenetic protein, or BMP. BMP can induce bone formation in extraskeletal sites through endochondral ossification. Many animal studies have shown when combined with some type of carrier, BMP is effective in healing segmental bone defects.[39,40] Patients with resistant nonunions including partial or complete segmental defects have been treated successfully with a composite alloimplant of human BMP and autolyzed, antigen-free, allogeneic bone.[41] The combination of BMP and autogenous cancellous grafts has been used to treat segmental defects in the tibia.[42] A graft composite bone substitute composed of a tricalcium phosphate cylinder, naturally occurring sheep bone morphogenetic protein, and type IV collagen has been found effective in the treatment of segmental tibial defects in sheep.[43] The routine clinical use of BMP still remains to be defined.

14.4.8 Distraction Osteogenesis

In the former Soviet Union, Gavriil Ilizarov developed the method of distraction osteogenesis to create new bone formation.[44-46] A circular external fixator was utilized to gradually separate (distract) osteotomized bone ends, creating new bone in the gap, mostly by intramembranous bone formation. Currently, this technique is used for the treatment of segmental nonunions, angular malunions and occasionally for the elective lengthening of congenitally short bones.

Distraction osteogenesis occurs through three phases: latency, distraction, and consolidation. The first phase occurs during the inflammatory phase of fracture healing and lasts 3 to 10 days. After this, distraction begins by intermittent lengthening, optimally at 1 mm/day in four increments (0.25 mm every 6 hours).[45] The final stage, consolidation, involves the stabilization of the construct after the appropriate amount of lengthening has been achieved. This generally lasts about as long as the initial lengthening time.

During the distraction phase, bone formation resembles intramembranous bone formation with only small amounts of endochondral ossification.[44] The newly formed trabeculae are oriented parallel to the direction of distraction. Mineralization and the formal bone organization occur during the consolidation phase. Weight bearing enhances this final phase.

SUGGESTED READING

Kasser, J.R., *Orthopaedic Knowledge Update V*, American Academy of Orthopaedic Surgeons, Rosemont, IL, 1996.

Simon, S.R., *Orthopaedic Basic Science*, American Academy of Orthopaedic Surgeons, Rosemont, IL, 1994.

Browner, B.D., *Skeletal Trauma*, 2nd Edition, W. B. Saunders Co., Philadelphia, 1998.

REFERENCES

1. Kasser, J.R. *Orthopaedic Knowledge Update V.* Rosemont, IL: American Academy of Orthopaedic Surgeons, 1995.
2. Cooper, R.R., Misol, S. Tendon and ligament insertion. A light and electron microscopic study. *Journal of Bone & Joint Surgery — American* Volume 1970; 52: 1-20.
3. Noyes, F.R., DeLucas, J.L., Torvik, P.J. Biomechanics of anterior cruciate ligament failure: an analysis of strain-rate sensitivity and mechanisms of failure in primates. *Journal of Bone & Joint Surgery — American* Volume 1974; 56: 236-53.
4. Fu, F.H., Harner, C.D., Johnson, D.L., Miller, M.D., Woo, S.L. Biomechanics of knee ligaments: basic concepts and clinical application. Instructional Course Lectures 1994; 43: 137-48.
5. Noyes, F.R., Torvik, P.J., Hyde, W.B., DeLucas, J.L. Biomechanics of ligament failure. II. An analysis of immobilization, exercise, and reconditioning effects in primates. *Journal of Bone & Joint Surgery — American* Volume 1974; 56: 1406-18.
6. Akeson, W.H., Amiel, D., LaViolette, D. The connective-tissue response to immobility: a study of the chondroitin-4 and 6-sulfate and dermatan sulfate changes in periarticular connective tissue of control and immobilized knees of dogs. *Clinical Orthopaedics & Related Research* 1967; 51: 183-97.
7. Klein, L., Player, J.S., Heiple, K.G., Bahniuk, E., Goldberg, V.M. Isotopic evidence for resorption of soft tissues and bone in immobilized dogs. *Journal of Bone & Joint Surgery — American* Volume 1982; 64: 225-30.
8. Noyes, F.R., Grood, E.S. The strength of the anterior cruciate ligament in humans and Rhesus monkeys. *Journal of Bone & Joint Surgery — American* Volume 1976; 58: 1074-82.
9. Engle, C.P., Noguchi, M., Ohland, K.J., Shelley, F.J., Woo, S.L. Healing of the rabbit medial collateral ligament following an O'Donoghue triad injury: effects of anterior cruciate ligament reconstruction. *Journal of Orthopaedic Research* 1994; 12: 357-64.
10. Jackson, D.W., Grood, E.S., Goldstein, J.D., Rosen, M.A., Kurzweil, P.R., Cummings, J.F., Simon, T.M. A comparison of patellar tendon autograft and allograft used for anterior cruciate ligament reconstruction in the goat model. *American Journal of Sports Medicine* 1993; 21: 176-85.

11. Potenza, A.D. Tendon healing within the flexor digital sheath in the dog. *Journal of Bone & Joint Surgery — American* Volume 1962; 44: 49-64.
12. Lundborg, G., Rank, F. Experimental intrinsic healing of flexor tendons based upon synovial fluid nutrition. *Journal of Hand Surgery — American* Volume 1978; 3: 21-31.
13. Manske, P.R., Gelberman, R.H., Vande Berg, J.S., Lesker, P.A. Intrinsic flexor-tendon repair. A morphological study in vitro. *Journal of Bone & Joint Surgery — American* Volume 1984; 66: 385-96.
14. Gelberman, R.H., Chu, C.R., Williams, C.S., Seiler, J.G., Amiel, D. Angiogenesis in healing autogenous flexor-tendon grafts. *Journal of Bone & Joint Surgery — American* Volume 1992; 74: 1207-16.
15. Gelberman, R.H., Vande Berg, J.S., Lundborg, G.N., Akeson, W.H. Flexor tendon healing and restoration of the gliding surface. An ultrastructural study in dogs. *Journal of Bone & Joint Surgery — American* Volume 1983; 65: 70-80.
16. Rodeo, S.A., Arnoczky, S.P., Torzilli, P.A., Hidaka, C., Warren, R.F. Tendon-healing in a bone tunnel. A biomechanical and histological study in the dog. *Journal of Bone & Joint Surgery — American* Volume 1993; 75: 1795-803.
17. Gothlin, G., Ericsson, J.L.E. The osteoclast: review of ultrastructure, origin, and structure-function relationship. *Clinical Orthopaedics & Related Research* 1976; 120: 201-31.
18. White, A.A., Panjabi, M.M., Southwick, W.O. The four biomechanical stages of fracture repair. *Journal of Bone & Joint Surgery — American* Volume 1977; 59: 188-92.
19. Allgower, M., Spiegel, P.G. Internal fixation of fractures: evolution of concepts. *Clinical Orthopaedics & Related Research* 1979: 26-9.
20. McKibbin, B. The biology of fracture healing in long bones. *Journal of Bone & Joint Surgery — British* Volume 1978; 60-B: 150-62.
21. Perren, S.M. Physical and biological aspects of fracture healing with special reference to internal fixation. *Clinical Orthopaedics & Related Research* 1979: 175-96.
22. Kenwright, J., Richardson, J.B., Cunningham, J.L., White, S.H., Goodship, A.E., Adams, M.A., Magnussen, P.A., Newman, J.H. Axial movement and tibial fractures. A controlled randomised trial of treatment. *Journal of Bone & Joint Surgery — British* Volume 1991; 73: 654-9.
23. Rand, J.A., An, K.N., Chao, E.Y., Kelly, P.J. A comparison of the effect of open intramedullary nailing and compression-plate fixation on fracture-site blood flow and fracture union. *Journal of Bone & Joint Surgery — American* Volume 1981; 63: 427-42.
24. Grundnes, O., Reikeras, O. Acute effects of intramedullary reaming on bone blood flow in rats. *Acta Orthopaedica Scandinavica* 1993; 64: 203-6.
25. Canalis, E., McCarthy, T., Centrella, M. Growth factors and the regulation of bone remodeling. *Journal of Clinical Investigation* 1988; 81: 277-81.
26. Einhorn, T.A., Lane, J.M., Burstein, A.H., Kopman, C.R., Vigorita, V.J. The healing of segmental bone defects induced by demineralized bone matrix. A radiographic and biomechanical study. *Journal of Bone & Joint Surgery — American* Volume 1984; 66: 274-9.
27. Friedenberg, Z.B., Brighton, C.T. Bioelectric potentials in bone. *Journal of Bone & Joint Surgery — American* Volume 1966; 48: 915-23.
28. Brighton, C.T., Hozack, W.J., Brager, M.D., Windsor, R.E., Pollack, S.R., Vreslovic, E.J., Kotwick, J.E. Fracture healing in the rabbit fibula when subjected to various capacitively coupled electrical fields. *Journal of Orthopaedic Research* 1985; 3: 331-40.
29. Scott, G., King, J.B. A prospective, double-blind trial of electrical capacitive coupling in the treatment of non-union of long bones [see comments]. *Journal of Bone & Joint Surgery — American* Volume 1994; 76: 820-6.

30. Burchardt, H. The biology of bone graft repair. *Clinical Orthopaedics & Related Research* 1983: 28-42.
31. Wilson, P.D., Jr. A clinical study of the biomechanical behavior of massive bone transplants used to reconstruct large bone defects. *Clinical Orthopaedics & Related Research* 1972; 87: 81-109.
32. Connolly, J., Guse, R., Lippiello, L., Dehne, R. Development of an osteogenic bone-marrow preparation. *Journal of Bone & Joint Surgery — American* Volume 1989; 71: 684-91.
33. Weiland, A.J., Moore, J.R., Daniel, R.K. Vascularized bone autografts. Experience with 41 cases. *Clinical Orthopaedics & Related Research* 1983: 87-95.
34. Jaffe, K.A., Morris, S.G., Sorrell, R.G., Gebhardt, M.C., Mankin, H.J. Massive bone allografts for traumatic skeletal defects. *Southern Medical Journal* 1991; 84: 975-82.
35. Beaver, R.J., Mahomed, M., Backstein, D., Davis, A., Zukor, D.J., Gross, A.E. Fresh osteochondral allografts for post-traumatic defects in the knee. A survivorship analysis. *Journal of Bone & Joint Surgery — British* Volume 1992; 74: 105-10.
36. Pelker, R.R., Friedlaender, G.E., Markham, T.C. Biomechanical properties of bone allografts. *Clinical Orthopaedics & Related Research* 1983: 54-7.
37. Urist, M.R., Silverman, B.F., Buring, K., Dubuc, F.L., Rosenberg, J.M. The bone induction principle. *Clinical Orthopaedics & Related Research* 1967; 53: 243-83.
38. Lind, M., Schumacker, B., Soballe, K., Keller, J., Melsen, F., Bunger, C. Transforming growth factor-beta enhances fracture healing in rabbit tibiae. *Acta Orthopaedica Scandinavica* 1993; 64: 553-6.
39. Johnson, E.E., Urist, M.R., Schmalzried, T.P., Chotivichit, A., Huang, H.K., Finerman, G.A. Autogeneic cancellous bone grafts in extensive segmental ulnar defects in dogs. Effects of xenogeneic bovine bone morphogenetic protein without and with interposition of soft tissues and interruption of blood supply. *Clinical Orthopaedics & Related Research* 1989: 254-65.
40. Yasko, A.W., Lane, J.M., Fellinger, E.J., Rosen, V., Wozney, J.M., Wang, E.A. The healing of segmental bone defects, induced by recombinant human bone morphogenetic protein (rhBMP-2). A radiographic, histological, and biomechanical study in rats [published erratum appears in *Journal of Bone & Joint Surgery — American* 1992 Aug;74(7):1111]. *Journal of Bone & Joint Surgery — American* Volume 1992; 74: 659-70.
41. Johnson, E.E., Urist, M.R., Finerman, G.A. Resistant nonunions and partial or complete segmental defects of long bones. Treatment with implants of a composite of human bone morphogenetic protein (BMP) and autolyzed, antigen-extracted, allogeneic (AAA) bone. *Clinical Orthopaedics & Related Research* 1992: 229-37.
42. Johnson, E.E., Urist, M.R., Finerman, G.A. Repair of segmental defects of the tibia with cancellous bone grafts augmented with human bone morphogenetic protein. A preliminary report. *Clinical Orthopaedics & Related Research* 1988: 249-57.
43. Gao, T.J., Lindholm, T.S., Kommonen, B., Ragni, P., Paronzini, A., Lindholm, T.C., Jamsa, T., Jalovaara, P. Enhanced healing of segmental tibial defects in sheep by a composite bone substitute composed of tricalcium phosphate cylinder, bone morphogenetic protein, and type IV collagen. *Journal of Biomedical Materials Research* 1996; 32: 505-12.
44. Ilizarov, G.A. The tension-stress effect on the genesis and growth of tissues. Part I. The influence of stability of fixation and soft-tissue preservation. *Clinical Orthopaedics & Related Research* 1989: 249-81.

45. Ilizarov, G.A. The tension-stress effect on the genesis and growth of tissues: Part II. The influence of the rate and frequency of distraction. *Clinical Orthopaedics & Related Research* 1989: 263-85.
46. Aronson, J., Johnson, E., Harp, J.H. Local bone transportation for treatment of intercalary defects by the Ilizarov technique. Biomechanical and clinical considerations. *Clinical Orthopaedics & Related Research* 1989: 71-9.

15 Tumors and Tumor-Like Lesions of Bone

Richard V. Worrell

CONTENTS

15.1 INTRODUCTION

Bone tumors are growths of cells from one or more tissues. These growths, also called neoplasms, are atypical, autonomous, and progressive.[1] They are usually designated as benign or malignant. Benign bone tumors grow more slowly than malignant ones. The tissue structures of benign tumors are much more orderly than those of malignant tumors.[1] In general terms, malignant tumors can metastasize. Benign tumors do not metastasize with the exception of the so-called "benign pulmonary implants" rarely seen in giant cell tumors or chondroblastomas.[6] There are tumor-like lesions of bone which contain many of the radiographic and histopathologic characteristics of bone tumors. The diagnoses of various tumors and tumor-like lesions are based on their clinical presentation, radiologic features, bone scan features, computed tomography, magnetic resonance imaging, microscopic findings and molecular data. Treatment of these tumors is facilitated by a staging procedure devised by Enneking.[8]

0-8493-9237-3/99/$0.00+$.50

15.2 CLASSIFICATION

The following classification of some of the most common bone tumors and tumor-like lesions is based on several contemporary classifications.[1,6,8,15]

BONE-FORMING TUMORS

Benign
Osteoma
Osteoid osteoma
Osteoblastoma

Malignant
Conventional osteosarcoma
Periosteal osteosarcoma
Parosteal osteosarcoma
Low-grade intraosseous osteosarcoma
Telangiectatic osteosarcoma

CARTILAGE-FORMING TUMORS

Benign
Osteochondroma
Hereditary multiplemexostoses
Enchondroma
Multiple chondromas (Ollier's, Maffucci's)
Chondroblastoma
Chondromyxoid fibroma

Malignant
Chondrosarcoma
Dedifferentiated chondrosarcoma
Mesenchymal chondrosarcoma
Clear cell chondrosarcoma

FIBROUS AND FIBROHISTIOCYTIC TUMORS

Benign
Desmoplastic fibroma
Benign fibrous histiocytoma

Malignant
Fibrosarcoma
Malignant fibrous histiocytoma

VASCULAR TUMORS

Benign
Hemangioma
Skeletal angiomatosis
Massive osteolysis

Malignant
Hemangioendothelioma
Hemangiosarcoma
Hemangiopericytoma

HEMATOPOIETIC LESIONS

Malignant
Non-Hodgkin's lymphoma of bone
Myeloma (solitary, multiple)

SMALL CELL SARCOMAS

Malignant
Ewing's sarcoma
Neuroectodermal tumor of bone

Tumors of Uncertain Origins

Benign	***Malignant***
Eosinophilic granuloma	*Adamantinoma*
Giant cell tumor	*Chordoma*

Tumor-like Lesions of Bone

Benign	***Malignant***
Unicameral bone cyst	*Metastatic carcinoma*
Aneurysmal bone cyst	
Nonossifying fibroma	
Fibrous cortical defect	
Fibrous dysplasia	
Osteofibrous dysplasia (ossifying fibroma)	
Giant cell reparative granuloma	

15.3 STAGING

The staging of bone tumors is of great importance for treatment planning and end-result evaluation. Peabody et al. state that "staging is the process of classifying a tumor, especially a malignant tumor, with respect to its degree of differentiation as well as its local and distant extent, in order to estimate the prognosis for the patient."[14] A current method of staging bone tumors adopted by the Musculoskeletal Tumor Society was described by Dr. William Enneking.[8] The following outline will summarize his method.

G represents the histologic or surgical grade of a tumor.

T is used to designate the site of the tumor.

M signifies the presence or absence of metastasis.

G is subdivided into three groups, i.e., $\mathbf{G_0}$ for **benign tumors**, $\mathbf{G_1}$ for **low-grade malignant tumors**, and $\mathbf{G_2}$ for **high-grade malignant tumors**.

T is subdivided into three groups, i.e., $\mathbf{T_0}$ for **intracapsular tumors**, $\mathbf{T_1}$ for **extracapsular, intracompartmental tumors**, and $\mathbf{T_2}$ for **extracapsular, extracompartmental tumors**.

M is subdivided into two groups, i.e., $\mathbf{M_0}$ for **no metastasis** and $\mathbf{M_1}$ for **regional** or **distant metastasis**.

Enneking defines a **compartment** as "an anatomic structure or space bounded by natural barriers to tumor extension." He states that "a whole bone is a compartment." A joint and "functional muscle groups bounded by major fascial septae" are compartments. He further states that "the interfascial planes containing the major neurovascular structures are **not** compartments since they have no proximal or distal barriers."

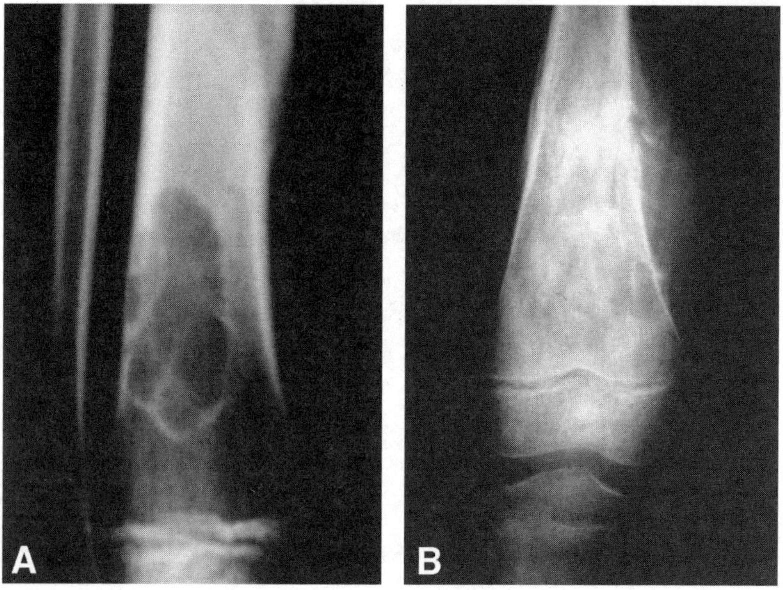

FIGURE 15.1 (A) A benign bone tumor, nonossifying fibroma. (B) A malignant bone tumor, osteosarcoma.

As tumors grow, normal connective tissue surrounding the tumor is compressed forming a **capsule**. Capsules are usually seen in benign tumors. Many malignant tumors grow rapidly and permeate surrounding soft tissues before a capsule can be fully formed. The presence or absence of a capsule can often be determined on a plain radiograph. Lesions that are well-encapsulated display sharp margins on a radiograph (Figure 15.1A). Rapidly growing malignant tumors usually appear as indistinct lesions which are poorly marginated on radiographs (Figure 15.1B).

Benign bone tumors are divided into three stages, i.e., **latent**, **active**, or **locally aggressive**. The giant cell tumor is a benign aggressive tumor that can metastasize to the lungs. According to Enneking,[8] the latent tumors "remain static or heal spontaneously." Active tumors display "progressive growth, not limited by natural barriers."

The staging of benign and malignant bone tumors can be summarized in the following chart derived from Enneking's textbook.[8]

Staging of Bone Tumors

Stage	Characteristics		
	Benign Stages		
1	G_0	T_0	M_0 Latent
2	G_0	T_0	M_0 Active
3	G_0	T_1	$M_{0\text{-}1}$ Aggressive

Stage	Characteristics		
	Malignant Stages		
I-A	G_1	T_1	M_0
I-B	G_1	T_2	M_0
II-A	G_2	T_1	M_0
II-B	G_2	T_2	M_0
III-A	$G_{1\text{-}2}$	T_1	M_1
III-B	$G_{1\text{-}2}$	T_2	M_1

15.4 DIAGNOSTIC STUDIES

15.4.1 Radiography

Radiographs depend on the use of X-rays, electromagnetic energy in the form of ionizing radiation. Radiographs give the best bony detail but very poor definition of soft tissue lesions. Benign and malignant tumors of bone as well as tumor-like lesions of bone all have specific radiographic features. Some tumors and tumor-like lesions have a predilection for certain bones, e.g., the spine, the long bones of the extremities, or the small bones of the hands and feet. Some lesions are characterized by their location in a particular bone, e.g., the epiphysis, metaphysis, or diaphysis. The radiographic appearance of a bony lesion will depend on its matrix (osteoblastic, fibroblastic, or chondroblastic). Certain tumors, usually malignant, will display a characteristic periosteal reaction on a radiograph, e.g., "onion skin" layering or solid. Certain tumors present radiographically with characteristic bone destruction, e.g., lytic, "moth-eaten," or permeative. In general terms, benign bone tumors are usually well defined on radiographs. The margins of the tumor are usually well defined and there is usually no evidence of a periosteal reaction. Malignant bone tumors, on the other hand, have poorly defined margins and often present with some type of periosteal reaction. It should be noted that some non-tumorous conditions of bone, e.g., osteomyelitis, can present with a periosteal reaction on radiographs.

15.4.2 Bone Scanning

When technetium 99m diphosphonate is injected into a patient, there will be an increase in the uptake of this radioisotope in the skeleton in areas of increased osteoblastic activity. Accordingly, this diagnostic technique is useful in detecting primary bone tumors, some tumor-like lesions of bone, and bone metastases.

15.4.3 Computed Tomography

This diagnostic technique depends on computer reconstruction of radiographs showing transaxial images of the anatomy. The CT scan provides excellent detail of bony lesions. However, it is often difficult to differentiate tissue types, e.g., fat, cartilage, fibrous tissue, or blood. Tissue types are more easily identified with the magnetic resonance image.

15.4.4 Magnetic Resonance Imaging

Magnetic resonance imaging has become a very important imaging modality, especially in the field of orthopaedic oncology. It overcomes the limitations of computed tomography in that coronal, sagittal, as well as transaxial images are provided. The MR signal depends on the number of mobile hydrogen atoms in a specific tissue. Fat, cartilage, blood and other body fluids contain an abundance of mobile hydrogen atoms and appear as bright signals on the MRI. Cortical bone has few mobile hydrogen atoms and, as a consequence, the signal appears dark or black. The MR signal depends on the repetition time (TR) and the echo time (TE). The repetition time is the time interval which occurs between the application of sequential radiofrequency pulses to the patient. The echo time is the time interval which occurs between applying a radiofrequency pulse and its return as an MR signal to a radio-antenna which has been placed next to the part of the body being examined. The T1-weighted image is produced when the TR and TE are relatively short. The T2-weighted image is produced when the TR and TE are relatively long. There appears to be better contrast between tissues containing different amounts of mobile hydrogen atoms in the T2-weighted image.

15.4.5 The Biopsy

The bone biopsy site should be placed so that it can be completely excised when the definitive surgical procedure is performed. Uninvolved compartments must not be contaminated by a biopsy. The bone biopsy hole should be small, round, or oval, with smooth edges. Bone becomes 40% weaker in torsion regardless of the size of the bone biopsy defect. Lesions involving the lateral aspect of the proximal femur should be approached through the greater trochanter. Whenever possible, the author uses a small trochar such a Rochester needle for performing bone biopsies. This method minimizes hematoma formation usually associated with open, incisional biopsies. A tourniquet is applied but it is not inflated. Hemostasis must be obtained at the time of wound closure to avoid dissemination of tumor cells. Occasionally, one can seal the bone biopsy hole with a small plug of acrylic cement used carefully.

A representative tissue sample is critically important for obtaining an accurate histopathological diagnosis. A frozen section is useful in determining whether residual tumor cells remain in the tissue margins following tumor resection. It is probably better to wait for the permanent section interpretations before undertaking major procedures, e.g., limb salvage surgery or amputations. There are currently many excellent bone pathology textbooks available for study.[1,4,6,8,9,12,15,20]

15.4.6 Molecular Biology

Current research in the field of molecular biology of neoplastic diseases of bone is adding to our understanding of how bone tumors develop and how they respond to drug therapy. Dorfman and Czerniak[6] divide malignant bone tumors into two distinct molecular groups: "(1) tumors that exhibit distinct molecular alterations that have been implicated as playing a significant role in tumor pathogenesis and (2) tumors with widespread genomic alterations that seem to develop by means of a multistep cumulative process." An important discovery has been the identification of the multidrug-resistant (mdr) gene. This gene is believed to be responsible for the resistance of certain bone tumors to chemotherapy. There are two types of mdr genes (mdr 1 and mdr 3) located on chromosome 7. P-glycoprotein is a product of the mdr gene. Accordingly, the presence of P-glycoprotein in a malignant tumor such as osteosarcoma suggests that the tumor will respond poorly to chemotherapy.

15.5 TREATMENT OPTIONS

Effective treatment of both benign and malignant bone tumors requires that the treating physician obtain a detailed history of the present illness and past medical history, including a profile of the immediate family. Every patient must have a complete physical examination. Appropriate diagnostic studies will then permit the staging of the tumor in question. Many latent and active benign bone tumors can be treated by simple curettage and grafting if necessary.

Aggressive benign bone tumors, e.g., giant cell tumor, may require wide or radical resection. Tumor-free surgical margins are especially important when treating benign bone tumors that have a high recurrence rate. Tumor-free surgical margins must be obtained when treating malignant bone tumors. The resection of many benign bone tumors may leave large defects in the involved bone. These defects may be filled with autografts (bone obtained from the patient), allografts (cadaveric bone), or bone substitutes, e.g., coralline hydroxyapatite. Acrylic cement (polymethyl-methacrylate) has been used to fill defects created by the resection of some bone tumors.

Dramatic advances have been made in the treatment of malignant bone tumors. The use of multiagent chemotherapy has made it possible to perform limb salvage surgery with long-term satisfactory results. The patients are usually given a course of neoadjuvant (preoperative) chemotherapy. A response to chemotherapy which results in greater than 90% tumor necrosis is considered to be a good response. Some of the patients with a good response to chemotherapy will be candidates for limb salvage surgery. A poor response to chemotherapy will usually lead to amputation. Surgery is followed by a course of postoperative chemotherapy. Limb-salvage surgery can involve the use of an allograft or endoprosthetic replacement following bone resection.[5,10,13,16,17] Allografts can result in successful replacement of resected bone. However, full recovery can take up to a year. It appears that the transplanted bone is never completely replaced by ingrowth from the host bone. The ingrowth of bone from the host bone is minimal when large long bone allografts are used. Small grafts are often completely incorporated.[16,17] Prosthetic replacement of bone after bone resection can be a relatively simple procedure.[5,13,16] Many of the prosthetic implants in current use have a modular design. Expandable modular implants are available for use in children.[3,17,18] Patients receiving prosthetic implants have immediate function. There is no disease transmission, e.g., HIV or hepatitis-C. Arthroplasty can be performed in conjunction with prosthetic replacement of resected bone, e.g., when tumors involve the distal or proximal ends of the femur. Some late complications related to the use of prosthetic implants are aseptic loosening, bearing failure, and fracture. Some technical problems related to muscle re-attachment may occur. Occasionally, there is bone stock loss. Patients with prosthetic implants are usually placed on prophylactic antibiotics prior to dental surgery. This is due to the fact that some dental procedures may cause a low-grade bacteremia which could result in an infection at the site of the prosthetic implant.

Amputation is necessary when it is impossible to obtain tumor-free margins at the time of bone tumor resection, or with a poor response to neoadjuvant chemotherapy. Amputation is sometimes required in the treatment of advanced aggressive benign tumors such as a giant cell tumor. Occasionally, amputation is necessary to facilitate nursing and to improve the quality of life in advanced, aggressive bone sarcomas.

Radiotherapy is sometimes used in combination with chemotherapy for tumor control, e.g., in the treatment of Ewing's sarcoma. It is commonly used in the treatment of multiple myeloma and metastatic bone disease.[2,7,11]

15.6 REPRESENTATIVE CASE STUDIES

Case 1

This 17-year-old male presented with a complaint of nine months' duration of pain in the lateral aspect of the proximal third of his left leg. There was no history of trauma. The pain was relieved when the patient took aspirin. Physical examination revealed no visible abnormalities referable to the left leg. There was slight tenderness noted on palpation over the proximal third of the fibula. Radiographs of the left tibia and fibula revealed a small lucent lesion in the cortex of the proximal third of the fibula. The lesion was surrounded by reactive cortical bone (Figure 15.2A). A whole body technetium bone scan revealed an increase in the uptake of the radioisotope at the site of the lesion (Figure 15.3A). An MRI revealed the lucent lesion surrounded by reactive cortical bone (Figure 15.3B). The patient was given tetracycline before surgery in order to identify the nidus in the surgical specimen with a Woods lamp. The lesion was completely excised (Figure 15.2B). The nidus appeared to be brightly fluorescent in the surgical specimen. The histopathology (Figure 15.4) revealed loose fibrovascular connective tissue with osteoid trabeculae surrounded by benign appearing osteoblasts. It should be noted that the spindle cells have a uniform appearance. A diagnosis of **osteoid osteoma**, a benign bone tumor, was established. The patient became completely asymptomatic following surgery.

This case is representative of a Stage 1 benign bone tumor. This tumor generally remains static.

Case 2

This 20-year-old female complained of excruciating right-knee pain and marked generalized swelling of her right knee. A review of her medical history revealed that ten months prior to our examination, she sustained an injury to her right knee while participating in a sports-related activity. She was treated by several physicians, but she failed to respond to prescribed treatment. It became apparent that she might have a malignant bone tumor. She was subsequently referred to our Cancer Center.

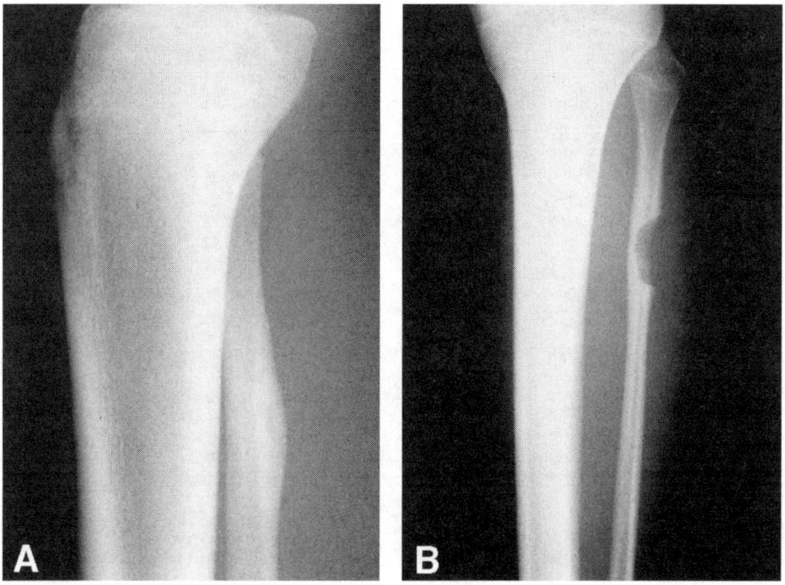

FIGURE 15.2 (A) Osteoid osteoma of the shaft of the fibula. (B) The osteoid osteoma has been resected.

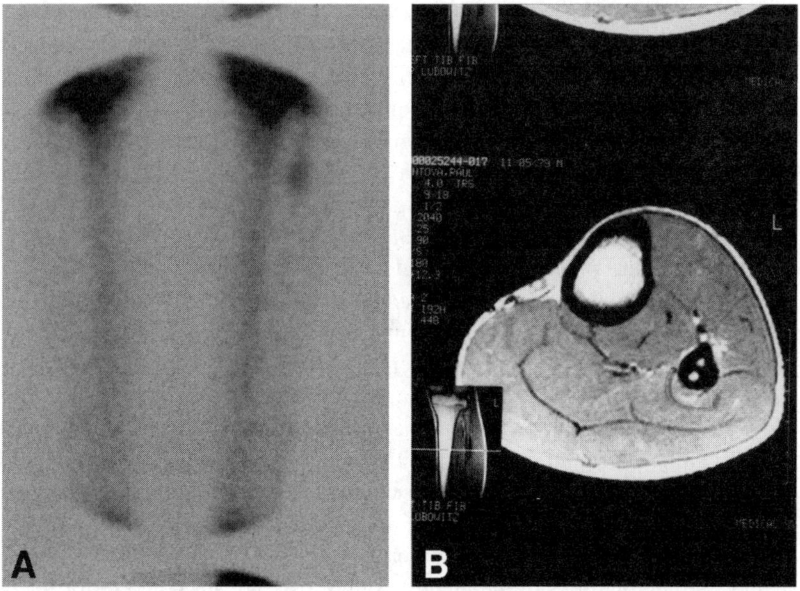

FIGURE 15.3 (A) There is an increase in the uptake of the radioisotope in the proximal left fibula. (B) An MRI reveals a lucent lesion involving the cortex of the fibula surrounded by reactive cortical bone.

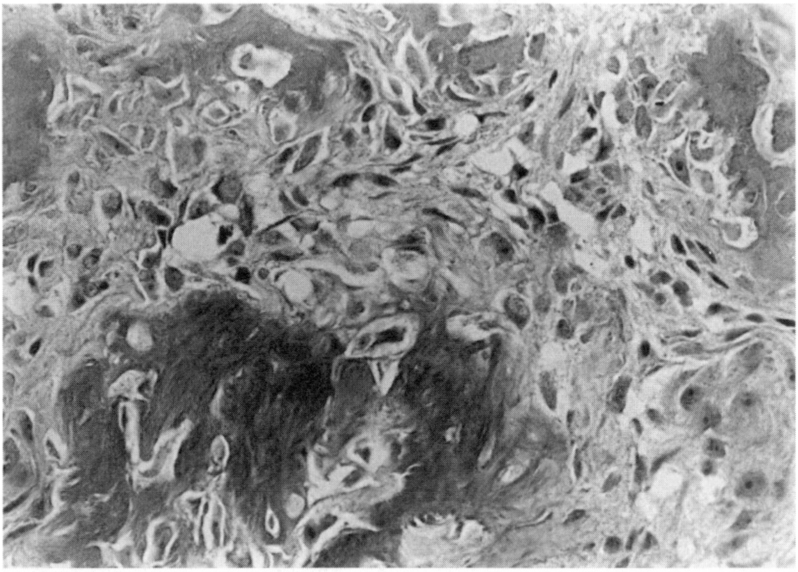

FIGURE 15.4 The histopathology reveals loose benign-appearing fibroblastic connective tissue with osteoid trabeculae surrounded by benign-appearing osteoblasts.

On our initial physical examination we noted marked swelling of the right knee (Figure 15.5A). The knee was fixed in 30 degrees of flexion. There was exquisite tenderness noted on palpation of the knee. The veins in the skin of the right knee and thigh were dilated. The patient had sensory deficits in all areas of her right foot. She had not been able to bear any weight on her right lower limb for several months. Auscultation of her chest revealed numerous rales. Radiographs of the right knee revealed a poorly marginated lesion with mixed bone destruction and production involving the distal femur. There was significant soft tissue extension. Periosteal reactions with a Codman's triangle were noted (Figure 15.6A,B). A radiograph of the chest revealed the presence of several metastases (Figure 15.5B). A biopsy of the tumor of the distal right femur revealed that this patient had a **high-grade osteosarcoma**. The patient was given a course of neoadjuvant chemotherapy. A post-chemotherapy biopsy was performed. There was tumor necrosis of 60%. It was the consensus that an above-knee amputation would improve this patient's quality of life. An above-knee amputation with immediate prosthetic fitting was accomplished without difficulty. The amputation specimen was examined (Figure 15.6C). The tumor involved all of the major neurovascular structures in the popliteal region of the knee. The histopathology of the tumor revealed that the tumor was hypercellular. The tumor cells showed marked pleomorphism (marked differences in the size, shape, and staining qualities of the nuclei). Tumor osteoid was noted to form a lace-like pattern (Figure 15.7).

Post operatively, this patient had obtained dramatic pain relief. She received a course of postoperative chemotherapy. Unfortunately, she failed to respond to this

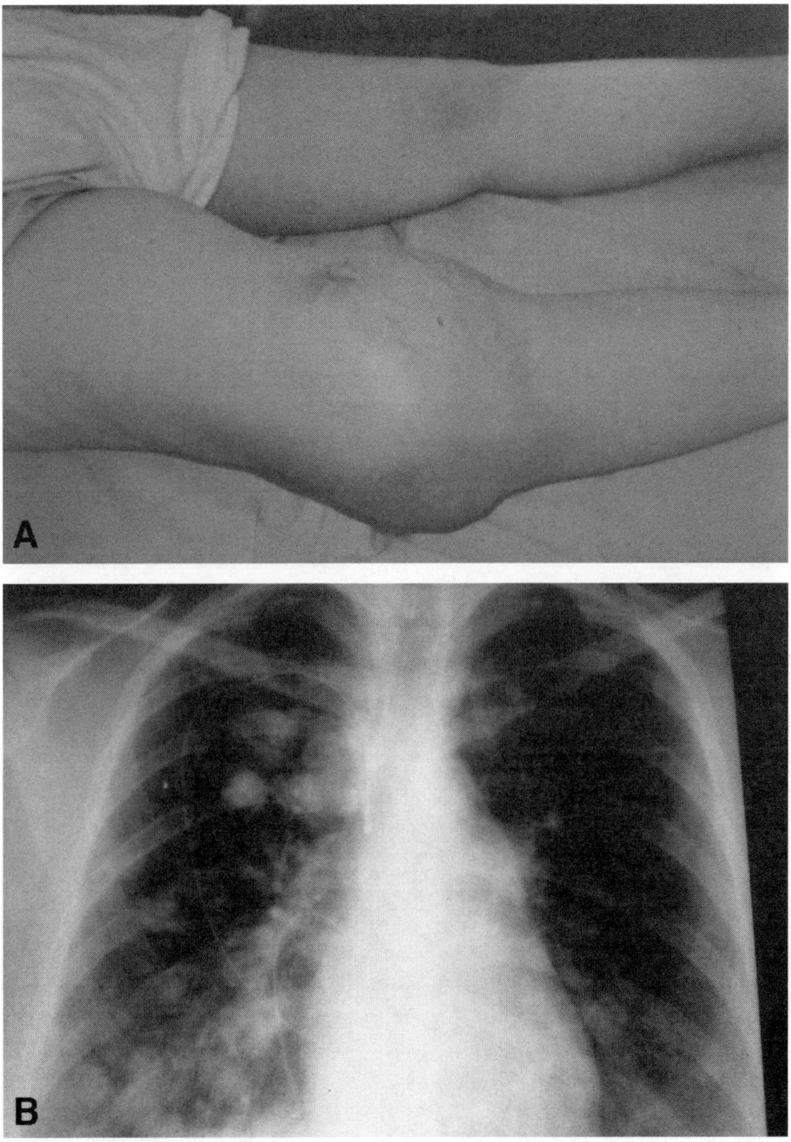

FIGURE 15.5 (A) There is marked swelling of the right knee. (B) The radiograph of the chest reveals the presence of multiple lung metastases.

treatment. There was a dramatic increase in the number of lung metastases in spite of the chemotherapy. She developed acute respiratory failure and died.

This case is representative of a Stage III-B malignant bone tumor.

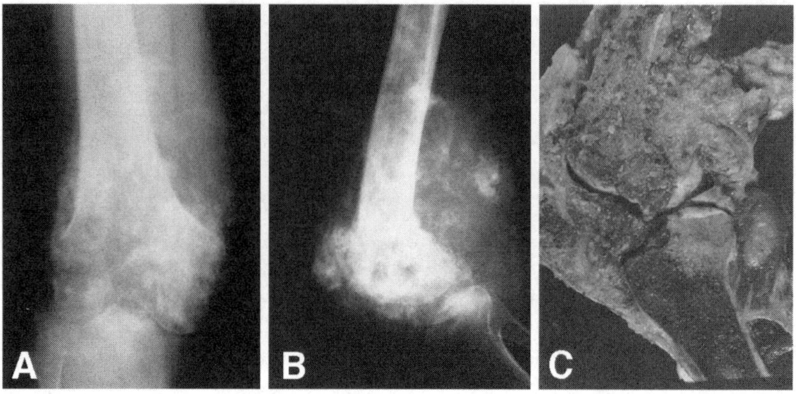

FIGURE 15.6 (A) An anteroposterior radiograph and (B) a lateral radiograph reveal a poorly marginated lesion with mixed bone destruction and production involving the distal femur. There is significant soft tissue extension. Periosteal reaction with a Codman's triangle is noted. (C) This is the amputation specimen.

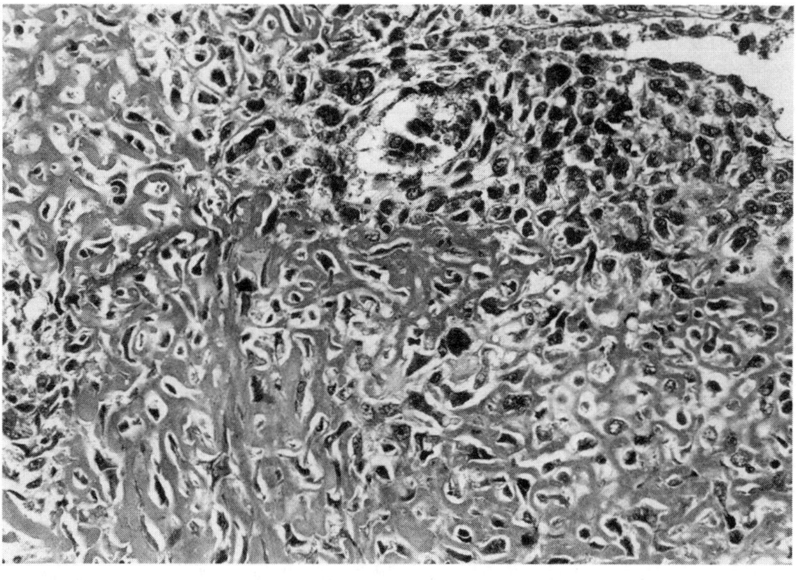

FIGURE 15.7 The histopathology of the tumor reveals that the tumor is hypercellular. The tumor cells showed marked pleomorphism (marked differences in the size, shape, and staining qualities of the nuclei). Tumor osteoid is noted to form a lace-like pattern.

Case 3

This 23-year-old male automobile mechanic presented with a complaint of inability to fully flex his right knee because of a mass behind his knee which appeared to block full flexion. He claimed that the mass had been increasing in size over several months prior to our examination. On physical examination, one could palpate a firm, nontender mass which appeared to be located on the posterior aspect of the distal aspect of the right femur. Radiographs of the right knee revealed a bony lesion involving the posterolateral aspect of the distal femur (Figure 15.8A). A whole body technetium bone scan revealed an increase in the uptake of the radioisotope in the distal portion of the right femur (Figure 15.8B). A CT scan of the right femur revealed a bony lesion on the surface of the posterolateral aspect of the distal portion of the femur (Figure 15.9A). A portion of the lesion appeared to be radiolucent. A biopsy of the lesion revealed benign-appearing bony trabeculae in a fibroblastic stroma containing minimal cytologic atypia. Some cartilaginous areas were noted (Figures 15.10). The histopathology had all of the characteristics of a low-grade neoplasm. A diagnosis of **parosteal osteosarcoma** was made. Due to the low-grade nature of the tumor, it was felt that the patient was not a candidate for chemotherapy. Limb-salvage surgery was performed. The distal portion of the right femur containing the bone tumor was resected with clean surgical margins (Figure 15.9B). A distal femoral allograft was used to replace the resected portion of the femur. Postoperative radiographs revealed satisfactory position and alignment of the allograft (Figure 15.11A). The patient's postoperative course was uneventful. By six months postoperatively, he had a full range of motion of his right knee. All ligaments of the knee were intact and taut. The patient has been followed on a yearly basis for the past seven years. Since surgery, he has completed college. When last examined, he was working as a computer engineer. Radiographs of the right femur made during his last visit revealed that the junction between the allograft and the proximal portion of the femur was not visible. The knee joint appeared to be intact (Figure 15.11B).

This case is representative of a Stage I-A malignant bone tumor.

Case 4

This 31-year-old female presented with a large, painful mass in the vicinity of the proximal end of her right fibula. She was in her second trimester of pregnancy. On examination an 8 cm × 6 cm tender, firm mass was noted in the vicinity of the proximal end of the right fibula. A radiograph of the right knee revealed a large, expansile, lytic lesion involving the proximal end of the fibula (Figure 15.12A). An MRI revealed a lytic, expansile lesion with an increased signal intensity on the T-2 weighted image (Figure 15.12B). A biopsy of the lesion was performed. The histopathology (Figure 15.13) revealed sheets of mononuclear cells, oval or round in shape, with scattered multinucleated giant cells. The nuclei of the giant cells resembled the nuclei of the mononuclear cells. A diagnosis of **giant cell tumor** of the proximal right fibula was made. The tumor was totally excised and the lateral collateral ligament of the knee was attached to the lateral condyle of the tibia.

Post operatively, this patient did well. Her pregnancy proceeded without any difficulty. She eventually delivered a normal baby boy.

This case is representative of an Stage 3 aggressive benign bone tumor.

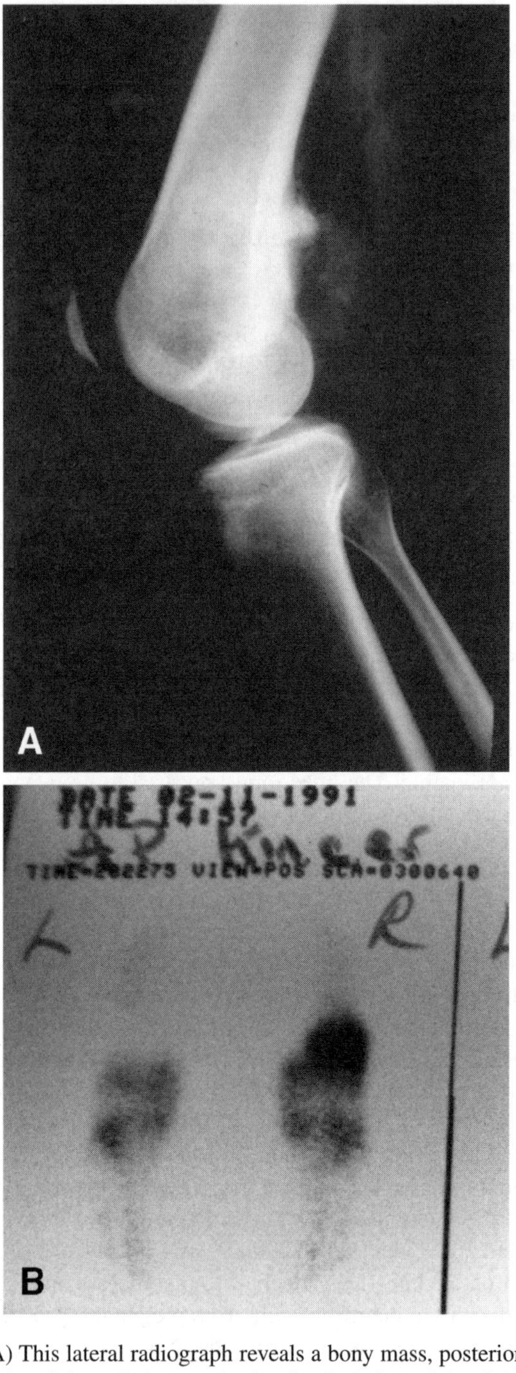

FIGURE 15.8 (A) This lateral radiograph reveals a bony mass, posteriorly. (B) There is an increase in the uptake of the radioisotope in the distal portion of the right femur.

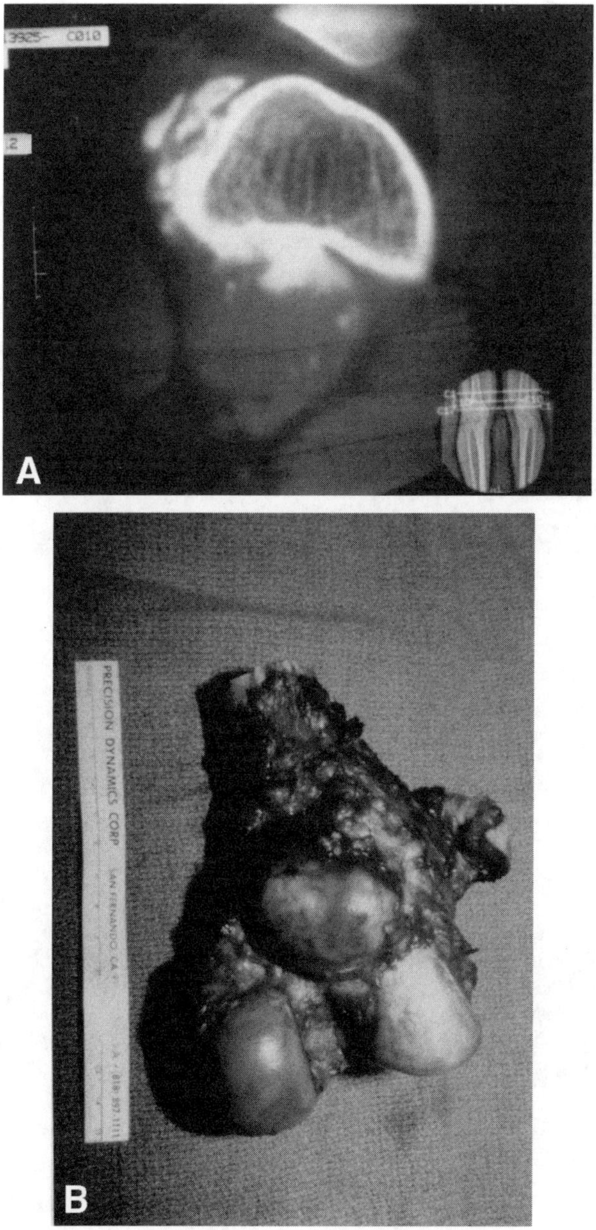

FIGURE 15.9 (A) The CT scan of the distal right femur reveals the lesion involving the posterolateral aspect of the femur. (B) The distal portion of the right femur containing the tumor.

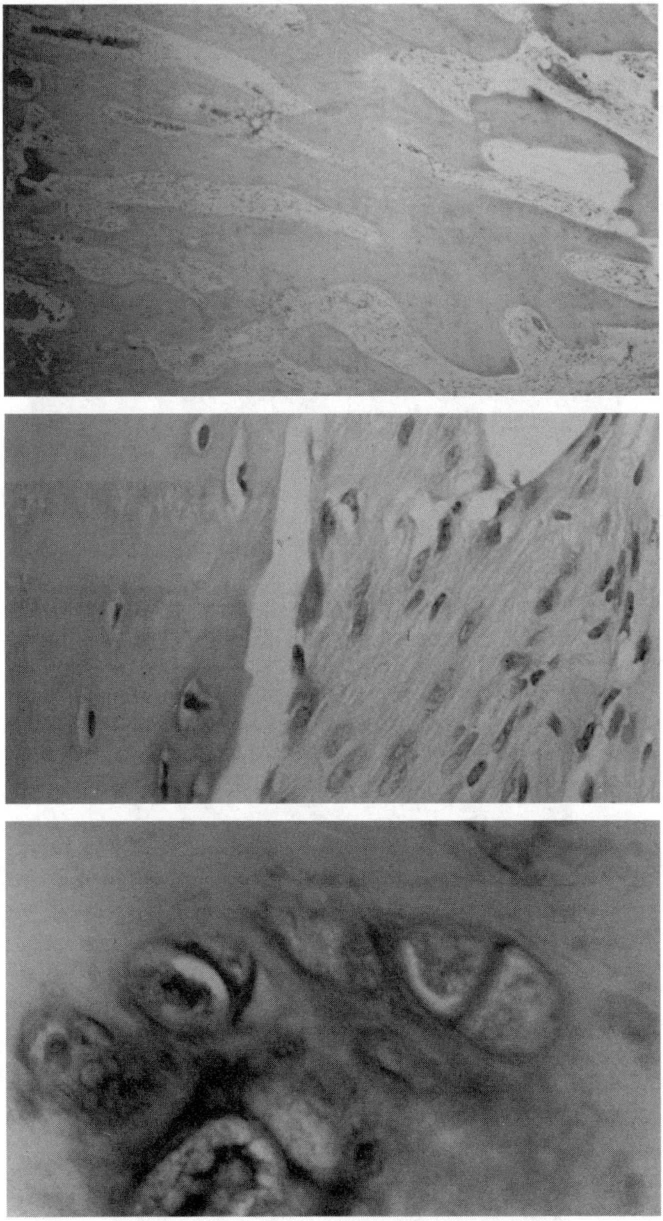

FIGURE 15.10 The histopathology revealed benign-appearing bony trabeculae in a fibroblastic stroma (upper photograph, low power and middle photograph, high power). Some cartilaginous areas are noted (lower photograph).

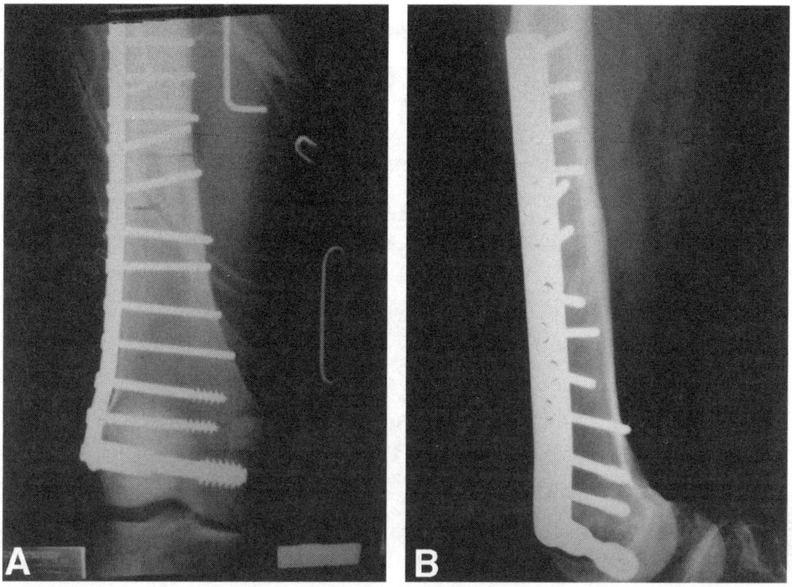

FIGURE 15.11 (A) A postoperative radiograph reveals satisfactory alignment of the allograft. (B) This lateral radiograph was made seven years after surgery. The junction between the allograft and proximal femur is no longer visible.

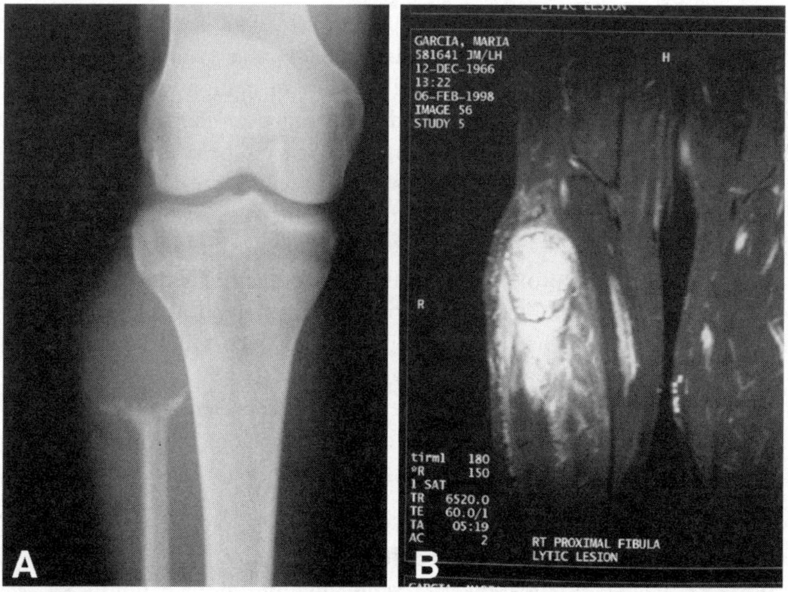

FIGURE 15.12 (A) This radiograph of the right knee reveals a large, expansile lesion involving the proximal end of the fibula. (B) The MRI reveals the lytic, expansile lesion with an increased signal intensity on the T-2 weighted image.

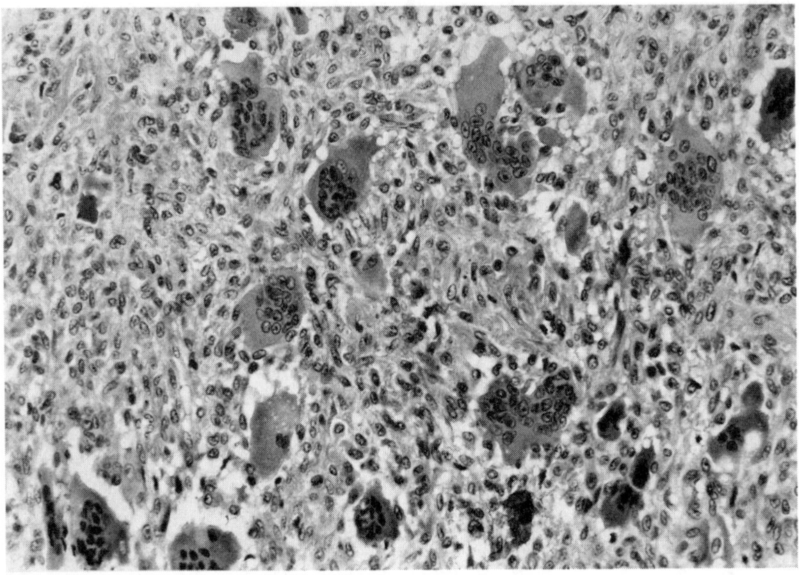

FIGURE 15.13 The histopathology reveals sheets of mononuclear cells, oval or round in shape, with scattered multinucleated giant cells.

Case 5

This 60-year-old female presented with pain in the lateral aspect of her right knee of six months duration. There was no history of trauma. Examination of the right knee revealed no visible abnormalities. The range of motion was normal. All ligaments were intact. There was slight tenderness noted on palpation of the head of the fibula. A radiograph revealed a lesion involving the head and neck of the right fibula with patchy calcification and endosteal erosion (Figure 15.14A). The histopathology (Figure 15.14B) from a biopsy revealed that the lesion was hypercellular with a chondroid matrix. Occasional binucleate cells were noted. A diagnosis of **chondrosarcoma** of the proximal right fibula was made. The proximal end of the right fibula was excised and the lateral collateral ligament of the knee was attached to the lateral condyle of the tibia. This patient has been followed for eight years. When last examined, she was doing very well.

This case is representative of a Stage I-A malignant bone tumor.

Case 6

This 10-year-old female presented with left leg pain, swelling, and fever of two weeks' duration. Examination of her left leg revealed mild generalized swelling. The tibia was tender to palpation. Her sedimentation rate was mildly elevated. A radiograph of the left leg revealed an indistinct lesion involving the proximal half of the diaphysis of the tibia with some lysis and an "onion skin" type periosteal reaction (Figure 15.15A). A whole body technetium bone scan revealed the uptake

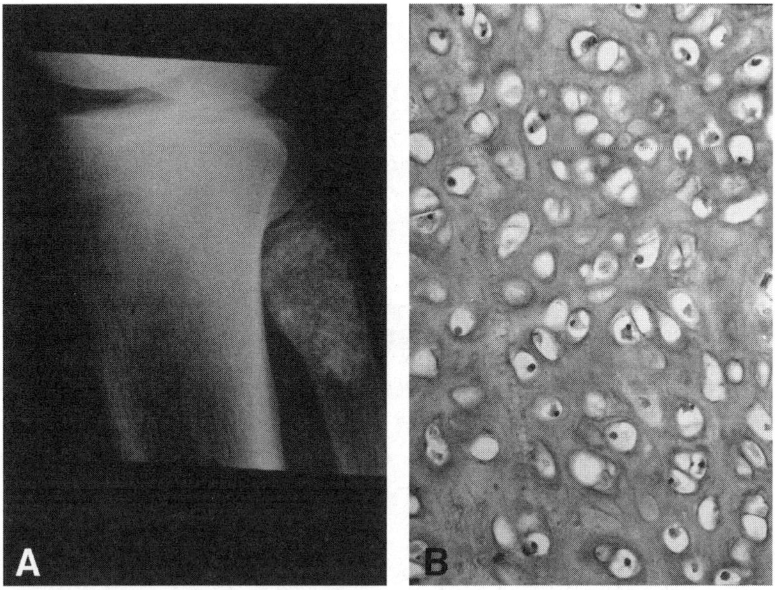

FIGURE 15.14 (A) A radiograph reveals a lesion involving the proximal end of the right fibula with patchy calcification and endosteal erosion. (B) The histopathology reveals that the lesion was hypercellular with a chondroid matrix.

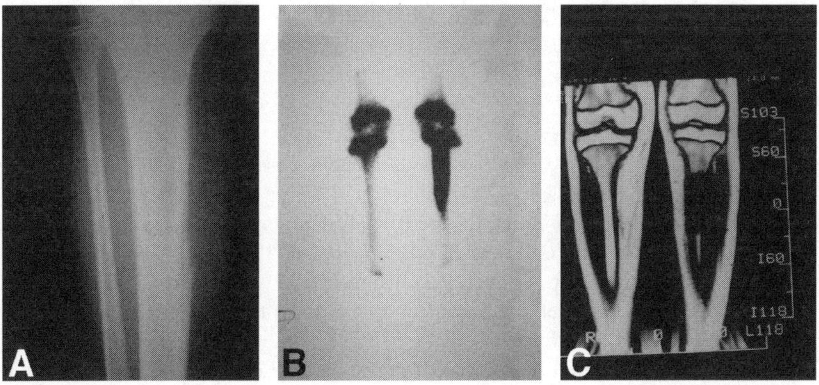

FIGURE 15.15 (A) The radiograph of the left tibia reveals an indistinct lesion in the diaphysis with "onion skin" type periosteal reaction. (B) There is an increase in the uptake of the radioisotope in the shaft of the tibia. (C) The MRI revealed a lesion in the diaphysis of the left tibia with a decreased signal intensity.

of the radioisotope in the left tibia (Figure 15.15B). The MRI revealed a lesion in the diaphysis of the left tibia with a decreased signal intensity (Figure 15.15C). A biopsy of the lesion revealed sheets of small, round, blue cells with little cytoplasm surrounding the nuclei (Figure 15.16). A diagnosis of **Ewing's** sarcoma was established. Treatment consisted of a combination of chemotherapy and radiation therapy.

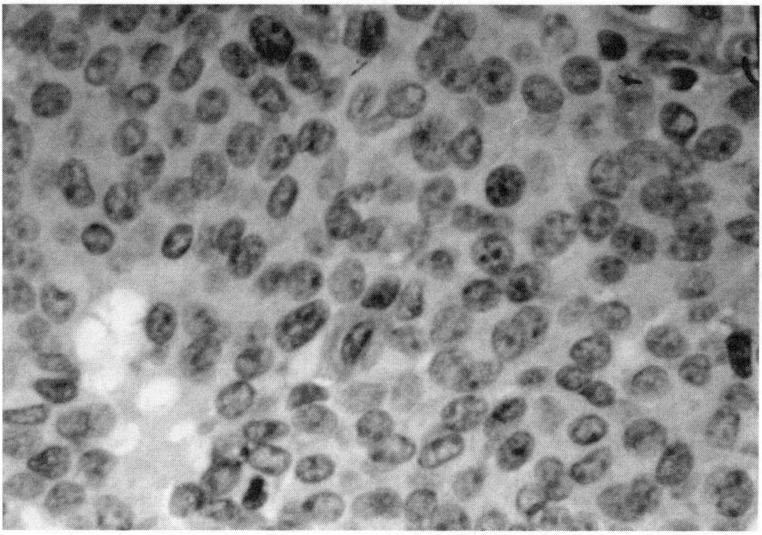

FIGURE 15.16 The histopathology reveals sheets of small round cells.

A biopsy of the left tibia was performed two years after the completion of her treatment. No tumor cells were found. This patient has been followed for the past eight years. The growth of her left tibia has been normal. When last examined, she was doing very well with no evidence of recurrence of her tumor.

This case is representative of a Stage II-B malignant bone tumor.

REFERENCES

1. Campanacci, M.: *Bone and Soft Tissue Tumors.* Springer-Verlag Wien, New York, 1990.
2. Carrie, C., Helfre, S., Bouffet, E., and Brunat-Mentigny, M.: Radiotherapy and Ewing tumor in children. *Bull. Cancer* 82(7): 527-30, Jul. 1995.
3. Cool, W.P., Carter, S.R., Grimer, R.J., Tillman, R.M., and Walker, P.S.: Growth after extendible endoprosthetic replacement of the distal femur. *J. Bone and Joint Surg. Br.* 79(6): 938-42, Nov. 1997.
4. Dahlin, D.C. and Unni, K.K.: *Bone Tumors.* 4th ed. Charles C. Thomas, Springfield, Illinois, 1990.
5. Damron, T.A.: Endoprosthetic replacement following limb-sparing resection of bone sarcoma. *Semin. Surg. Oncol.* 13(1): 3-10, Jan.–Feb. 1997.
6. Dorfman, H.D. and Czerniak, B.: *Bone Tumors.* Mosby, St. Louis, 1998.
7. Dunst, J., Hoffman, C., Ahrens, S., and Jurgens, H.: Surgery versus radiotherapy in Ewing's sarcoma with good prognosis. *Strahlenther Onkol.* 172(5): 244-8; discussion 249, May 1996.
8. Enneking, W.F.: Musculoskeletal Tumor Surgery. Churchill Livingstone, New York, 1983.
9. Fechner, R.E. and Mills, S.E.: *Tumors of the Bones and Joints.* Third Series. Fascicle 8. Armed Forces Institute of Pathology, Washington, D.C., 1993.

10. Frassica, F.J., Chao, E.Y., and Sim, F.H.: Special problems in limb-salvage surgery. *Semin. Surg. Oncol.* 13(1): 55-63, Jan.–Feb. 1997.
11. Jyothirmayi, R., Gangadharan, V.P., Nair, M.K., and Rajan, B.: Radiotherapy in treatment of solitary plasmacytoma. *Br. J. Radiol.* 70(833): 511-6, May 1997.
12. Mirra, J.M.: *Bone Tumors*. Lea and Febiger, Philadelphia, 1989.
13. Morris, H.: The role of prostheses after resection of primary sarcomas of bone. *Acta Orthop. Scand. Suppl.* 273: 86-8, Feb. 1997.
14. Peabody, T.D., Gibbs, C.P., and Simon, M.A.: Evaluation and staging of musculoskeletal neoplasms. *J. Bone And Joint Surg.* 80-A(8): 1204-17, Aug. 1998.
15. Schajowicz, F.: *Tumors and Tumorlike Lesions of Bone: Pathology, Radiology and Treatment*, 2nd ed. Springer-Verlag, New York, 1994.
16. Simon, M.A. and Springfield, D., eds.: *Surgery for Bone and Soft-Tissue Tumors*. Lippincott-Raven, Philadelphia, 1998.
17. Springfield, D.S.: Allograft reconstructions. *Semin. Surg. Oncol.* 13(1): 41-8, Jan.–Feb. 1997.
18. Tillman, R.M., Grimes, R.J., Carter, S.R., Cool, W.P., and Sneath, R.S.: Growing endoprostheses for primary malignant bone tumors. *Semin. Surg. Oncol.* 13(1): 41-8, Jan.–Feb. 1997.
19. Ward, W.G., Yang, R.-S., and Eckardt, J.J.: Endoprosthetic bone reconstruction following malignant tumor resection in skeletally immature patients. *Orthop. Clin. North Am.* 27(3): 493-5502, Jul. 1996.
20. Wold, L.E., McLeod, R.A., Sim, F.H., and Unni, K.K.: *Atlas of Orthopaedic Pathology*. W.B. Saunders, Philadelphia, 1990.

16 Infectious Diseases of Bone

Richard V. Worrell

CONTENTS

0-8493-9237-3/99/$0.00+$.50

16.1 INTRODUCTION

The term osteomyelitis was used initially with reference to pyogenic (pus-forming) infections of bone. Today, it is also used with reference to nonpyogenic infections of bone. The origin of the term has been linked to Nelaton (1844) and Chassignac (1854). Osteomyelitis may be acute, subacute, or chronic. Causative agents can be bacteria, fungi, parasites and (rarely) viruses. Causative agents can spread to bone via the bloodstream (hematogenous spread) or from a contiguous focus of infection. In the latter category, open fractures can be complicated by bone infection. Open reduction with internal fixation of closed fractures and total hip, knee, and shoulder arthroplasties with implantation of biomaterials can all be complicated by bone infections. Lastly, osteomyelitis can occur as a complication in patients with peripheral vascular disease secondary to disorders such as atherosclerosis or diabetes mellitus.

There are several classifications of osteomyelitis. Waldvogel[12,13] divides osteomyelitis into three categories, i.e., hematogenous osteomyelitis, osteomyelitis secondary to a contiguous infection, and osteomyelitis secondary to vascular insufficiency. The Cierny-Nader classification[2,3] is "based on the anatomy of the bone infection and the physiology of the host." Several other classification systems have been developed to address various clinical aspects of osteomyelitis.[5,8-10]

16.2 PYOGENIC OSTEOMYELITIS

16.2.1 Acute Hematogenous Osteomyelitis

The clinical and pathological manifestations of acute hematogenous osteomyelitis are determined in part by the age of the patient. In infancy, metaphyseal arterioles in the long bones penetrate the growth plate and pass into the epiphysis. As these vessels leave the epiphysis they enter venous sinusoids in the metaphysis. Accordingly, bacteria may pass in vascular channels in long bones of an infant from the metaphysis to the epiphysis. In adults, the growth plates in long bones are closed and there is continuity of vascular channels in the metaphyseal portions of the bones to the epiphyses. There is a common blood supply between the vessels of the epiphysis and the vessels of synovium in infants and adults. Accordingly, bacteria can spread from the epiphysis to the joint space, giving rise to septic arthritis in infants and adults. In children older than one year, with intact growth plates, metaphyseal blood vessels do not penetrate the growth plates; therefore, bacteria cannot pass from the metaphysis to the epiphysis via these vessels. Septic arthritis of the hip joint and shoulder joint can occur in older children because the metaphysis of the proximal femur and proximal humerus are in an intraarticular location due to the attachment of the joint capsules. Bacteria, therefore, can leave the metaphysis and enter the joint space, giving rise to a septic arthritis. Hematogenous osteomyelitis occurring in a child over one year old usually begins in the metaphysis of a long bone. The metaphyseal blood vessels in these children form vascular loops just beneath the last intact transverse septa of the growth plates. As noted above, these vessels do not penetrate the growth plate.

According to Waldvogel,[12] bacterial involvement in osteomyelitis is related to the age of the patient. *Staphylococcus aureus* and group B streptococci are frequently isolated in neonates. *Staphylococcus aureus*, coagulase-negative staphylococci, various streptococci, and *Hemophilus influenzae* are frequently isolated in infants. Osteomyelitis in adults involves mostly S. aureus. In elderly patients with gram-negative bacteremias, vertebral osteomyelitis may develop in which gram-negative bacteria are isolated. S. aureus is rarely isolated in these patients. Drug addicts often develop hematogenous osteomyelitis, due to *Pseudomonas aeruginosa*.

According to Vassilopoulos et al.,[11] osteomyelitis occurring in half of their patients with human immunodeficiency virus (HIV) involved atypical mycobacteria.

The pathogenesis of acute and chronic hematogenous, pyogenic osteomyelitis is quite interesting. If, for example, a child older than one year develops a bacteremia, bacteria may find their way via a nutrient artery into the intramedullary vessels of a long bone. The bacteria then travel via a metaphyseal arteriole toward the growth plate. Once the metaphyseal arteriole reaches the last intact transverse septum of the growth plate, it makes a 180-degree turn to join a venous sinusoid. Experimental studies indicate that there is a relatively high rate of blood flow through these vascular loops. This high flow rate is probably responsible for delivery of large amounts of bacteria to the metaphysis. The mechanism of bacterial deposition in the metaphysis is not yet understood. This concept of a high flow rate in the metaphyseal vascular loops is at variance with the older concept of a sluggish blood flow through the vascular loops.

Once bacteria have been deposited in the metaphysis, the immune response is triggered and many polymorphonuclear leukocytes rush to the area where bacterial multiplication is occurring. Many leukocytes die and pus is formed. The pus builds up in the metaphyseal region, then follows the path of least resistance from the metaphysis through the Volkmann's and Haversian canals of the cortex to the subperiosteal region of the bone. In a child, the periosteum is thick and is easily stripped away from the bone. The subperiosteal accumulation of pus causes the periosteum to be stripped away from the underlying bone. Accordingly, a subperiosteal abscess is formed. It should be noted that in the proximal ends of the femur and humerus, the growth plate is intracapsular. A subperiosteal abscess in the metaphyseal area of either the proximal femur or humerus may therefore give rise to septic arthritis.

The presence of pus in a subperiosteal location stimulates the osteogenic layer of the periosteum to form new bone. This is seen as a periosteal reaction on radiographs. The pressure of pus within the medullary cavity of bone coupled with the pressure of pus in the subperiosteal area causes vascular compromise of the involved area of bone, leading to bone death. The dead bone is called a *sequestrum*. The periosteal new bone surrounding the dead bone is called the *involucrum*. The involucrum contains many small holes or *cloacae* through which pass pus, necrotic debris, and small particles of dead bone, entering sinus tracts in the soft tissues that lead to the skin surface.

In reviewing the sequence of events, it should be noted that the subperiosteal abscess is formed during the acute stage of hematogenous osteomyelitis. The formation of sequestrated bone surrounded by the involucrum occurs during the chronic stage of osteomyelitis. Bacteria appear to reach the spine by way of peripheral and periosteal arteries of the spine and the venous plexus of Batson. It should be noted that the intervertebral disc is avascular in the skeletally mature adult. Accordingly, the disc space is not primarily involved in the adult. By contrast, in the infant, the cartilaginous end-plates of the intervertebral disc space contain small blood vessels. Infection will, therefore, spread to the disc space primarily in the infant.

16.2.2 Bacterial Adhesion, Colonization of Substrata, and the Formation of Biofilm

It is now appropriate to discuss how bacteria interact with organic substances and biomaterials with regard to the development of osteomyelitis.[6] A substratum is a substance to which bacteria can adhere and which they can colonize. Substrata can be organic, e.g., living or dead bone, allografts or soft tissues, or non-organic biomaterials, e.g., metals, synthetic polymers, and ceramics. Almost all bacteria have the ability to adhere to and colonize substrata. Bacteria may reach various substrata during a surgical procedure, as a result of trauma, from a contiguous focus of infection, or through the bloodstream. Once in contact with a particular substratum, bacteria secrete proteinaceous adhesins and exopolysaccharide polymers that help the bacteria to adhere to the substratum, once repelling charges on the bacteria and substratum are overcome. The bacterial exopolysaccharide polymer ("slime" or glycocalyx) along with bacteria and associated colonies form, in large part, the *biofilm*. Bacterial glycocalyx has been visualized in its natural, highly hydrated state by means of scanning electron microscopy.[4] The biofilm offers the bacteria some form of resistance from antibiotics and the agents of the immune response. Within the biofilm is the *microzone*, the environment that promotes growth of bacteria.

16.2.3 Osteomyelitis Occurring from a Contiguous Focus of Infection

An untreated subcutaneous abscess may spread toward an adjacent bone and cause it to become infected.[12] Treatment failures related to open fractures can lead to the development of osteomyelitis. Tragically, the acute stage may become chronic. Animal bites, human bites, and puncture wounds can result in the development of acute osteomyelitis.

16.2.4 Osteomyelitis Resulting from Implantation of Biomaterials[6]

Osteomyelitis can occur as a complication when biomaterials, e.g., metals or synthetic polymers, are used in the open treatment of fractures or in total joint arthroplasties. Bacteria can adhere to and colonize metallic surfaces of synthetic polymers such as polyethylene, polypropylene, or methylmethacrylate. The bacteria and exopolysaccharide polymers (glycocalyx) form a biofilm which helps to protect the bacteria from antibiotic therapy and the natural defense mechanisms of the host. The presence of bacteria that can adhere to metal and form a biofilm may explain why some infections related to bones that have been internally fixed with plates and screws or intramedullary rods are resistant to antibiotic therapy until the hardware is removed.

S. aureus has a predilection for adhering to and colonizing metals used as surgical implants. S. epidermidis is often associated with bacterial colonization of synthetic polymers.

16.2.5 Subacute Osteomyelitis

In some instances of acute hematogenous osteomyelitis, the host defense mechanisms can contain the infection within a well-circumscribed area in a particular bone. This area is usually located in the metaphysis of a long bone in a child over the age of one year, and is called a *Brodie's abscess*. This abscess represents a subacute manifestation of osteomyelitis.

16.2.6 Chronic Osteomyelitis

Chronic osteomyelitis remains one of the most difficult and frustrating disease entities that the orthopaedic surgeon and the infectious disease specialist are called upon to treat. There are no universally accepted criteria used to designate a particular bone infection as being chronic. However, chronic osteomyelitis can be considered a complication of acute osteomyelitis. It occurs as a result of treatment failure from inadequate antibiotic therapy, failure to remove dead bone or infected granulation tissue, or failure of treatment in persons with depressed immune systems. Some bone infections such as those caused by Mycobacterium tuberculosis are characterized by a chronic course. Persons with diabetes mellitus often develop a polymicrobial form of chronic osteomyelitis that may involve one or more bones of the foot. A complication of chronic osteomyelitis is the late development (20 to 40 years) of squamous cell carcinoma in a chronic draining sinus tract. This occurs in one percent of those patients with chronic infection. Presently, amyloidosis is no longer considered to be a complication of chronic osteomyelitis.

16.2.7 Osteomyelitis Associated with the Hemoglobinopathies

Salmonella has been isolated in patients with hemoglobin SS and hemoglobin SC types of sickle cell disease complicated by osteomyelitis.[12] However, S. aureus is still the most common pathogen isolated in these patients.

16.2.8 Osteomyelitis Associated with Peripheral Vascular Disease or Diabetes Mellitus

Patients in this category have marginal peripheral circulation, especially in their feet. Patients with atherosclerosis develop atheromatous plaques in major vessels of the extremities. Many of these vessels become occluded, giving rise to diminished peripheral circulation. Patients with diabetes mellitus develop microangiopathy (small vessel disease). These patients have marginal perfusion of peripheral soft tissues, giving rise to a relative ischemia. Minor lacerations and abrasions, especially of the feet, have a tendency to heal very slowly if at all. These indolent wounds sometimes become secondarily infected with the formation of chronic draining ulcers. These ulcers represent a contiguous focus of infection, which can lead to the development of osteomyelitis in adjacent bones. Most of these infections are polymicrobial.

16.2.9 Diagnostic Findings in Pyogenic Osteomyelitis

16.2.9.1 Clinical Findings

In acute hematogenous osteomyelitis there is usually severe pain in the affected limb associated with a fever. Muscle spasm may be present as a protective mechanism, i.e., to prevent movement of the limb. In subacute osteomyelitis or in osteomyelitis secondary to or contiguous to infection, pain will be present. However, many of these patients will remain afebrile. In patients with chronic osteomyelitis, pain may range from mild to severe. These patients may or may not be febrile. Many of these patients frequently complain of foul-smelling drainage arising from one or more sinus tracts.

16.2.9.2 Sedimentation Rate

The sedimentation rate may be normal in initial stages of acute hematogenous osteomyelitis. In subacute and chronic forms of osteomyelitis, the sedimentation rate may or may not be elevated. Accordingly, the diagnosis of osteomyelitis should not be excluded because a patient has a normal sedimentation rate. Response to therapy can be followed in a patient with an elevated sedimentation rate. As the patient shows clinical improvement, the sedimentation rate should decrease.

16.2.9.3 Radiographic Findings

According to Boutin et al.[1] "radiography is insentive to the detection of early osteomyelitis." Bone destruction and periostitis may not be detected for approximately two weeks after the initiation of a pyogenic infection. The earliest radiographic sign of acute hematogenous osteomyelitis is blurring of the fascial planes of the involved limb. This may not be present until three days following the onset of symptoms. The radiographic changes in long bones of a child with acute hematogenous osteomyelitis include a mottled, lytic destruction of bone in the metaphyseal area associated with periosteal reaction in the area of involvement. If the infection becomes chronic, destructive changes progress to the point of sequestration of bone. The periosteum makes new bone, the involucrum, which surrounds the sequestrum. In subacute osteomyelitis (Brodie's abscess) there is a well-circumscribed area of lysis, usually in the metaphyseal area of a long bone. An interesting radiographic finding in sickle cell disease patients with Salmonella osteomyelitis is cortical fissuring. This finding has also been seen in patients with leukemia complicated by pyogenic osteomyelitis.

16.2.9.4 Computed Tomography

The CT scan can provide a detailed transaxial visualization of cortical bone. It is useful in detecting cortical destruction, sequestra and involucra. The cloacae of the involucra are very well visualized with the CT scan.

16.2.9.5 Magnetic Resonance Imaging

The MR signal depends on the hydrogen ion content of a specific tissue. MR imaging can detect early changes in the bone marrow of infected bone. However, MRI findings seen in osteomyelitis are often seen in bone tumors or metabolic disorders among other entities. The lack of specificity is one of the drawbacks to the use of the MRI as a diagnostic tool in osteomyelitis.[1]

16.2.9.6 Bone Scans

Technetium, gallium, and indium bone scans are positive long before radiographic changes become visible in cases of acute hematogenous osteomyelitis. Increased radionuclide uptake will be seen as early as 24 hours following the onset of symptoms. Bone scans are useful in detecting an exacerbation of infection in cases of quiescent chronic osteomyelitis. Bone scans are not reliable in patients with peripheral vascular disease or diabetes mellitus complicated by osteomyelitis.

16.2.9.7 Blood Cultures

Blood cultures are positive in approximately half of the patients with acute hematogenous osteomyelitis. Blood cultures may be of little value in subacute, chronic, and contiguous forms of osteomyelitis. In patients with peripheral vascular disease or diabetes mellitus complicated by osteomyelitis, blood cultures are of little value. These patients often have polymicrobial infections, and specific pathogens can be identified by cultures of bone biopsies.

16.2.9.8 Bone Biopsy

Bone biopsy cultures will enable the clinician to identify the offending pathogen in all forms of pyogenic osteomyelitis. This is particularly true in cases of polymicrobial infections seen in patients with osteomyelitis associated with peripheral vascular disease or diabetes mellitus.

16.2.9.9 Histopathology

In acute pyogenic osteomyelitis, the inflammatory exudate consists of fields of living and dead polymorphonuclear leukocytes. In chronic pyogenic osteomyelitis, the fields contain a mixture of lymphocytes, plasma cells, and histiocytes. Areas of dead bone are noted. Fibroblastic activity and reactive new bone are also seen. In subacute osteomyelitis, an inflammatory exudate consisting of polymorphonuclear leukocytes, lymphocytes, plasma cells, and histiocytes is surrounded by a dense fibrous capsule.

16.2.10 Treatment Strategies in Pyogenic Osteomyelitis

Antibiotics are most effective before bacteria adhere to substrata. Accordingly, methods of preventing bacterial adhesion would be useful in preventing infection. Once adhesion colonization of bacteria is initiated, antibiotics that penetrate the biofilm could abort the process. Normal tissue cells attempt to grow over implanted biomaterials. These cells (epithelium and endothelium) inhibit bacterial adhesion on implants. Therefore, any method of promoting the growth of normal tissue cells covering biomaterial implants before bacterial adhesion can occur will help to prevent infection.

Along with the use of antibiotics, surgery is an important component of the treatment of pyogenic osteomyelitis. Surgical debridement of the infected bone, drainage, the implantation of antibiotic beads, and the removal of implanted biomaterials when necessary are useful in controlling and eradicating infection.[6]

16.3 NONPYOGENIC OSTEOMYELITIS

Tuberculosis, syphylitic, fungal, and parasitic infections of bone usually result in the formation of granulomas in response to the pathogen. These bone infections form the category often referred to as nonpyogenic.

16.3.1 Tuberculous Osteomyelitis

Tuberculous infection of bone develops as a result of lymphohematogenous spread, usually from an infected lung or a gastrointestinal focus of infection.[6] Approximately one percent of patients with pulmonary tuberculosis develop bony involvement. The spine is involved in 50 to 60 percent of all patients with tuberculous osteomyelitis. The next area of predilection is the hip, followed by the knee. However, any bone or joint may be involved with tuberculous infection.

Osseous tuberculosis is characterized by a chronic course. The patients with this disease usually present with pain in the affected area of the body. This may be accompanied by fever and malaise. The sedimentation rate may be normal. These patients may have a positive skin test.

Radiographic changes involving the long bones may reveal epiphyseal involvement in children with tuberculous osteomyelitis who are over one year of age. This is distinctly different from pyogenic osteomyelitis in which the epiphysis is usually spared. With regard to the short tubular bones of the hands and feet, destruction of the diaphyseal areas of these bones gives rise to a radiographic appearance called tuberculous dactylitis. Another finding is fusiform enlargement of the diaphyses of these bones called *spina ventosa*. In tuberculous spondylitis (Pott's disease), bony destruction begins in a vertebral body. The disc space is subsequently involved, followed by the involvement of an adjacent vertebra. The vertebral destruction often results in gibbus formation due to anterior angulation with a severe kyphosis. This severe deformity in the thoracic area may result in spinal cord compression giving rise to paraplegia (Pott's paraplegia). The areas of predilection with regard to tuberculous infection of the spine are the lower thoracic and upper lumbar areas.

The histopathology is characteristic. In the typical case of tuberculous osteomyelitis or spondylitis, one can usually identify the tuberculous granuloma. Tubercle bacilli are found in only 50 percent of untreated cases and rarely in treated cases. The typical granuloma consists of several Langhans'-type giant cells. These cells are characterized by the peripheral location of their nuclei. Surrounding each giant cell is a zone of histiocytes, which are called epithelioid cells because of their tendency to line up in a row of parallel cells. Among the epithelioid cells are varying amounts of lymphocytes. Surrounding this zone is a zone comprised of fibroblasts. As the disease progresses, the cells comprising the granuloma are killed. The death of cells comprising several granulomas leads to the formation of necrotic debris called *caseation necrosis*. In the area surrounding the caseation necrosis, epithelioid cells coalesce to form new Langhans'-type giant cells. New granulomas are formed, which in turn undergo necrosis. Accordingly, as the disease progresses the amount of caseation necrosis increases.

Treatment of tuberculosis involving the skeleton usually involves the use of two chemotherapeutic agents, namely, isoniazid and rifampin. Surgical debridement of abscesses may be necessary. In advanced tubercular spondylitis, spinal fusion may be necessary.

16.3.2 Brucella Osteomyelitis

Approximately ten percent of patients who develop chronic brucellosis develop bone lesions. Many of these patients are farmers, meat packers, and individuals who drink unpasteurized milk. Three-quarters of those patients with brucella osteomyelitis have vertebral involvement. The pathogens most commonly isolated are *B. melitensis* and *B. suis*. Less commonly involved is *B. abortus*. Clinically, these patients may have pain, fever, and weight loss. There is a leukocytosis and an increase in the sedimentation rate. Radiographically, there may be destructive changes in one or more vertebrae. Histopathologically, the infected tissue resembles chronic pyogenic osteomyelitis associated with abundant fibrosis and reactive bone formation. Occasionally, granuloma-like lesions may be seen.

Treatment of brucella osteomyelitis involves the use of a combination of antibiotics such as doxycycline and streptomycin. Single agent therapy can result in a relapse.

16.3.3 Actinomycosis

Actinomyces israeli is a Gram-positive filamentous bacterium responsible for the development of actinomycosis. Bone involvement occurs in cervicofacial actinomycosis. There may be mandibular involvement, especially after tooth extraction. Involvement of the second rib and the thoracic spine has been reported. Clinically, the patient may present with fever, chills, weight loss, trismus, or with a pneumonitis. Radiographically, areas of nonspecific bone destruction will be noted in the mandible, ribs, and thoracic vertebrae. Histopathologically, bone abscesses are connected by sinuses. The sinuses are formed by liquefaction necrosis. The walls of the sinuses contain granulomatous tissue made of histiocytes, epithelioid cells, lymphocytes, polymorphonuclear leukocytes, and giant cells. The actinomyces bacteria present as amorphous yellow granules, the so-called sulfur granules.

Treatment consists of incision and drainage of abscesses and debridement when necessary. The antibiotics recommended for use in the treatment of actinomycosis are penicillin or tetracycline.

16.3.4 Fungal Infections

16.3.4.1 Blastomycosis

The causal agent is the fungus *Blastomyces dermatitidis*. This fungus is found in the soil, especially along the Ohio and Mississippi Rivers. Persons who work with soil, such as farmers, may develop this disease by inhaling the fungus. In the acute phase, there may be pulmonary involvement manifested by chills, fever, cough, fatigue, and chest pain. Radiographs of the chest may be abnormal. A sputum culture may be used to identify the pathogen. Approximately one third of patients who have chronic blastomycosis will develop bone infections. The spine, ribs, long bones, and skull may be involved. Radiographically, the lesions that involve cancellous bone may be well-circumscribed, lytic, or diffuse, with or without periosteal reaction. Histopathologically, one sees a granuloma consisting of histiocytes, epithelioid cells, lymphocytes, polymorphonuclear leukocytes, and giant cells. Doubly refractile blastomyces may be noted to be free in the tissues and in the giant cells. Numerous fibroblasts are also seen.

Treatment of blastomycosis consists of the use of surgical debridement and the administration antifungal agents such as ketoconazole or amphotericin B.[6]

16.3.4.2 Coccidioidomycosis

Coccidioidomycosis occurs mainly in the San Joaquin Valley region of the southwestern part of the United States. The fungus responsible for this disease is *Coccidioides immitis*. The fungus is usually inhaled, resulting in a pulmonary infection or disseminated coccidioidomycosis. Bone involvement can occur as a manifestation of the disseminated disease. Usually the ribs, spine, and skull are involved. Distal ends of long bones may be involved.

Clinically, these patients present initially with fever, cough, dyspnea, and chest pain. A skin rash may be present. Chest radiographs are abnormal. Sputum cultures and serological tests may be useful in making the diagnosis. Radiographically, the bone lesions which involve cancellous bone are lytic with little periosteal reaction or new bone formation. Histopathologically, the characteristic granuloma contains histiocytes, epithelioid cells, lymphocytes, polymorphonuclear leukocytes, and doubly refractile, thick-walled coccidioides spherules. The spherules are seen in giant cells and are also free in the tissues. A fibroblastic reaction is also noted.

Treatment consists of the use of antifungal agents such as amphotericin B or ketoconazole plus surgical debridement when necessary.[6]

16.3.4.3 Sporotrichosis

The offending pathogen is the fungus *Sporothrix schenckii*. This fungus is found in the north-central part of the United States. The portal of entry is usually through a break in the skin that may be considered trivial, e.g., a thorn prick from a rose bush. Accordingly, the disease is often seen in gardeners, florists, and farmers. The two major forms of this disease are the cutaneous and disseminated. Bone and joint involvement occurs in 80 percent of patients with disseminated sporotrichosis. Clinical findings are minimal. There may be some weight loss or a low-grade fever. The white cell count may be normal or slightly elevated. Diagnosis can be established with cultures from cutaneous drainage and serological tests.

Radiographically, the epiphyseal ends of long bones are usually involved along with adjacent joints. The skull, ribs, and phalanges may be involved. There are no characteristic radiographic findings. Histopathologically, granulomas containing histiocytes and giant cells without necrosis are seen.

Treatment consists of the use of potassium iodide in the cutaneous form or amphotericin B in the disseminated disease.[6] Surgical debridement is used when necessary.

16.3.5 Parasitic Infestation of Bone

The rare infestation of bones by the parasite *Echinococcus granulosus* in its hydatid form has been reported.[7] The infected ova are found in the fecal matter of dogs. Outbreaks occur periodically in some Third-World countries, e.g., in certain areas of Kenya.

In long bones, hydatid disease is characterized by the presence of multiple intramedullary cysts. Radiographical findings mimic those of neoplastic diseases of bone. Histopathological studies reveal reactive fibrosis surrounding a hydatid cyst.

Treatment consists of surgical excision of the cysts and the use of benzimidazole carbamates.

REFERENCES

1. Boutin, R.D., Brossmann, J., Sartoris, D.J., Reilly, D., and Resnick, D.: Update on imaging of orthopaedic infections. *Orthop. Clin. North Am.* 29(1): 41-66, 1998.
2. Cierny, G. and Mader, J.T.: Adult chronic osteomyelitis. *Orthopedics* (7): 1557-64, 1984.
3. Cierny, G., Mader, J.T., and Pennick, H.: A clincial staging system of adult osteomyelitis. *Contemp. Orthop.* (10): 10-37, 1985.
4. Evans, R.P., Nelson, C.L., Bowen, W.R., Kleve, M.G., and Hickmon, S.G.: Visualization of bacterial glycocalyx with a scanning electron microscope. *Clin. Orthop.* (347): 243-49, 1998.
5. Gordon, L. and Chiu, E.J.: Treatment of infected non-unions and segmental defects of the tibia with staged microvascular muscle transplantation and bone-grafting. *J. Bone Joint Surg.* 70-A: 377-86, 1988.

6. Gustilo, R.B., Gruninger, R.P., and Tsukayama, D.T.: *Orthopaedic Infection: Diagnosis and Treatment*. W.B. Saunders Co., Philadelphia, 1989.
7. Hooper, J. and McLean, I.: Hydatid disease of the femur. *J. Bone Joint Surg.* 59-A: 974, 1977.
8. Kelly, P.J.: Infected nonunion of the femur and tibia. *Orthop. Clin. North Am.* (15): 481-90, 1984.
9. Mader, J.T., Shirtliff, M., and Calhoun, J.H.: Staging and staging application in osteomyelitis. *Clin. Infectious Dis.* (25): 1303-9, 1997.
10. May, J.W., Jupiter, J.B., and Weiland, A.J.: Current concepts review: clinical classification of post-traumatic tibial osteomyelitis. *J. Bone Joint Surg.* 71-A: 1422-8, 1989.
11. Vassilopoulos, D., Chalasani, P., Jurado, R.L., Workowski, K., and Agudelo, C.A.: Musculo-skeletal infections in patients with human immunodeficiency virus infection. *Medicine* 76 (4): 284-94, 1997.
12. Waldvogel, F.A.: Osteomyelitis. In: *Infectious Diseases,* 2nd ed., Gorbach, S.L., Bartlett, J.G., and Blacklow, N.R., Eds., W.B. Saunders Co., Philadelphia, 1998.
13. Waldvogel, F.A., Medoff, G., and Swartz, M.M.: Osteomyelitis, a review of clinical features, therapeutic considerations, and unusual aspects. *N. Engl. J. Med.* (282): 198-206, 260-6, 316-22, 1970.

17 The Foot

Richard A. Miller and David M. Bloome

CONTENTS

17.1 INTRODUCTION

The goal of this chapter is to familiarize the reader with the anatomy and radiography of the foot, in addition to the diagnosis and treatment of common pathologies of the foot.

17.2 ANATOMY AND BIOMECHANICS

The foot provides support for standing and walking, and can be divided into three regions: the hindfoot, midfoot, and forefoot. The bones of the hindfoot are the talus and calcaneus. The cuboid, navicular, and three cuneiforms constitute the midfoot. The forefoot bones are the five metatarsals and phalanges of the toes. In addition, two major sesamoid bones underlie the first metatarsal head.

The foot has both extrinsic tendons attaching to it and intrinsic musculotendinous units. The extrinsic tendons can be classified according to their location with respect to the ankle axis. Posteriorly is the Achilles tendon which is a strong plantarflexor

0-8493-9237-3/99/$0.00+$.50

of the foot. Posterolaterally are the peroneus longus and brevis tendons which both plantarflex and evert the foot. Posteromedially are the tibialis posterior, flexor digitorum longus, and flexor hallucis longus tendons. The tibialis posterior tendon plantarflexes and inverts the foot while providing support to the medial longitudinal arch. Anteriorly lie the tibialis anterior, extensor digitorum longus, and extensor hallucis longus tendons. The tibialis anterior tendon dorsiflexes and inverts the foot. In addition to the extrinsic tendons, the intrinsic foot muscles provide support and balance to the foot and toes.[1]

The arterial supply to the foot comes from the terminal branches of the posterior tibial artery which branches into the medial and lateral plantar arteries, and from the anterior tibial artery which branches into the dorsalis pedis artery. The main venous drainage of the foot consists of the great saphenous vein medially and the small saphenous vein laterally.

Five nerves contribute to the sensation in the foot. The tibial nerve branches into the medial and lateral plantar nerves which supply sensation to the plantar foot and toes. In addition, the tibial nerve has a medial calcaneal branch which goes to the heel. The superficial peroneal nerve supplies sensation to the majority of the dorsum of the foot, while the deep peroneal nerve is responsible for sensation to the first dorsal web space. The sural nerve supplies the lateral foot and heel, and the saphenous nerve provides sensation to the medial aspect of the foot.

The subtalar joint consists of anterior, middle, and posterior facets. This joint is important in providing inversion and eversion to the hindfoot. When the heel is inverted, the transverse tarsal joint is locked. The transverse tarsal joint contains the talonavicular and calcaneocuboid joints. During normal gait, when the heel rises in the last portion of the stance phase, the hindfoot inverts to provide stability to the transverse tarsal joint. This stability allows the foot to carry the body weight forward. Early in the gait cycle, when the heel strikes and the foot subsequently lies flat to the ground, the hindfoot is everted to allow the transverse tarsal joint to be supple. This motion allows the foot to absorb the shock of weight-bearing and adapt to the terrain.[2]

The Lisfranc joint is the tarsal-metatarsal joint complex. A small amount of motion is present at each of these joints. The second metatarsal articulates with the middle cuneiform proximal to the first and third metatarsal-cuneiform articulations. This recessed position provides further stability to this region of the foot. The Lisfranc ligament attaches the medial cuneiform to the second metatarsal base.

17.3 RADIOGRAPHY

The standard radiographic views of the foot are the antero/posterior (AP), lateral, and oblique views. Weight-bearing X-rays are helpful in certain conditions to evaluate the bony alignment and to demonstrate the maximal deformity present.[3] X-rays of the contralateral foot can be used to assess subtle injuries such as those to the Lisfranc joint. In the normal situation, the base of the second metatarsal should align with the middle cuneiform on the AP view, and the base of the fourth metatarsal should be

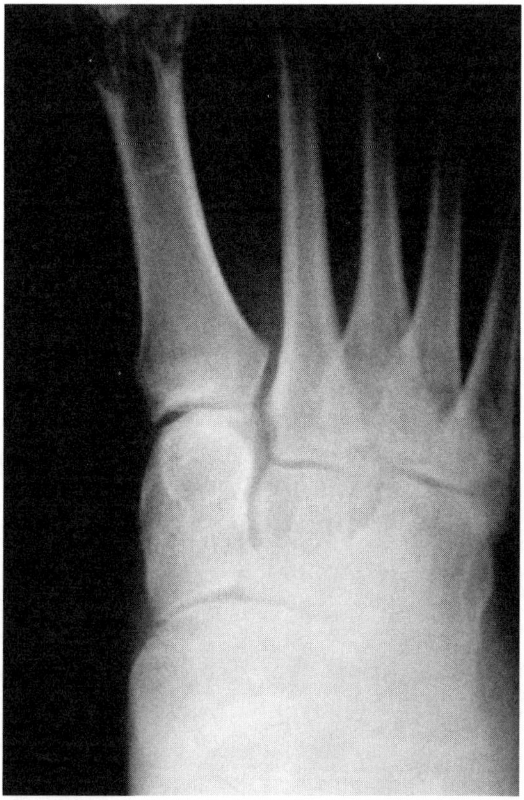

FIGURE 17.1 Normal AP radiograph of the foot. The medial aspect of the second metatarsal aligns with the edge of the middle cuneiform.

congruous with the medial aspect of the cuboid on the oblique view. These relationships become disrupted when there is injury to the Lisfranc joint (Figures 17.1 and 17.2).

Computed tomography (CT) is helpful when more bony detail is required and can be used to assess fractures, tarsal coalition, arthritis, and tumors. Technetium and Indium labeled bone scans are useful for the evaluation of the presence or absence of infections, occult fractures, inflammatory disorders, and tumors. Magnetic resonance imaging (MRI) also aids in the diagnosis of tumors, injuries, osteonecrosis, and infection.

17.4 TRAUMATIC DISORDERS OF THE FOOT

Restoring maximum function to the foot is the primary goal in the treatment of foot trauma. To accomplish this goal, the injured structure must heal in proper alignment, swelling must be brought under control, and motion of the injured region must be restored.

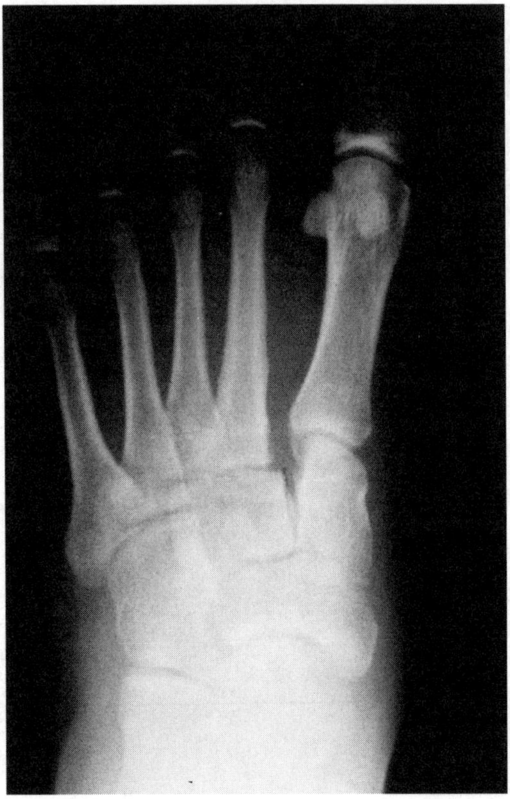

FIGURE 17.2 Injured Lisfranc joint. The base of the second metatarsal is shifted lateral to the edge of the cuneiform.

17.4.1 Talus Fractures

The talus has no tendinous attachments and is largely covered by cartilage. Any portion of the talus may be fractured, and due to the importance of the talus to both ankle and subtalar joint motion, even minor fractures may result in a poor outcome.

Osteochondral fractures of the talar dome may be difficult to visualize on plain radiographs. CT-scan images of the ankle best delineate the size and displacement of the fractures (Figure 17.3). Generally, nondisplaced fractures may be treated with a cast and non-weight-bearing. Small, displaced fractures are treated with arthroscopic or open ankle debridement. Larger fractures may be reduced and internally fixed.

Fractures of the lateral process of the talus are often mistaken for an ankle sprain. Close inspection of the radiographs will help in evaluating for this injury. Due to the fact that the lateral process involves a portion of the subtalar joint, posttraumatic arthritis of this joint may be a sequela of lateral process fractures.

Talus neck fractures are usually the result of forced dorsiflexion of the ankle. These fractures have been classified by Hawkins according to the amount of displacement present.[4] With increased displacement, a higher percentage of patients

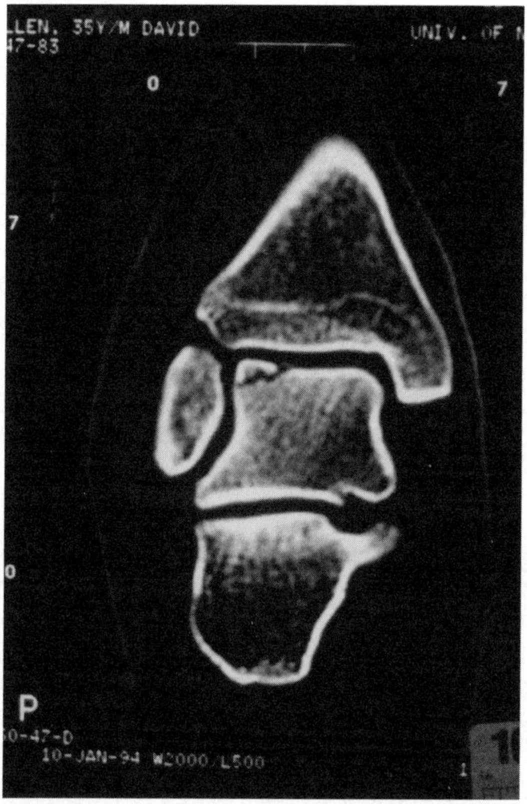

FIGURE 17.3 CT scan demonstrating an osteochondral fracture of the talar dome.

will ultimately develop avascular necrosis of the body of the talus which may lead to arthritis of the ankle and/or subtalar joint. Open reduction and internal fixation of displaced talar neck fractures are recommended.

17.4.2 Calcaneus Fractures

Major fractures of the calcaneus usually result from a fall. Associated injury to the spine needs to be ruled out. Calcaneal fractures often involve the subtalar joint, and posttraumatic arthritis of this joint is a frequent sequela. Generally, best results occur in those fractures which have minimal displacement of the fragments. Operative reduction and fixation are gaining popularity in attempts to improve the results of displaced calcaneus fractures.[5] Fusion of the subtalar joint may be used to treat symptomatic posttraumatic arthritis.

17.4.3 Stress Fractures

The foot is a common location for stress fractures. Patients present with pain that is exacerbated by activity and is often associated with swelling. Plain radiographs may be normal initially and may not show signs of a stress fracture for weeks. Bone scan or MRI is useful to detect stress fractures prior to radiographically detected changes.

The calcaneus and metatarsal shafts are common locations for stress fractures. These can be treated with activity modification and/or casting. Stress fractures of the proximal fifth metatarsal in the area between the metaphysis and diaphysis are associated with a high rate of nonunion. Early operative fixation is often recommended to promote healing with a shorter recovery time.[6]

17.5 INFECTIOUS DISORDERS OF THE FOOT

Infections of the foot may take one of many forms. Athlete's foot, for instance, is a fungal infection of the skin. More serious life- or limb-threatening infections may occur in association with diabetes mellitus. In this section, some of the most common foot infections for which patients seek medical care will be discussed.

17.5.1 Nail Puncture Wounds

Puncture wounds to the foot are relatively common. Patients may seek medical care acutely after the injury or later if infection has developed. Upon presentation, radiographs should be obtained to look for bone involvement and radiopaque foreign bodies. Tetanus prophylaxis should be updated as necessary.

If early presentation occurs without overt signs of infection, local wound debridement and irrigation should be performed. Removal of foreign bodies, if present, is important and may require formal operative treatment. Bone involvement should also be treated with operative debridement. Antibiotics are useful against Staphylococcus, Streptococcus, and Pseudomonas bacteria.

Patients may present with ongoing infection days to weeks after the injury. Pain, swelling, warmth, redness, and drainage may be present. Operative debridement should be performed including tendon sheaths, joints, and bone if involved. Wound culture, antibiotics, and open packing of the wound are necessary.[7]

17.5.2 Toenail Infections

Fungal infections of the toenails are common in adults and may be present in 90% of diabetic patients. The organism invades the hard nail plate, resulting in its destruction. The nail subsequently becomes thickened, discolored, and brittle. Patients may complain of the appearance or because of difficulty in trimming the thick nail. The nail may also interfere with shoewear. For mild asymptomatic cases, no treatment is necessary. In more advanced cases, treatment options include periodic debridement and trimming of the nail to decrease its thickness. Nail removal and ablation of the nail germinal matrix may also be performed. Oral and topical antifungal medications have variable success in alleviating the infection.

Ingrown toenails result when the distal nail edge grows into the skin of the nail fold. This most commonly results from improper trimming of the nail, leaving rounded edges which are short of the distal nail fold. As the nail grows in, irritation and trauma to the skin lead to a bacterial infection with pain, swelling, erythema, and drainage.

When acute infection is present, decompression of the ingrowing nail by removal of a portion of the nail plate is performed. Soaking the foot and providing oral antibiotics may also help alleviate the problem. Unfortunately, recurrence of ingrown toenails is high as the nail continues to grow. For this problem, the germinal matrix may have to be removed after the infection has resolved. Matrixectomy may be partial or complete depending on whether one or both sides of the nail are affected by ingrowing. The procedure may be performed with surgical excision or chemical ablation using phenol. Generally, a digital nerve block of the toe using lidocaine without epinephrine gives adequate anesthesia for these procedures.[8]

17.5.3 Diabetes Mellitus

Ulceration with subsequent infection of the foot is the most common reason for hospital admissions in diabetic patients. Diabetic foot infections are also the most common cause of amputation in the United States. Peripheral neuropathy, vascular insufficiency, and an impaired immune response predispose diabetics to these problems.[9]

Neuropathy leads to decreased protective sensation such that minor or repetitive trauma may go unnoticed until skin breakdown occurs. In addition, neuropathy may lead to an imbalance among the musculature of the foot, resulting in deformities. Bony prominences may cause increased pressure and lead to skin irritation and breakdown.

Vascular insufficiency may involve large and/or small vessels of the extremities. Evaluation of the patient must include an exam for diminished pulses and may include determination of segmental pressures and transcutaneous oxygenation. A diminished vascular supply correlates with a decreased chance of healing.

Preventative measures can decrease the number of foot complications in diabetes. The most important of these measures is instruction to the patient regarding the potential problems and foot care. Frequent self examinations, proper skin and nail care, and accommodating shoes with pressure-relieving orthotics are stressed.

Lesions of the foot have been classified by their depth.[10] Ulcers without deep involvement or infection can be treated with local wound care or a series of total contact casts. When infection develops, surgical debridement of the infection and systemic administration of an antibiotic are necessary. The infection often involves multiple organisms. Osteomyelitis and gangrene frequently require amputation. The primary goal is to amputate at a level where the infection will be eradicated and the skin will heal. Whenever possible, amputations that spare a portion of the foot should be performed. The advantage of partial foot amputations over higher-level amputations (e.g., below knee amputations) is that the patient may be able to walk better when the foot has been partially salvaged.

17.6 ARTHRITIC CONDITIONS OF THE FOOT

Arthritis can affect any joint of the foot. It may be primary degenerative or secondary to rheumatoid disease, gout, prior trauma, or other causes. Patients may complain

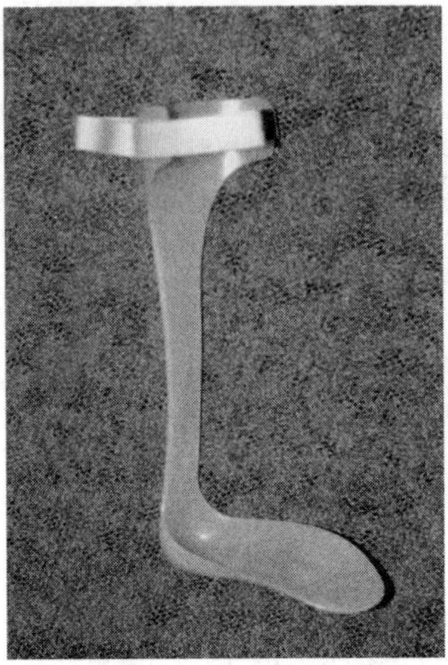

FIGURE 17.4 An ankle-foot-orthosis (AFO). This brace fits in a shoe and can benefit patients with ankle and foot arthritis by unloading the painful joint.

of pain, swelling, crepitation, and/or deformity. Nonoperative treatment consists of nonsteroidal anti-inflammatory medication, activity modification, walking supports such as canes, shoewear changes, and orthotics. A firm supportive shoe with a rocker bottom sole may facilitate transfer of weight during ambulation to unload the painful joint. Orthotics are devices placed in the shoe to support, cushion, or unload areas of the foot. For painful hindfoot arthritic conditions, an ankle-foot-orthosis (AFO) is most useful for unloading the affected joint and decreasing pain (Figure 17.4). The most common surgical treatment for advanced foot arthritis is fusion of the affected joints to alleviate pain.

Hallux rigidus is an arthritic condition which affects the great toe metatarsophalangeal joint. Initially, spurs develop on the dorsal side of the joint which may produce a prominence and limit joint dorsiflexion (Figure 17.5). Over time, joint space narrowing and further degenerative changes occur. When nonoperative treatment measures fail to relieve the pain, cheilectomy (removal of spurs) is useful in the early stages of the disease. After significant degenerative changes have developed, joint fusion is indicated.[11]

17.7 COMMON FOOT PATHOLOGIES

17.7.1 Heel Pain

The most common cause of heel pain is plantar fasciitis or the "heel spur syndrome." These two terms are used synonymously, although a heel spur is seen on X-ray in 60% of cases and may also be present in asymptomatic individuals (Figure 17.6). Patients complain of pain in the plantar medial heel around the origin of the plantar fascia. The pain is generally worse upon first arising in the morning and with activity. Patients often have a history of increased activity or overuse.

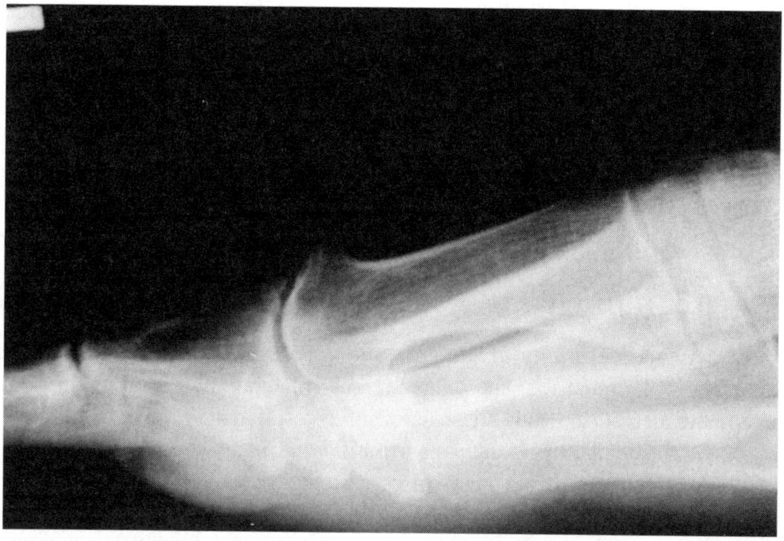

FIGURE 17.5 Lateral radiograph of the great toe in hallux rigidus. There is spur formation dorsal to the first metatarsal head.

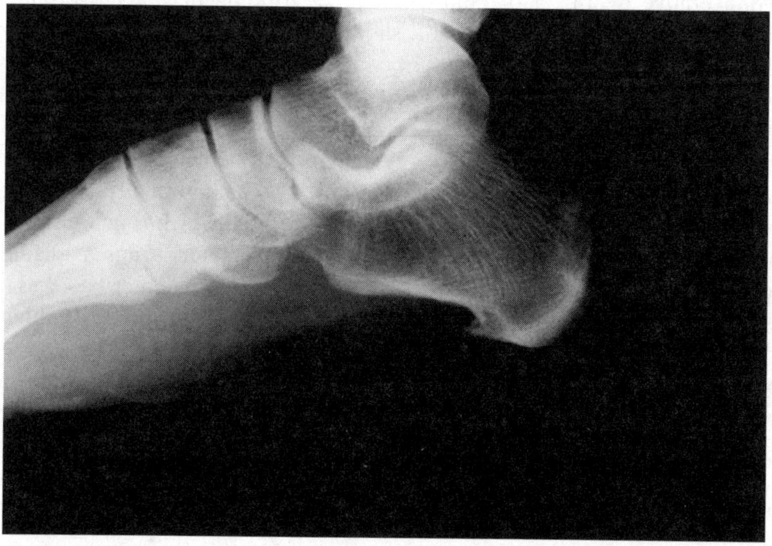

FIGURE 17.6 Lateral radiograph demonstrating the heel spur beneath the calcaneus that is commonly associated with plantar fasciitis.

The majority of patients with plantar fasciitis respond to nonoperative treatment, although the course may be prolonged, lasting months to years. Treatment methods which have been reported to be of benefit include stretching, casting, heel cushions, steroid injections, and night splints. Surgical release of a portion of the plantar fascia with or without removal of the heel spur is not universally successful. Surgery is generally not recommended prior to a prolonged course of nonoperative treatment.[12]

Calcaneal stress fractures also cause activity-related pain; however, patients often have swelling and pain with medial and lateral compression of the posterior heel. Tarsal tunnel syndrome may also result in medial heel pain as a result of tibial nerve compression posterior to the medial malleolus. Patients with tarsal tunnel syndrome usually have a Tinel's sign over the nerve and diminished sensation on the plantar foot.[13]

17.7.2 Toe Deformities

The most common deformity of the great toe is hallux valgus or bunion deformity. Hallux refers to the great toe, and valgus refers to lateral angulation of the proximal phalanx on the metatarsal head. These deformities result in a prominence of the medial portion of the metatarsal head, causing irritation and pain when in contact with the shoe. Bunions may result from years of constrictive shoewear. Other causes include genetic predisposition, rheumatoid disease, trauma, and neurologic conditions.

Some of the common radiographic features of bunion deformity are an increased angle between the first and second metatarsal shafts (normal <9 degrees), and increased angle between the first metatarsal and the great toe proximal phalanx (normal <15 degrees), and lateral subluxation of the sesamoids.

Nonoperative treatment of bunions includes padding the medial prominence, anti-inflammatory medication, and soft shoewear with a wider toe box. Numerous operative procedures have been described for bunions. Most operations involve removal of the medial bony prominence and an osteotomy of the metatarsal to decrease the width of the forefoot.[14]

Deformities of the lesser toes may result from any condition that changes the delicate balance between the tendons and ligaments which normally align the toes. These include congenital conditions such as the curly toe which is caused by a tight flexor tendon. Other causes for lesser toe deformities include trauma, rheumatoid disease, and neurologic conditions. Toe deformities such as hammer toes and mallet toes are most commonly idiopathic. Pain results from the deformed toe rubbing the shoe.

Nonoperative treatment of lesser toe deformities includes padding the prominence of the deformity and accommodative shoewear. Operative fixation includes realigning fixed bone deformities and release of deforming tendons and ligaments.

17.7.3 Metatarsalgia

Metatarsalgia is defined as pain about the metatarsals. There are a number of entities which can cause this complaint, including metatarsal stress fractures, Morton's neuromas, rheumatoid synovitis, plantar calluses, and avascular necrosis of the metatarsal head (Freiberg's disease).

Morton's neuroma is caused by compression of the common plantar digital nerve about the level of the metatarsal heads. Patients complain of pain in this location and often have symptoms of numbness or tingling in the adjacent toes. The third web space is affected most commonly, with the second web space the second most common site.

Shoes with a wider toe box, metatarsal pads, nonsteroidal anti-inflammatory medication, and a steroid injection placed about the nerve are nonoperative treatments which can be useful for Morton's neuroma. Excision of the neuroma gives a good result in approximately 80% of cases.[15]

REFERENCES

1. Moore, K., *Clinically Oriented Anatomy*, 3rd edition, Williams and Wilkins, Baltimore, 1992, Chap. 5.
2. Donatelli, R., *The Biomechanics of the Foot and Ankle*, F.A. Davis Co., Philadelphia, 1996, Chap. 1.
3. Long, B. and Rafert, J., *Orthopaedic Radiography*, W.B. Saunders, Philadelphia, 1995, 380-391.
4. Canale, S.T. and Kelly, F.B., Jr., Fractures of the neck of the talus, *Journal of Bone and Joint Surgery*, 60A, 143, 1978.
5. Macey, L.R., Benirsschke, S.K., Sangeorzan, B.J., and Hansen, S.T., Acute calcaneal fractures: treatment options and results, *Journal of the American Academy of Orthopaedic Surgeons*, 2, 36, 1994.
6. Lawrence, S.J. and Botte, M.J., Jones fractures and related fractures of the proximal fifth metatarsal, *Foot Ankle*, 13, 358, 1993.
7. DeCoster, T.A. and Miller, R.A., Management of traumatic foot wounds, *Journal of the American Academy of Orthopaedic Surgeons*, 2, 226, 1994.
8. Dixon, G.L., Treatment of ingrown toenail, *Foot Ankle*, 3, 254, 1983.
9. Brodsky, J.W., The diabetic foot, *Surgery of the Foot and Ankle*, 6th edition, Mann, R.A. and Coughlin, M.J., Eds., Mosby, St. Louis, 1993, 887.
10. Wagner, F.W., A classification and treatment program for diabetic, neuropathic, and dysvascular foot problems, *Instructional Course Lectures*, American Academy Orthopaedic Surgeons, Volume XXVIII, Mosby, St. Louis, 1979, 143.
11. Pedowitz, W.J., Deformities of the first ray, *Orthopaedic Knowledge Update, Foot and Ankle*, Lutter, L.D., Mizel, M.S., and Pfeffer, G.B., Eds., American Academy of Orthopaedic Surgeons, Rosemont, 1994, 141.
12. DeMaio, M., Paine, R., Mangine, R.E., and Drez, D., Plantar fasciitis, *Orthopaedics*, 16, 1153, 1993.
13. Bailie, D.S. and Kelikian, A.S., Tarsal tunnel syndrome: diagnosis, surgical technique, and functional outcome, *Foot Ankle*, 19, 65, 1998.
14. Mann, R.A., Decision making in bunion surgery, *Instructional Course Lectures*, Volume XXXIX, Greene, W.B., Ed., American Academy of Orthopaedic Surgeons, Park Ridge, 1990, 3.
15. Mann, R.A. and Reynolds, J.C., Interdigital neuroma: a critical analysis, *Foot Ankle*, 3, 238, 1983.

18 The Hand

Charles R. Pribyl and Moheb S. Moneim

CONTENTS

18.1 ANATOMY OF HAND AND WRIST

18.1.1 Bones and Joints

The tubular bones of the hand are the phalanges and metacarpals. Each finger has a metacarpal and three phalanges (proximal, middle, and distal). The long finger ray is the most stable and considered the center of the hand. The index ray is also very stable and along with the long ray is used with the thumb for prehension (pinch) activities. The ring and small rays are more mobile and provide power grip. This mobility is at the carpometacarpal (CMC) joints.

The interphalangeal (IP) joints are hinge joints that have bony stability to resist radioulnar stresses. A thick ligamentous capsule supports these joints in the form of collateral ligaments and volar plate. This contrasts with the metacarpal-phalangeal (MP) joints which allow radioulnar motion in extension, but not in flexion. This concept allows the finger, while extended at the MP joint, to be positioned easily, but when flexed, as in power grip, provides stability. This mechanical phenomenon is accomplished through a cam effect in the metacarpal head. Due to its eccentric shape, the distance from the attachment of the collateral ligament on the head to the joint surface is longer in flexion than in extension. Thus, the collateral ligament is lax (longer relatively) in extension, and shorter (tight) in flexion.

0-8493-9237-3/99/$0.00+$.50

The thumb IP and MP joints are similar to those of the fingers. Thumb MP joint stability is critical for pinch. Disruption of the ulnar collateral ligament of this joint leads to weak and ineffective pinch. This injury can be acute or chronic. The acute type is often seen in skiers and is known as skier's thumb.

The thumb CMC joint is a complex double-saddle shaped joint that provides stability for the thumb ray, but is also mobile to allow the necessary thumb motion for our unique opposable thumb. This joint frequently becomes arthritic, especially in middle-aged females, and is the subject of much study in an attempt to describe its biomechanics in definitive fashion.

18.1.1.1 Wrist Bones

The distal row of the wrist is made up of these bones: capitate, hamate, trapezoid, and trapezium. Capitate (captain) is the stable, center of the wrist and is flanked by the hamate (ulnar side) and trapezoid (radial side). These bones are held together relatively tightly by their ligaments and have little relative motion. The trapezium is anterior to the other bones and provides the takeoff for the thumb ray.

The proximal row consists of the lunate, scaphoid, triquetrum, and pisiform. The intrinsically unstable lunate is held in place by ligamentous attachments to the scaphoid and triquetrum. Loss of scapholunate ligament integrity results in a dorsal tilting of the lunate (dorsal intercalated segmental instability [DISI] pattern). Similarly, loss of lunotriquetral ligament integrity results in a volar tilt of the lunate (volar intercalated segmental instability [VISI] pattern). The scaphoid bone links the proximal and distal rows and is best thought of as a peanut-shaped bone with its proximal half in the proximal row of the wrist and the distal half in the distal row. The waist of the scaphoid, between the two parts, is susceptible to fracture when the wrist is hyper-dorsiflexed as in a fall on an outstretched hand. The pisiform is a sesamoid bone within the flexor carpi ulnaris tendon which, much like the patella, lies within the quadriceps tendon of the lower extremity.

In the wrist joint, approximately one half of wrist flexion and extension occurs at the radiocarpal joint and the other half at the midcarpal joints. Most radioulnar deviation occurs at the radiocarpal joint. Pronation and supination occur at the distal and proximal radioulnar joints.

Wrist stability is provided by extrinsic (capsular) ligaments and intrinsic (between carpal bones) ligaments. The volar ligaments are more important than the dorsal extrinsic ligaments. The radioscaphocapitate ligament is the strongest of these. Less strong extrinsic dorsal ligaments add to stability. Intrinsic ligaments, such as the above-mentioned scapholunate ligament, are also very important.

18.1.2 Tendons and Muscles

Flexor tendons arise from muscles in the volar forearm. The palmaris longus and flexor carpi radialis and ulnaris are more superficial and their tendons pass outside the carpal canal. The palmaris longus inserts on the superficial palmar fascia. The flexor carpi radialis passes volar to the scaphoid and trapezium to insert on the second metacarpal base. The flexor carpi ulnaris incorporates the pisiform bone as a sesamoid on its way to insert into the base of the fifth metacarpal. The flexor pollicis longus to the thumb distal phalanx, the flexor digitorum superficialis (or sublimis) to each finger's middle phalanx, and the flexor digitorum profundus (FDP) to each finger's distal phalanx pass through the carpal canal along with the median nerve.

The flexor tendons to the fingers and thumb are enclosed in a sheath from the distal palmar flexion crease to the insertions on the distal phalanges. The sheath has thickenings, called pulleys, to hold the tendons close to the bones. Each finger has five annular and three cruciate pulleys.

Extensor tendons also arise from muscles in the forearm. At the wrist they are separated into six compartments beneath the extensor retinaculum. Most radial, in the first dorsal compartment, are the abductor pollicis longus and the extensor pollicis brevis, which insert on the bases of the first metacarpal and proximal phalanx of the thumb, respectively. The extensor carpi radialis longus and brevis are in the second dorsal compartment on their way to the second and third metacarpal bases. The extensor pollicis longus goes around a bony prominence on the distal radius called Lister's tubercle as it passes through the third dorsal compartment on the way to the distal phalanx of the thumb. The finger extensors, the extensor indicis proprius and extensor digitorum communis pass through the fifth dorsal compartment. The extensor digiti minimi passes through the fifth dorsal compartment and on to the small finger. Lastly, the extensor carpi ulnaris passes through a fibrous tunnel over the distal ulna in the sixth dorsal compartment en route to the base of the fifth metacarpal.

Thumb intrinsic muscles include the median innervated abductor pollicis brevis, opponens, and usually one half of the flexor pollicis brevis. The ulnarly innervated half of the flexor pollicis brevis and adductor pollicis complete the thumb musculature.

Each finger has an interosseous muscle for radial and ulnar deviation at the MP joint. Dorsal interossei abduct, while volar interossei adduct the index, ring, and small fingers. Volar interossei radially and ulnarly deviate the long finger. Lumbricals originate from the radial side of each FDP tendon and pass volar to the volar transverse intermetacarpal ligament to insert on the radial lateral band of each finger. The radial two lumbricals are median innervated, while the ulnar lumbricals and all the interossei are innervated by the ulnar nerve.

Finger extension is a complex motion carried out by the intrinsic and extrinsic tendons. The extrinsic tendons form a sling via the sagittal bands to extend the MP joints. They continue on and contribute to the central slip and lateral bands to aid in IP joint extension. The interossei insert on the proximal phalanx base to provide MP flexion and also carry on as the lateral band to provide IP extension. Thus, the flexor system is relatively simple with a tendon flexing each joint: MP-intrinsics, PIP-FDS, and DIP-FDP. The extensor system is more complex with the extrinsic tendons extending the MP joints and contributing to PIP joint extension. The intrinsics provide most of the power to extend the IP joints and this system is linked, i.e., the power to PIP and DIP joints is shared. This explains the boutonniere and swan neck deformities seen in extensor tendon injuries.

18.1.3 Nerves

The radial nerve (some via the posterior interosseous nerve) innervates all of the extrinsic extensors of the wrist, thumb, and fingers. In addition, the radial nerve provides sensation to the back of the entire thumb, the back of the radial half of the hand, and the back of the index and long finger as far distal as the PIP joint.

The median nerve innervates the extrinsic flexors except for the FCU and the ulnar half of the FDP which are ulnarly innervated. The median nerve provides sensation to the volar thumb, index, long, and radial half of ring, as well as the dorsal same fingers distal to the PIP joints. The ulnar nerve provides sensation to the ulnar half of the ring and the entire small finger. The sensation to the ulnar half of the dorsal hand and the proximal portions of the small and ulnar half of the ring fingers is provided by the dorsal branch of the ulnar nerve which comes off the ulnar nerve about nine centimeters above the wrist and winds dorsally just distal to the ulnar head.

Skin and nails: The palmar skin of the hand is thicker, has more sweat gland, and has fingerprints as compared to dorsal skin. The nailbed has two parts, a germinal, proximal portion responsible for generation of the nail plate and a sterile, distal portion which is supported by the distal phalanx. The skin around the nail plate is called the epinychium and the nail plate sits in the nail fold.

Blood supply: Most hands have both a radial and an ulnar artery. The radial artery passes under the first dorsal compartment, between the first and second metacarpal bases, and then forms the deep palmar arch. The ulnar artery passes into the hand with the ulnar nerve via Guyon's canal, between the pisiform and hamate, and then crosses the palm as the superficial palmar arch. Off of this arch come the digital arteries, one each on the radial and ulnar sides of each digit. Communications and anastomoses are many and variable in each hand.

18.2 AMPUTATIONS, ARTHRODESIS, AND ARTHROPLASTY

Injury to the hand is the most common cause of amputation of digits and the hand. Tumors and unreconstructable deformities rarely lead to amputation. Using current microvascular techniques, many amputated parts can be successfully reattached. Sharp injuries with narrow zones of injury are most successfully replanted, while injuries with extensive soft tissue or avulsion injuries, such as rodeo roper's thumb, have a much poorer prognosis. Indications for replantation are based on the amount of function returned to the hand by reattachment of the part. Thus, thumb replantation is always attempted. Other strong indications for replantation include multiple digit amputation, whole hand amputations, and functional loss in children. Relative contraindications include other life-threatening injuries, multiple levels of amputation in the same part, and amputated border digits where reattachment would not add significant function to the hand and may compromise further function due to stiffness.

Clinical considerations in digital and hand amputation include providing tough, stable skin in the amputated area to prevent pain and skin breakdown during use, as well as resecting or removing amputated nerve ends away from high contact areas to lessen the likelihood of symptomatic post-traumatic neuromas.

Reconstruction after amputation is most frequently performed to recreate a thumb. Techniques include lengthening of the existing thumb; transposition of a finger, usually the index (pollicization); and toe-to-thumb transfer. Patient needs and desires, level of previous injury, and surgeon experience are important factors in selecting the reconstructive technique. Toe-to-hand transfer for finger replacement is technically possible, but only indicated in exceptional cases where all fingers are lost or absent. Motion, sensibility, and cosmesis are less than optimal in toes attempting to perform as fingers.

Finger prostheses are available and are very cosmetic. Due to lack of motion and sensibility, they are not very functional. A small number of patients who are self-conscious about the loss of fingers are grateful users of these prosthetics.

The wrist joint and small joints of the hand provide motion, stability, and are pain-free. If a joint is painful or unstable, a fusion of that joint will provide pain relief and stability for the trade-off of motion. This trade-off is particularly good at the MP joint of the thumb, and IP joints of the fingers, as well as for the wrist. Retention of motion would be ideal; however, joint replacement in the fingers and wrist has not yet been perfected (see below). Arthrodesis of the MP joint of the thumb restores a stable, pain-free thumb, when done for pain, instability, or deformity. The CMC joint of the thumb is seldom fused, as the loss of mobility here constitutes a significant functional loss, and soft tissue reconstruction performs well. Fusion of the MP joints of the fingers causes a significant loss and soft tissue or silastic joint reconstruction are usually performed. In patients with inflammatory diseases the demands on the crippled hand are less, and silastic joints in the MP and IP joints are acceptable. In the post-traumatic or osteoarthritic joint of a patient with otherwise normal function, the silastic joints tend to break down and form particles which may incite an inflammatory response and lead to bone destruction. Therefore, IP joint fusions are performed in these patients when surgery is indicated. By the time these patients present for surgery, they usually have little motion left in their arthritic joints and have adapted to this change. They are grateful for the pain relief.

18.2.1 Arthroplasty

When joint surfaces are eroded or destroyed by local or systemic factors, arthroplasty, or joint replacement, can be considered. After joint resection, three types of arthroplasty are available in the hand and wrist. The resected area is replaced with either soft-tissue, foreign material to act as a spacer, or a formal artificial joint which attempts to recreate the original structure.

The ideal joint replacement restores joint surfaces and motion with a durable result. Unfortunately, due to the small bones, limiting fixation area, and poor bone quality in systemic disease, such as rheumatoid arthritis, traditional cemented and uncemented metal and polyethylene total joint constructs like those used in the hip and knee have not been successful in the hand and wrist. Research in this area continues.

In the thumb CMC joint, soft tissue arthroplasty that uses a rolled-up tendon spacer with or without ligament reconstruction has been shown to relieve pain and restore motion. Maximum strength is not restored, but at present this construct provides the best clinical result. Soft tissue arthroplasty is sometimes used in MP and IP joints of the fingers where motion is deemed necessary, precluding fusion, but silastic spacers are contraindicated. Although motion is maintained by this method, pain relief is not as consistent as with silastic spacers.

In patients with systemic disease such as rheumatoid arthritis, where many joints are affected, it is necessary to preserve motion since multi-joint fusions are less functional. Silastic spacers work well in these patients. They are primarily used in the MP and IP joints to restore motion and provide significant pain relief and return of function when accompanied by soft tissue rebalancing. Silastic is reserved for low-stress joints in relatively low-demand patients, as the silastic will fracture and fragment under larger loads. Silastic particles released during this process can cause a bone-destroying synovitis.

The ideal wrist joint is stable, painless, and has a functional range of motion. When a wrist is painful and/or unstable, motion can be sacrificed by fusing the wrist. The result is a painless fusion which provides a stable platform for the hand. Alternatives include partial wrist fusions, eliminating painful joints, but preserving some motion, and excision of the proximal row of carpal bones (proximal row carpectomy, or PRC). These alternatives are useful when the wrist is not entirely destroyed. Silastic and formal total joint arthroplasty have not proven effective in the wrist due to silicon synovitis in the former and problems with loosening in the latter.

18.3 MANAGEMENT PRINCIPLES FOR FRACTURES, DISLOCATIONS, INFECTIONS, AND TENDON INJURIES

18.3.1 Fractures

Fractures in the hand are generally the result of trauma. Specific history, and directed physical examination to areas of tenderness, and posterior-anterior, lateral, and oblique X-rays are generally sufficient for the diagnosis. Special views are sometimes needed for particular bones. A post-anterior (PA) view in ulnar deviation aids in diagnosis of scaphoid fractures. A reverse oblique view of the hand aids in diagnosis of the base of the fifth metacarpal fracture and fractures around the MP joints of the fingers are aided by a Brewerton view, which is taken to put these joints more in profile.

Important principles in treatment of fractures of the hand include anatomic alignment of fractures that involve joint surfaces and adequate alignment of other fractures to minimize their interference later with function. Fractures are immobilized long enough to provide stability, but mobilization is important in the hand to prevent stiffness and subsequent contractures. In general, metaphyseal bone heals in three to six weeks, whereas diaphyseal bone takes six to eight weeks. Open fractures, that is, fractures that communicate with the external environment, require irrigation and debridement; on the whole, these take longer to heal because of the greater energy imparted to cause such fractures, inasmuch as soft tissue has been stripped off and the blood supply has been impaired. Internal fixation, closed reduction and percutaneous pinning (CRPP) or open reduction internal fixation (ORIF), is used to stabilize fractures that are either unstable or irreducible (after reduction).

In general, fractures should be classified as: nondisplaced; displaced but reducible and stable after reduction; reducible but unstable; or irreducible on the known fracture pattern and anatomy around the fracture.

Some principles regarding specific bones of the hand follow.

Distal phalanges: In fractures of the distal phalanx, dorsal surface, the reduction of the surface must be smooth in order minimize nail deformity.

Phalanges: Fractures into the joint that are displaced must be reduced and stabilized to provide a congruent joint to prevent post-traumatic arthritis. Fractures of the shaft of the phalanges generally deform in an apex volar fashion, that is, on the lateral radiographic view, the base of the V points volar. This is due to the intrinsic tendon forces across these joints. These displaced fractures are frequently unstable due to their oblique or spiral nature and require internal fixation. In general, closed reduction and percutaneous pinning is preferred to open reduction, as the dissection and bulk of a plate frequently lead to post-operative stiffness and difficulty in tendon gliding in these areas. In stable and minimally displaced fractures, a technique of dorsal block splinting using the extensor hood as a internal splint by flexing the wrist and MP joints and then allowing some minimal motion of the IP joints is an acceptable way to treat stable phalangeal shaft fractures.

Metacarpals: A common fracture encountered is a metacarpal neck fracture. This is also known as a boxer's fracture and frequently occurs after a patient strikes either a fixed object such as a wall, car, or a jaw, and usually occurs in the fifth metacarpal neck. Fortunately, due to the mobility of the fourth and fifth rays, some deformity can be accepted in this area. After reduction, the MP joint should be held flexed with the IP joints straight to prevent joint contacture. In general, motion should be started by post-injury week three or four to prevent MP joint stiffness. In unstable fractures, percutaneous pinning may be necessary.

Bennett's fracture: Fractures of the base of the thumb metacarpal frequently occur through the CMC joint. These fractures leave a small triangular piece of bone on the volar ulnar side of the joint and the rest of the metacarpal is pulled dorsally and proximally by the abductor pollicis longus tendon. This fracture is mentioned because it is intrinsically unstable due to the pull of this tendon, and internal fixation is required to hold it during healing. A similar situation occurs on the base of the fifth metacarpal where the extensor carpi ulnaris tendon will pull the fifth metacarpal proximally and dorsally.

Carpal bones: The most frequently fractured carpal bone is the scaphoid. If at all displaced, it requires internal fixation for healing. A frequent complication of this fracture is avascular necrosis of the proximal pole of the scaphoid; nonunion is common if the fracture is not immobilized. The blood supply of the scaphoid enters distally and proceeds to the proximal pole. Thus, a fracture may interrupt the blood supply to the proximal pole. This impedes healing and may result in early post-traumatic arthritis of the wrist.

Dorsal triquetral fractures frequently occur in wrist trauma. These are seen on the lateral view and are small capsular avulsion fractures that require three to four weeks of immobilization.

18.3.2 Dislocations

In general, when treating dislocations of the small joints of the hand, it is advisable to get pre-reduction X-rays. This ascertains that the dislocation is not a periarticular fracture. After adequate anesthesia and reduction of the joint, it is most important to check the joint for stability in various planes. For instance, a PIP joint should be checked for stability of the collateral ligaments as well as the volar plate. In addition, after reduction, active motion should be documented to ensure that there has not been a tendon injury.

If interphalangeal joints are dislocated, they can generally be relocated by gently recreating the deformity and then moving the joint back into a reduced position. If the joint is stable, minimal immobilization should be used and early protected motion begun to prevent contractures. The PIP joint is particularly prone to a flexion contracture and any length of immobilization is prone to encourage this difficult-to-treat contracture. If a collateral ligament joint is injured without a bony avulsion, these will heal with three to four weeks of protected motion. If a volar plate injury is encountered, these too will heal and it is more common to have a flexion contracture after this injury than to have dorsal instability of the joint.

In metacarpal phalangeal joint dislocations of the fingers, when the proximal phalanx is parallel to the metacarpal, this complete dislocation may be difficult to reduce due to interposition of the volar plate between the joint surfaces. This frequently requires open reduction. Again, in finger MP joint dislocations, stiffness is more of a problem than laxity, so after reduction, early motion is encouraged.

In the MP joint of the thumb, the most frequent joint injury is to the ulnar collateral ligament of the thumb in a skier's or gamekeeper's thumb. In this injury, the thumb is hyper-abducted, tearing the ulnar collateral ligament which may become superficial to the adductor aponeurosis upon reduction of the joint, thus leaving it in a position where it cannot possibly heal. This Stenner lesion can result in chronic disability if not openly repaired. Therefore, complete ulnar collateral ligament injuries of the MP joint of the thumb should be openly repaired. Frequently, the volar plate or dorsal capsule can be injured with collateral ligament injuries and this should be looked for at the time of examination.

The CMC joints of the fourth and fifth finger can be dislocated as a result of axial trauma with or without subsequent fracture. A closed reduction should be attained and, if stable, immobilized for approximately four weeks. If the reduction is not stable, the joints should be pinned for approximately one month.

The most common wrist ligament injury is a scapholunate ligament rupture. This taut, tough interosseous ligament between the scaphoid and lunate is frequently diagnosed as a wrist sprain. Careful examination of radiographs, paying particular attention to the relationship between the scaphoid and lunate, will avoid missing this important diagnosis. Treatment of these injuries is open repair or reconstruction of the ligament.

18.3.3 Infections

Infections of the hand can be extremely painful and debilitating, and result in permanent loss of function if not treated early and adequately. It is important to distinguish between the presence of cellulitis, which should be treated with local treatments and antibiotics, and the presence of pus which requires incision and drainage. Cultures should be obtained of any purulent material. In acute infections, aerobic and anaerobic cultures should be taken. In any chronic infection, examination for mycobacterium and fungi should also be undertaken. Treatment of these patients should be initiated with a broad spectrum antibiotic covering *Staphylococcus aureus,* plus any additional antibiotics if there is suspicion of other organisms. It is most important to observe these patients frequently for worsening or the presence of pus. It is inappropriate to skip seeing these patients for several days to a week, as their conditions can rapidly deteriorate.

Infections frequently occur in the hand. Proceeding distally to proximally, the first of these is a paronychia which involves an infection around the nail. These infections frequently are caused by *Staphylococcus aureus* and range from a mild inflammation to frank pus lifting the nail off the nail bed. The presence of pus requires open drainage.

A felon occurs in the pulp space. These are particularly painful because fibrous septi bind the skin to the bone to allow firm gripping of objects without sliding around. This, however, creates great pressure when there is inflammation or infection in the pulp. A felon will frequently produce pus early and incision and drainage are required for these lesions.

A subcutaneous abscess can occur anywhere on the hand. These are usually associated with minor penetrating trauma.

A particularly feared infection in the hand is that of the flexor tendon sheath. This closed synovial space, which allows gliding of the flexor tendons between the pulleys and between themselves, is a delicate structure that, once harmed by the inflammation and trauma of an infection, frequently leads to a very stiff finger. The history of an individual with a flexor tendon sheath infection is generally that of a penetrating injury over the flexor tendon 24 to 72 hours prior to presentation. The patient will frequently state that suddenly, within the last four to six hours, the finger became extremely swollen, painful, and became impossible to move. Kanavel has described the four cardinal signs of flexor tendon sheath infections. These include a sausage-shaped finger, a finger held in a semi-flexed position, a finger that has pain along the flexor tendon sheath, and a finger which is exquisitely painful to any forced extension of the finger. These infections need to have operative irrigation and debridement. When caught early, normal function of the finger may be expected; however, once pus has accumulated within the flexor tendon sheath, some stiffness and a difficult post-operative course may result.

The thenar space is deep to the muscles on the volar aspect of the thumb side of the hand. A penetrating injury to this area or an extension of infection in a flexor tendon sheath has usually preceded infection of the mid-palmar space.

A mid-palmar space infection occurs in the same fashion. The mid-palmar space and thenar space are separated by the muscular attachment of the adductor pollicis to the volar aspect of the third metacarpal.

Joint infections usually occur secondary to penetrating trauma. Irrigation and debridement are required in the case of these injuries and early motion should be begun to minimize cartilage damage.

Bites to the hand frequently occur. Human bites are the result of a patient having been bitten or when a patient strikes another individual's mouth with a closed fist. These injuries frequently result in penetration through the extensor mechanism into the MP joint of the fingers and are often known as "fight bites". They require emergent irrigation and debridement, as the human mouth is a haven for many bacteria and these injuries will frequently produce pus within four to six hours after a joint has become inoculated. *Staphylococcus aureus* is the most common infection from human bites; however, *Eickenella corrodens*, a facultative anaerobe that is sensitive to penicillin, is also common. Cat and dog bites frequently inoculate *Pasteurella multocida* into the wound. The *Pasteurella* is sensitive to penicillin. Dog bites are frequently a tearing-type bite with some potential soft tissue loss; however, they are generally open and are easily debrided. Cat bites are frequently penetrating and needle-like, inoculating deep tissues and are suspiciously benign in nature until several days after the bite when infection is rip-roaring and well under way in a closed space.

Post-operative care for infections includes close observation of the patient. If the patient states that he/she does not feel better after incision and drainage of an abscess, one must be suspicious that more abscess area remains or that the host may be compromised and not fighting the infection as well as a normal patient, or that the patient is infected with an organism with less-than-usual susceptibility to antibiotics. Whirlpool or other cleansing of the wound is advised. When the wound is clean, dressing changes, range of motion, and rehabilitation of the hand should be started as wound healing progresses. Incisions made to drain infections should seldom be closed. Healing should be left to secondary intention in most cases.

18.3.4 Tendon Injuries

Tendon injuries in the hand can be divided into flexor and extensor tendon injuries. In general, tendon injuries should be repaired within seven to ten days. The sooner repaired, the more easily the repair will be accomplished. Repairs attempted after three weeks generally are unsuccessful due to tissue immobility and early healing which prevents satisfactory repair. Tendon repairs should be accomplished within good vascular beds, free of infection, and in the presence of a tidy wound. Failure to adhere to these principles will result in increased rates of tendon adhesions and/or rupture of repairs.

The flexor tendons are divided into five areas or zones as described by Verdan. Zone 1 is the area of the flexor tendon sheath from the sublimis insertion on the middle phalanx to the insertion of the profundus tendon on the distal phalanx. Zone 2 is the area proximal to the sublimis insertion to the end of the fiberosseus canal, approximately at the level of the flexor crease of the palm. In this area both tendons are encased in a fiberosseus sheath lined with synovia that has little tolerance for scarring or adhesion. Zone 3 is from the start of the synovial sheath proximal to the distal end of the transverse carpal ligament. Zone 4 is underneath the transverse carpal ligament. Zonc 5 is proximal to the transverse carpal ligament.

Injuries in Zone 1 include profundus tendon ruptures from hyperextension injuries, most commonly occurring in the ring finger, or traumatic lacerations distal to the sublimis insertion. These should be repaired promptly, and may be treated by three to four weeks of immobilization with the wrist and MP joints in flexion and the IP joints in extension or in an early mobilization program as described by Kleinert. The latter uses a rubber band traction system to allow active extension, but with the rubber band providing passive flexion of the digit to minimize the pulling force across the tendon. Another type of early mobilization program was described by Duran. It involves passive mobilization of the digit to provide some motion to prevent tendon adhesions at the repair site.

These mobilization programs are now accepted treatment for Zone 2 injuries. With rare exceptions, both flexor tendons should be repaired if lacerated and an early mobilization program started. In Zones 3, 4, and 5 the repairs are carried out and then either immobilized or begun on an early mobilization program, the choice being left to the operating surgeon on a case-by-case basis.

Extensor tendon injuries can be more complicated and debilitating than flexor tendon injuries as the extensor system is less forgiving of adhesion and repairs than the flexor system. An avulsion or laceration of the terminal tendon as it inserts into the distal phalanx will result in a mallet finger, i.e., is an inability to extend the DIP joint. If these injuries are closed, the joint may be splinted in extension for eight weeks followed by night splinting for another three to four weeks, provided there is not significant drop of the distal phalanx. Lacerations or avulsions of the central slip insertion into the middle phalanx frequently are obscured by swelling at the PIP joint. One to two weeks later, the patient may notice inability to extend the PIP joint and a hyperextension deformity at the DIP joint. This hyperextension deformity is caused by the transfer of extensor force from the PIP joint through the intact lateral bands to the DIP joint. This deformity is called a boutonnière or buttonhole deformity. Treatment of acute injuries involves splinting the PIP joint in extension or surgical repair of lacerated tendons followed by careful rehabilitation of the PIP and DIP joint motion.

Lacerations over the MP joint frequently involve the extensor tendon; however, they do not retract significantly due to the presence of the sagittal bands holding the extensor tendons in place over the MP joints. These may be treated by repair and a short period of immobilization, followed by mobilization to prevent stiffness of the MP joints. These lacerations are most frequently encountered in "fight bites" and treatment to prevent or treat infection takes priority over treating the tendon injury.

Lacerations proximal to the MP joints over the metacarpals or under the extensor retinaculum frequently result in retraction of the tendon into the forearm. These should be approached carefully in the emergency room, as frequently extensive exploration is required to find the retracted ends. This is probably best done in the operating room.

Wrist flexor and extensor tendons can also be lacerated. These require stout sutures for repairs, as these are powerful tendons which require immobilization for four to six weeks.

FURTHER INFORMATION — ANATOMY OF HAND AND WRIST

1. Berger, R.A. *General Anatomy.* In: *The Wrist: Diagnosis and Operative Repair*; Cooney, W.P.; Linscheid, R.L.; Dobyns, J.H., Eds. Mosby: St. Louis, 1998; pp 32-60.
2. Berger, R.A. *Ligament Anatomy.* In: *The Wrist: Diagnosis and Operative Treatment*; Cooney, W.P.; Linscheid, R.L.; Dobyns, J.H., Eds. Mosby: St. Louis, 1998; pp 73-105.
3. Brand, P.W.; Hollister, A. *Clinical Mechanics of the Hand*; Mosby Year Book: St. Louis, MO, 1993.
4. Garci-Elias, M.; Dobyns, J.H. *Bones and Joints.* In: *The Wrist: Diagnosis and Operative Treatment*; Cooney, W.P.; Linscheid, R.L.; Dobyns, J.H., Eds. Mosby: St. Louis, 1998; pp 61-72.
5. Johnson, M.K.; Cohen, M.J. *The hand atlas*; Thomas: Springfield, IL, 1975.
6. Kaplan, E.B. *Functional and Surgical Anatomy of the Hand*; Lippincott: Philadelphia, PA, 1965.
7. McGrouther, D.A.; Higgins, P.O. *Interactive Hand Anatomy.* version 1.0.0. London UK: Primal Pictures. 1997, CD-ROM.
8. Taleisnik, J. *The Wrist*; Churchill Livingstone: New York, 1985.
9. Tountas, C.P.; Bergman, R.A. *Anatomic Variations of the Upper Extremity*; Churchill Livingstone: New York, 1993.
10. Zancolli, E.A. *Structural and Dynamic Bases of Hand Surgery*; J.B. Lippincott Company: Philadelphia, 1979.
11. Zancolli, E.A.; Cozzi, E.P. *Atlas of Surgical Anatomy of the Hand*; Churchill Livingstone: New York, 1992.

FURTHER INFORMATION — AMPUTATION, ARTHRODESIS, AND ARTHROPLASTY

1. Beckenbaugh, R.D.; Linscheid, R.L. *Arthroplasty in the Hand and Wrist.* In: *Operative Hand Surgery*; Green, D.P., Ed. Churchill Livingstone: New York, 1993; pp 143-188.
2. Bednar, J.M. *Wrist Joint Arthroplasties.* In: *Surgery of the Hand and Upper Extremity*; Peimer, C.A., Ed. McGraw-Hill: New York, 1996; pp 795-828.
3. Brockman, R.; Weiland, A.J. *Small Joint Arthrodeses.* In: *Operative Hand Surgery*; Green, D.P., Ed. Churchill Livingstone: New York, 1993; pp 99-112.
4. Dick, H.M. *Wrist Arthrodesis.* In: *Operative Hand Surgery*; Green, D.P., Ed. Churchill Livingstone: New York, 1993; pp 131-142.
5. Goldner, R.D.; Howson, M.P.; Nunley, J.A., One hundred eleven thumb amputations: Replantation vs. Revision. *Microsurgery* 1990, 11, 243-250.
6. Gould, J. *Arthroplasty of the Metacarpophalangeal and Interphalangeal Joints of the Digits and Thumb.* In: *Surgery of the Hand and Upper Extremity*; Peimer, C.A., Ed. McGraw-Hill: New York, 1996; pp 1677-1690.
7. Kleinert, J.M. *Amputations and Prosthetics.* In: *Hand Surgery Update*; Manske, P.R., Ed. American Academy of Orthopedic Surgeons: Rosemont, IL, 1996; pp 437-447.

8. Leclerq, C.; Brunelli, F. *Treatment of Fingertip Amputations*. In: *Surgery of the Hand and Upper Extremity*; Peimer, C.A., Ed. McGraw-Hill: New York, 1996; pp 1069-1100.
9. Louis, D.S. *Amputations*. In: *Operative Hand Surgery*; Green, D.P., Ed. Churchill Livingstone: New York, 1993; pp 53-98.
10. Luchetti, R. *Wrist and Forearm Amputations*. In: *Surgery of the Hand and Upper Extremity*; Peimer, C.A., Ed. McGraw-Hill: New York, 1996; pp 853-866.
11. Moneim, M.S.; Pribyl, C.R.; Garst, J.R. *Clinical Orthopaedics and Related Research* 1997, 341, 23-29.
12. Pellegrini, V.D., Jr. *The Basal Articulations of the Thumb: Pain, Instability, and Osteoarthritis*. In: *Surgery of the Hand and Upper Extremity*; Peimer, C.A., Ed. McGraw-Hill: New York, 1996; pp 1019-1042.
13. Pribyl, C.R.; Omer, G.E. Effectiveness of the chevron arthrodesis in small joints of the hand. *Journal of Hand Surgery* 1996, 21A, 1052-1058.
14. Rockwell, W.B.; Wray, R.C., Jr. *Nail Bed Injuries and Reconstruction*. In: *Surgery of the Hand and Upper Extremity*; Peimer, C.A., Ed. McGraw-Hill: New York, 1996; pp 1101-1112.
15. Sennwald, F.R.; Zdravkovic, V. *Wrist Joint Arthrodeses*. In: *Surgery of the Hand and Upper Extremity*; Peimer, C.A., Ed. McGraw-Hill: New York, 1996; pp 795-828.
16. Sennwald, G.R.; Zdravkovic, V. *Wrist Joint Arthrodeses*. In: *Surgery of the Hand and Upper Extremity*; Peimer, C.A., Ed. McGraw-Hill: New York, 1996; pp 795-828.
17. Sotereanos, D.F.; Schmidt, C.C. *Hand and Digital Amputations*. In: *Surgery of the Hand and Upper Extremity*; Peimer, C.A., Ed. McGraw-Hill: New York, 1996; pp 999-1018.
18. Thompson, J.S. *Small Joint Arthrodeses*. In: *Surgery of the Hand and Upper Extremity*; Peimer, C.A., Ed. McGraw-Hill: New York, 1996; pp 973-998.
19. Watson, H.K.; Dhillon, H.S. *Intercarpal Arthrodisis*. In: *Operative Hand Surgery*; Green, D.P., Ed. Churchill Livingstone: New York, 1993; pp 113-130.

FURTHER INFORMATION — FRACTURES, DISLOCATIONS, INFECTIONS, AND TENDON INJURIES

1. Amadio, P.C.; Taleisnik, J. *Fractures of the Carpal Bones*. In: *Operative Hand Surgery*; Green, D.P., Ed. Churchill Livingstone: New York, 1993; pp 799-860.
2. Apicella, M.A. *Musculoskeletal Infections and Antibiotic Prophylaxis*. In: *Surgery of the Hand and Upper Extremity*; Peimer, C.A., Ed. McGraw-Hill: New York, 1996; pp 1723-1730.
3. Bishop, A.T. *Infections*. In: *Hand Surgery Update*; Manske, P.R., Ed. American Academy of Orthopaedic Surgeons: Rosemont, IL, 1996; pp 395-404.
4. Brennwald, J. *Principles and Techniques of AO/ASIF Fracture Fixation*. In: *Operative Hand Surgery*; Green, D.P., Ed. Churchill Livingstone: New York, 1993; pp 759-766.
5. Britton, E.N.; Kleinert, J.M. *Acute Flexor Tendon Injury: Repair and Rehabilitation*. In: *Surgery of the Hand and Upper Extremity*; Peimer, C.A., Ed. McGraw-Hill: New York, 1996; pp 1113-1132.
6. Doyle, J.R. *Extensor Tendons — Acute Injuries*. In: *Operative Hand Surgery*; Green, D.P., Ed. Churchill Livingstone: New York, 1993; pp 1925-1954.
7. Doyle, J.R. *Extensor Tendon Injuries*. In: *Hand Surgery Update*; Manske, P.R., Ed. American Academy of Orthopaedic Surgeons: Rosemont, IL, 1996; pp 149-160.

8. Dray, G.J.; Eaton, R.G. *Dislocations and Ligament Injuries in the Digits*. In: *Operative Hand Surgery*; Green, D.P., Ed. Churchill Livingstone: New York, 1993; pp 767-798.
9. Fischer, T.J. *Phalangeal Fractures*. In: *Hand Surgery Update*; Manske, P.R., Ed. American Academy of Orthopaedic Surgeons: Rosemont, IL, 1996; pp 3-10.
10. Floyd, W.E.I.; Troum, S.; Frankle, M.A. *Acute and Chronic Sepsis*. In: *Surgery of the Hand and Upper Extremity*; Peimer, C.A., Ed. McGraw-Hill: New York, 1996; pp 1731-1762.
11. Floyd, W.E.I.; Foulkes, G.D. *Tuberculosis, Mycotic, and Granulomatous Diseases*. In: *Surgery of the Hand and Upper Extremity*; Peimer, C.A., Ed. McGraw-Hill: New York, 1996; pp 1763-1786.
12. Freeland, A.E.; Sennett, B.J. *Phalangeal Fractures*. In: *Surgery of the Hand and Upper Extremity*; Peimer, C.A., Ed. McGraw-Hill: New York, 1996; pp 921-938.
13. Glickel, S.Z. *Metacarpophalangeal and Interphalangeal Joint Injuries and Instabilities*. In: *Surgery of the Hand and Upper Extremity*; Peimer, C.A., Ed. McGraw-Hill: New York, 1996; pp 1043-1068.
14. Green, D.P. *Carpal Dislocations and Instabilities*. In: *Operative Hand Surgery*; Green, D.P., Ed. Churchill Livingstone: New York, 1993; pp 861-928.
15. Greene, T.L. *Metacarpal Fractures*. In: *Hand Surgery Update*; Manske, P.R., Ed. American Academy of Orthopaedic Surgeons: Rosemont, IL, 1996; pp 11-16.
16. Hewitt, R.G. *Manifestations of HIV Infection in the Upper Extremity*. In: *Surgery of the Hand and Upper Extremity*; Peimer, C.A., Ed. McGraw-Hill: New York, 1996; pp 1787-1796.
17. Hotchkiss, R.N. *Fractures and Dislocations of the Thumb*. In: *Hand Surgery Update*; Manske, P.R., Ed. American Academy of Orthopaedic Surgeons: Rosemont, IL, 1996; pp 29-32.
18. Jupiter, J.B. *Scaphoid Fractures*. In: *Hand Surgery Update*; Manske, P.R., Ed. American Academy of Orthopaedic Surgeons: Rosemont, IL, 1996; pp 77-84.
19. Kiefhaber, T.R. *Intra-articular Fractures in Joint Injuries*. In: *Hand Surgery Update*; Manske, P.R., Ed. American Academy of Orthopaedic Surgeons: Rosemont, IL, 1996; pp 17-28.
20. Kiefhaber, T.R. *Phalangeal Dislocations/Periarticular Trauma*. In: *Surgery of the Hand and Upper Extremity*; Peimer, C.A., Ed. McGraw-Hill: New York, 1996; pp 939-972.
21. Leddy, J.P. *Flexor Tendons — Acute Injuries*. In: *Operative Hand Surgery*; Green, D.P., Ed. Churchill Livingstone: New York, 1993; pp 1823-1852.
22. Minamikawa, Y. *Extensor Repair and Rehabilitation*. In: *Surgery of the Hand and Upper Extremity*; Peimer, C.A., Ed. McGraw-Hill: New York, 1996; pp 1163-1188.
23. Neviaser, R.J. *Infections*. In: *Operative Hand Surgery*; Green, D.P., Ed. Churchill Livingstone: New York, 1993; pp 1021-1038.
24. Schneider, L.H. *Flexor Tendon Injuries*. In: *Hand Surgery Update*; Manske, P.R., Ed. American Academy of Orthopaedic Surgeons: Rosemont, IL, 1996; pp 141-148.
25. Stern, P.J. *Fractures of the Metacarpals and Phalanges*. In: *Operative Hand Surgery*; Green, D.P., Ed. Churchill Livingstone: New York, 1993; pp 695-758.
26. Szabo, R.M.; Sutherland, T.B. *Acute Carpal Fractures and Dislocations*. In: *Surgery of the Hand and Upper Extremity*; Peimer, C.A., Ed. McGraw-Hill: New York, 1996; pp 711-726.
27. Viegas, S.F. *Carpal Instabilities*. In: *Hand Surgery Update*; Manske, P.R., Ed. American Academy of Orthopaedic Surgeons: Rosemont, IL, 1996; pp 93-104.
28. Wolfe, S.W.; Elliott, A.J. *Metacarpal and Carpometacarpal Trauma*. In: *Surgery of the Hand and Upper Extremity*; Peimer, C.A., Ed. McGraw-Hill: New York, 1996; pp 883-920.

19 Prosthetic Implants and Total Joint Arthroplasty

Richard V. Worrell

CONTENTS

19.1 INTRODUCTION

The restoration of function and stability along with the relief of pain in a joint that has been destroyed by trauma, degenerative changes related to aging or neoplastic disease, can be accomplished by means of arthroplasty. The most common joints to be treated with arthroplastic procedures are the hip, knee, and shoulder joints. Arthroplastic procedures have also been used to treat diseased joints of the hand and foot.

The first arthroplastic procedures were performed in the mid-19th century. The science of arthroplasty has evolved since. The original procedures involved the interposition of tissues, e.g., skin, muscle, fat, or fascia, between resected bone ends. Eventually, joint arthroplasty involved resurfacing of damaged joints with metallic and plastic materials. Hemiarthroplasty involves replacing of one side of a joint. Total joint arthroplasty involves the replacement or resurfacing of both sides of a joint.

Current methods of total hip arthroplasty were first described by Sir John Charnley in 1961. He designed a method of replacing both sides of a hip joint that utilized a stainless steel prosthetic femoral head and a high density polyethylene acetabulum. Ten years later, Gunston described the polycentric knee arthroplasty. Over the past quarter century, of total arthroplasties, both hip and knee have been significantly refined. At the present time, metallic components are made of cobalt-chromium-molybdenum alloy instead of stainless steel. Ultrahigh molecular weight polyethylene has replaced high-density polyethylene. Design improvements have increased the survival of the implants and have provided better stability and ranges of motion.

0-8493-9237-3/99/$0.00+$.50

19.2 HIP ARTHROPLASTY

The design of total hip prosthetic implants must take into account that the implants need to withstand cyclic loading that approximates 3 to 12 times the body weight. The usual cyclic load associated with the activities of daily living is 4 times the body weight. Running or jumping will increase the cyclic load to approximately 10 times the body weight.

Among many factors related to successful total hip arthroplasty are the diameter of the head of the femoral component, the coefficient of friction and frictional torque, and factors related to the wear of the metallic and plastic components. The prosthetic components must be designed to promote joint stability with minimal wear. Some implants are held in place with cement whereas in some implants, the fixation is cementless.

The indication for total hip arthroplasty is replacement of the hip joint in elderly patients who have symptomatic severe osteoarthritis and are no longer responding to nonsurgical therapy. Total hip arthroplasty is often used in the treatment of hip joints damaged by trauma or neoplastic disease in both elderly and younger patients. Total joint surgery or hemiarthroplasty is sometimes used in patients with advanced, symptomatic avascular necrosis of the femoral head or nonunions of fractures of the femoral neck. Following successful treatment of infectious diseases involving the hip joint, total hip arthroplasty may be considered. In many younger patients, arhrodesis of the hip joint is still an acceptable procedure.

The major complications related to total hip arthroplasty are prosthetic loosening or infection. In spite of possible complications and technical considerations, the long-term durability of total hip arthroplasty has been established. Callaghan et al. reported the findings of total joint arthroplasty in patients less than 50 years old who had been followed for 20 to 25 years. Their findings confirmed the long-term durability of total hip arthroplasty in relatively young patients whose activity levels are much higher than those of elderly patients.

19.3 KNEE ARTHROPLASTY

Many attempts have been made in the past century to resurface diseased knee joints. Interposition arthroplasty using skin, muscle, fat and fascia has been attempted without measurable success. The original hinged prosthetic knee implants had a single axis of flexion and extension which failed to duplicate the normal flexion, extension, and axial rotation of the normal knee. The current hinged total knee implants duplicate the complex flexion, extension, and axial rotation of the normal knee.

The current total knee prosthetic implants that operate without a hinge are based on the implant developed by Gunston in 1971. Insall et al. developed the total condylar prosthesis in 1973. In the course of its development, two implant designs emerged. One design was designated as a posterior cruciate ligament (PCL)-retaining implant. An alternate design was designated as a posterior cruciate ligament-substituting prosthetic implant. Currently, there is a debate regarding the merits of either the PCL-retaining or the PCL-substituting prosthetic implants. In spite of the differences in technology of each implant, failure rates in 10-year follow-up studies appear to be the same in each group. Insall et al. modified the PCL-substituting implant by creating the constrained condylar knee. This prosthetic implant is used most often for revision total knee arthroplasties.

Some total knee prosthetic implants are cemented in place. There are, however, advocates of cementless prosthetic implants.

As with total hip arthroplasty, loosening and infection represent the major complications.

19.4 SUMMARY

In summary, total joint arthroplasty of either the hip or knee joint can be of value in elderly patients with advanced symptomatic arthritis, or in younger patients with symptomatic traumatic arthritis. Modular total joint arthroplasty is currently being used in many patients with neoplastic disease involving shoulder, elbow, hip, and knee joints.

RECOMMENDED READING

1. Callaghan, J.J., Forest, E.E., Olejniczak, B.A., Goetz, D.D., and Johnston, R.C.: Charnley total hip arthroplasty in patients less than fifty years old. A twenty to twenty-five-year follow-up note. *J. Bone and Joint Surg.* 80-A: 704, 1998.
2. Camnasio, F. and Ravasi, F.: Modular prostheses in metastatic bone disease of the proximal femur. *Bulletin-Hospital for Joint Diseases* 54(4): 211, 1996.
3. Charnley, J.: Arthroplasty of the hip: a new operation. *Lancet* 1: 1129, 1961.
4. Charnley, J. and Cupic, Z.: The nine and ten-year results of low friction arthroplasty of the hip. *Clin. Orthop.* 95: 9, 1973.
5. Gunston, F.H.: Polycentric knee arthroplasty: prosthetic simulation of normal knee movement. *J. Bone and Joint Surg.* 53-B: 272, 1971.
6. Guyton, J.L.: Arthroplasty of ankle and knee. In: *Campbell's Operative Orthopaedics,* 9th ed., Canale, S.T., Ed., Mosby, St. Louis, 1998, p. 232.
7. Harkess, J.W.: Arthroplasty of the hip. In: *Campbell's Operative Orthopaedics,* 9th ed., Canale, S.T., Ed., Mosby, St. Louis, 1998, p. 296.
8. Insall, J.N., Ranawat, C.S., Scott, W.N., and Walker, P.: Total condylar knee replacement. Preliminary report. *Clin. Orthop.* 120:149, 1976.
9. Kelsey, D. and Goodman, S.B.: Design of the femoral component for cementless hip replacement: the surgeon's perspective. *Am. J. Orthop.* 26(6): 407, 1997.
10. Sledge, C.B.: Polyethylene: is the enemy of good, better? *Orthopaedics* 19(9): 805, 1996.

Index

C

D

E

F

G

H

I

N

P

S

T

U

V

W

Y